The Handbook of Contraception

CURRENT CLINICAL PRACTICE

NEIL S. SKOLNIK, MD, SERIES EDITOR

The Handbook of Contraception: *A Guide for Practical Management,* edited by *DONNA SHOUPE AND SIRI L. KJOS,* 2006

Obstetrics in Family Medicine: *A Practical Guide, PAUL LYONS,* 2006

Psychiatric Disorders in Pregnancy and the Postpartum: *Principles and Treatment, VICTORIA HENDRICK,* 2006

Disorders of the Respiratory Tract: *Common Challenges in Primary Care, MATTHEW L. MINTZ,* 2006

Sexually Transmitted Diseases: *A Practical Guide for Primary Care,* edited by *ANITA NELSON AND JOANN WOODWARD,* 2006

Cardiology in Family Practice: *A Practical Guide, STEVEN M. HOLLENBERG AND TRACY WALKER,* 2006

Bronchial Asthma: *A Guide for Practical Understanding and Treatment, Fifth Edition,* edited by *M. ERIC GERSHWIN AND TIMOTHY E. ALBERTSON,* 2006

Dermatology Skills for Primary Care: *An Illustrated Guide, DANIEL J. TROZAK, DAN J. TENNENHOUSE, AND JOHN J. RUSSELL,* 2006

Thyroid Disease: *A Case-Based and Practical Guide for Primary Care, EMANUEL O. BRAMS,* 2005

Type 2 Diabetes, Pre-Diabetes, and the Metabolic Syndrome: *The Primary Care Guide to Diagnosis and Management, RONALD A. CODARIO,* 2005

Chronic Pain: *A Primary Care Guide to Practical Management, DAWN A. MARCUS,* 2005

Bone Densitometry in Clinical Practice: *Application and Interpretation, Second Edition, SYDNEY LOU BONNICK,* 2004

Cancer Screening: *A Practical Guide for Physicians,* edited by *KHALID AZIZ AND GEORGE Y. WU,* 2001

Hypertension Medicine, edited by *MICHAEL A. WEBER,* 2001

Allergic Diseases: *Diagnosis and Treatment, Second Edition,* edited by *PHIL LIEBERMAN AND JOHN A. ANDERSON,* 2000

The Handbook of Contraception

A Guide for Practical Management

Edited by

Donna Shoupe, MD

Division of Reproductive Endocrinology and Infertility
Departments of Obstetrics and Gynecology and Family Medicine
Keck School of Medicine
at the University of Southern California
Los Angeles, CA

Siri L. Kjos, MD

Department of Obstetrics and Gynecology
David Geffen School of Medicine
at University of California at Los Angeles
Los Angeles, CA
and
Harbor-UCLA Medical Center
Torrance, CA

HUMANA PRESS ✻ TOTOWA, NEW JERSEY

999 Riverview Drive, Suite 208
Totowa, New Jersey 07512

humanapress.com

This publication is printed on acid-free paper. ∞
ANSI Z39.48-1984 (American Standards Institute) Permanence of Paper for Printed Library Materials.

Cover Illustration: Fig. 1, Chapter 3, "Oral Contraceptives: *Patient Screening and Counseling, Pill Selection, and Managing Side Effects*," by Donna Shoupe.

Cover design by Patricia F. Cleary

Production Editor: Amy Thau

For additional copies, pricing for bulk purchases, and/or information about other Humana titles, contact Humana at the above address or at any of the following numbers: Tel.: 973-256-1699; Fax: 973-256-8314; E-mail: orders@humanapr.com, or visit our Website: http://humanapress.com

Printed in the United States of America. 10 9 8 7 6 5 4 3 2 1
eISBN: 1-59745-150-9
Library of Congress Cataloging in Publication Data
The handbook of contraception : a guide for practical management /
edited by Donna Shoupe, Siri L. Kjos.
p. ; cm. -- (Current clinical practice)
Includes bibliographical references and index.
ISBN 1-58829-599-0 (alk. paper)
1. Contraception--Handbooks, manuals, etc. 2.
Contraceptives--Handbooks, manuals, etc.
[DNLM: 1. Contraception--methods. 2. Contraception--standards.
3. Contraceptive Devices. 4. Practice Management,
Medical--standards. WP 630 H236 2006] I. Shoupe, Donna. II. Kjos,
Siri L. III. Series.
RG136.H28 2006
613.9'43--dc22

2006000941

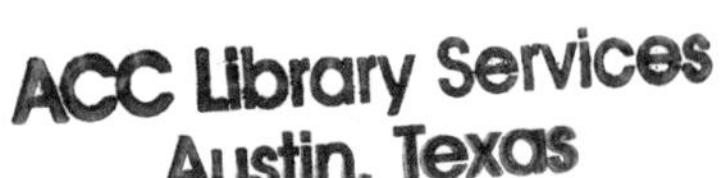

Dedication

This book is dedicated to Wendene Wilson Shoupe

Series Editor Introduction

I opened my series editor manuscript of *The Handbook of Contraception: A Guide for Practical Management*, edited by Drs. Donna Shoupe and Siri Kjos, on a tiny plane on the way to giving a lecture in Albany, NY. I expected to peruse the manuscript, and found that I could not put it down. *The Handbook of Contraception: A Guide for Practical Management* is an incredibly informative and enjoyable read. In keeping with the objective of this series for primary care clinicians, there is a quality in this title that is uncommon among medical textbooks.

The chapters of this book are written with extraordinary intelligence and understanding, and with attention to practical considerations in the selection and management of contraceptive options. The authors have reviewed the science behind contraception, including the chemical structure and effects of hormonal contraception, physiology of contraception, efficacy rates, and side effects, as well as the practical considerations that are relevant in helping patients choose between different contraceptive options. They do this with a clarity of language and intent that lets the book cover with sufficient detail the full range of questions that any primary care clinician will have regarding any of the traditional or new contraceptive options. Also included in each chapter is a section on "counseling tips," which explicitly answers many of the questions that clinicians and their patients often have when discussing contraceptive options. For a book so useful and well done, the editors and authors deserve our thanks.

***Neil Skolnik,** MD*

Preface

With so many contraceptive options currently available, and such a broad scope of issues to address, matching a patient to her best contraceptive method is more challenging today than it has ever been. To address this challenge, *The Handbook of Contraception: A Guide for Practical Management* is designed to give the modern health care provider up-to-date information on safety, side effects, advantages, and disadvantages of each method, as well as guidance in selecting appropriate users and practical counseling tools. An effort has been made to cover the currently available methods and those that are expected to be available shortly, and to emphasize the growing list of noncontraceptive benefits associated with each method. An extensive reference list allows interested readers to further investigate issues of interest.

The first chapter in *The Handbook of Contraception: A Guide for Practical Management* is an overview of current contraceptive use in the United States, with a comparison of the effectiveness and cost of the various methods. Chapters 2 through 8 discuss hormonal methods of contraception, including combination oral contraceptives, the contraceptive patch, the contraceptive vaginal ring, progestin-only pills, and the new progestin implant. Chapter 7 on long-acting injectable contraceptives and Chapter 8 on intrauterine devices compare the two current options in each category. Chapter 10 on barriers separately covers male condoms and vaginal spermicides, and then compares, as a group, the various cervical barrier methods. Chapter 11 covers behavioral methods of contraception including abstinence, and Chapter 12 discusses emergency contraceptive options. Chapter 13 reviews the research methods of sterilization that are currently under investigation, and the many methods that have been abandoned for various insurmountable reasons, as well as an extensive review and description of current methods of sterilization, including the newly approved hysteroscopic method. Chapters 14 and 15 are designed to guide the reader on factors to consider when selecting the correct contraceptive method for adolescents, perimenopausal women, postpartum mothers, and medically compromised women.

I dedicate this book to my mother, Wendene Wilson Shoupe, who backed me when I needed it the most. When I was living in Boston and applying to medical school, I became fascinated by the menstrual cycle and developed a deep desire to know everything I could about estrogen. But even more, I dreamed of developing the perfect birth control method. Many years later, I am awed by the difficulty of such a task, but I am honored to put together this compilation of how far contraceptive technology has come. Thank you, Mom, for giving me the support, financial help, drive, and love that got me through the tough days in Boston and allowed me to work toward my dreams.

My grateful thanks to Lee Hellmuth, Richard Montz, Rene B. Allen, MD, Marc Kalan, MD, for technical assistance; to Sherry Cochran, Rph, Director of Pharmacy,

USC Medical Plaza Pharmacy; Eunju Lee Kwak, RN, Midwife; Blanca Ovalee, Research Coordinator Women and Children's Hospital Family Planning for access to contraceptive supplies; and to Diane Quan for her excellent coordinating efforts.

Lastly, I support and echo the statements of Felicia Stewart, MD, writing for the authors of the latest edition of *Contraceptive Technology*, that the commitment and courage of our colleagues is deeply appreciated, and that when dealing with the challenges that we face in reproductive health, working together is the best way to ensure success.

Donna Shoupe, MD
Siri L. Kjos, MD

Contents

Contributors

SUSIE BALDWIN, MD, MPH • Department of Obstetrics and Gynecology, David Geffen School of Medicine at the University of California at Los Angeles, Los Angeles, CA

SUSAN A. BALLAGH, MD • Conrad Clinical Research Center, Jones Institute for Reproductive Medicine; Department of Obstetrics and Gynecology, Eastern Virginia Medical School, and Jones Institute for Reproductive Medicine, Norfolk, VA

ANGELA Y. CHEN, MD, MPH • Department of Obstetrics and Gynecology, David Geffen School of Medicine at the University of California at Los Angeles, Los Angeles, CA

PHILIP D. DARNEY, MD, MSc • Chief, Obstetrics, Gynecology, and Reproductive Sciences, San Francisco General Hospital, University of California, San Francisco, CA

RONNA JUROW, MD • Department of Obstetrics and Gynecology, Keck School of Medicine at the University of Southern California, Los Angeles, CA

SIRI L. KJOS, MD • Department of Obstetrics and Gynecology, David Geffen School of Medicine at the University of California at Los Angeles, Los Angeles, CA; and Harbor-UCLA Medical Center, Torrance, CA

CHARLES M. MARCH, MD • California Fertility Partners, Division of Gynecology, Department of Obstetrics and Gynecology, Keck School of Medicine at the University of Southern California, Los Angeles, CA

DANIEL R. MISHELL, JR., MD • Department of Obstetrics and Gynecology, Keck School of Medicine at the University of Southern California, Los Angeles, CA

ANITA L. NELSON, MD • Department of Obstetrics and Gynecology, David Geffen School of Medicine at the University of California at Los Angeles, Los Angeles, CA; Medical Director, Women's Health Care Programs, Harbor-UCLA Medical Center, Torrance, CA

JENNEFER A. RUSSO, MD • Department of Obstetrics and Gynecology, David Geffen School of Medicine at the University of California at Los Angeles, Los Angeles, CA; and Harbor-UCLA Medical Center, Torrance, CA

DONNA SHOUPE, MD • Division of Reproductive Endocrinology and Infertility, Departments of Obstetrics and Gynecology and Family Medicine, Keck School of Medicine at the University of Southern California, Los Angeles, CA

1 Contraceptive Overview

Donna Shoupe, MD

Contents

INTRODUCTION

Despite improvements in contraceptive technology and a growing market of effective and safe contraceptive options, unintended pregnancy continues to be a significant public health issue in the United States. The more than 2.5 million unintended pregnancies in the United States each year make up nearly half (49%) of all pregnancies. During their reproductive years, 48% of women will have an unintended pregnancy. Adolescents and women in poverty are at highest risk of having an unplanned birth *(1)*, an event that may further challenge their ability to obtain an education, appropriate job training, and a meaningful job.

In the United States, more than 98% of sexually active women ages 15–44 report they have used at least one contraceptive method *(2)*. In fact, in 2002, 90% of sexually experienced women reported having had a male partner use a male condom and 82% reported using an oral contraceptive (OC) at some time *(2)*. Although these figures reflect a high degree of awareness and experience with contraceptive methods, unfortunately they do not reflect the number of users who used such methods properly and consistently for every sexual exposure. The large disparity between the reported high contraceptive use and the high unintended pregnancy rate in the United States is not primarily caused by a lack of effectiveness of a chosen method, but rather in large part results from poor adherence to a method.

From: *Current Clinical Practice: The Handbook of Contraception: A Guide for Practical Management*
Edited by: D. Shoupe and S. L. Kjos © Humana Press, Totowa, NJ

GOALS OF THE HEALTH CARE PROVIDER

> *The goal of the health care provider is to match a user with a contraceptive method that will be used safely, correctly, and consistently.*

To match the user with the optimum contraceptive method, the provider should consider the age, motivation, sexual practices, financial ability, religious beliefs, reproductive history and plans, and overall health status of the user. Appropriate, accurate provider counseling includes giving information on the user requirements of various methods along with availability, costs, possible side effects, and possible health benefits. As the user narrows her selections, more detailed information is given on each these issues. After a patient has selected the method that fits her lifestyle and health status, further information on use of the method is detailed. Finally, information on when to use and the availability of emergency backup protection, as well as the warning signs to look out for, are explained.

Screening Considerations

- Age. Young users have high fecundity rates, higher risk for sexually transmitted infection (STI) transmission, and lower risk of having serious illnesses.
- Motivation and knowledge level of user.
  - Following initiation, the implant, intrauterine device (IUD), and sterilization require little, if any, user intervention.
  - The barrier methods demand user intervention with every sexual act.
- User's ability to address upfront and ongoing costs of a method.
  - For sexually active women, long-term costs of any method are significantly lower than costs of an unintended pregnancy (as shown in Table 1), but upfront costs may discourage or prevent use of some methods to low-income, non-health-insured women.
- User's health and presence of cardiovascular risk factors including smoking status may preclude some hormonal methods.
  - Progestin-only methods contraindications (*see* Chapters 4, 7, 8, and 14 for more details).
    - Active liver disease is a contraindication to progestin- and estrogen-containing contraceptives.
  - Estrogen plus progestin methods (*see* Chapters 3, 5, 6, and 14 for more details).
    - Thrombogenic events and risk factors are often contraindications to estrogen-plus-progestin methods.
    - Known cardiovascular disease or significant risk factors are often contraindications to estrogen-plus-progestin methods.
- The presence of health problems that may benefit from use of a hormonal method, such as bleeding problems, acne, premenstrual syndrome (PMS), dysmenorrhea, or perimenopausal symptoms.
- STI risk and need for condom protection.

Table 1
Direct Costs of Various Contraceptives

	Contraceptive method	*Average cost per month (or per cycle)*	*Average upfront and ongoing costs*
Combined estrogen and progestin	COC	$20–50 (can run as low as $0–1.50 for covered users)	$50–200 (initial and yearly office visits)
	COC (extended cycle)	$120 (3 months)	$50–200 (initial and yearly office visits; often some insurance coverage)
	Contraceptive patch	$38–40	$50–200 (initial and yearly office visits; often some insurance coverage)
	Vaginal ring	$35–40	$50–200 (initial and yearly office visits; often some insurance coverage)
Progestin only	Injectable progestin (DMPA, and depo sub-Q provera 104™)	$30–100 (3 months) including injection fee	Initial and periodic office visits; covered by some insurance carriers; among the least expensive contraceptives
	Progestin-only pill	$9–50	$50–200 (initial and yearly office visits)
Implant	Progestin implant Implanon® (availability expected in United States shortly)		$500–600 (insertion and cost of Norplant®; plus $100–200 for removal; covered by some insurers)
Intrauterine device (IUDs)	Progestin containing IUD Mirena®		$300–1000 (insertion, removal, and cost of device [over 5 years is less expensive than other contraceptives]; may be covered by insurance)
	Copper IUD (ParaGard®)		$300–1000 (insertion, removal, and cost of device [over 10 years is less expensive than other contraceptives]; may be covered by insurance)

(continued)

Table 1 *(Continued)*
Direct Costs of Various Contraceptives

	Contraceptive method	*Average cost per month (or per cycle)*	*Average upfront and ongoing costs*
Barriers	Spermicides	$10–20 (box of film), $10–20 (tube of gel), $10–20 (package of suppositories)	
	Diaphragm	$15–75 (diaphragm replaced every 2 years plus $8–17 for cost of spermicide)	$50–200 (initial visit for fitting)
	Male condom	$1–3 per condom	
	Female condom	$2–3 per condom; sold in packs of 3 or 6	
	Cervical cap and shield	$15–75 (plus $8–17 for cost of spermicide if using a cap)	$50–200 (initial visit for prescription)
	Sponge	$1.50 per sponge	
Female sterilization			$1000–5000 or more (may be covered by insurance)

IUD, intrauterine device; COC, combination oral contraceptive; DMPA, depo-medroxyprogesterone acetate.

- Consideration of a user's weight if more than 160–200 lb; the contraceptive effectiveness of combination OCs, progestin-only OCs, and the contraceptive patch may be decreased.
  - Long-acting injectable progestin, the contraceptive ring, barrier methods, or IUDs may be better choices for heavier women.

Counseling Considerations

Supply pertinent information about proper use of a method, safety issues, and what to do in case of misuse.

- Counseling tips on how to handle common problems associated with a particular method.
- When to use a backup method.
  - Information on emergency contraceptives when appropriate.
- Warning signals.

TRENDS OF CONTRACEPTIVE USE AND STERILIZATION

In 2002, only 7.4% of sexually active US women ages 15–44 reported using no method of contraception (Table 2).

The most popular forms of contraception in the United States in 2002 were contraceptive pills (11.6 million), female sterilization (10.3 million), and male condoms (6.8 million). The distribution of contraceptive use among reproductive-aged women in the United States in 2002, using some form of contraception, is shown in Fig. 1.

The male condom is the most popular method used at first intercourse and the pill is the leading contraceptive method for women under 30 *(2)*. Female sterilization is used most commonly in women over 35. The number of women ages 14–55 in the United States and the percent distribution of contraceptive and non-contraceptive use is shown in Table 2 *(2)*. Since 1982, the percentage of women who have ever had a male partner use a male condom has risen from 52 to 90%. This is largely owing to the increased awareness of STIs and HIV transmission. There has also been an increase in women who report ever having used withdrawal (from 25 to 56%) and decreases in the use of the IUD, diaphragm, calendar rhythm, and spermicidal foam.

In 2002, the percentage of women using contraception who were using OC pills was 53% in those 15–19 years of age and 11% in those 40–44 years of age *(2)*. Less educated women were more likely to rely on female sterilization, whereas more educated women rely more heavily on OC pills. Only 11% of women without a high school degree who used some form of contraception, whereas 42% of contraceptive users with a high school degree used the pill. Female sterilization was the choice in 55% of users without a high school degree compared with only 13% of women with a 4-year college degree *(2)*.

Table 2
Number and Percentage of US Women Ages 15–44 Using Current Contraceptive Methods and Not Using Contraception

	All women ages 15–44
Total number	**61,561,000**
Percentage using a contraceptive method	61.9%
Pill	18.9%
Female sterilization	16.7%
Condom	11.1%
Male sterilization	5.7%
3-Month injectable Depo-Provera®	3.3%
Withdrawal	2.5%
Intrauterine device	1.3%
Implant, Lunelle, patch	0.8%
Periodic abstinence/calendar rhythm	0.7%
Periodic abstinence/natural family planning	0.2%
Diaphragm	0.2%
Other methods including sponge, cervical cap, and female condom	0.6%
Percentage not using a contraceptive method	38.1%
Never had intercourse or no intercourse in 3 months	18.1%
Had intercourse within 3 months of interview	7.4%
Pregnant or postpartum	5.35%
Trying to get pregnant	4.2%
Nonsurgically sterile: female or male	1.6%
Surgically sterile: female non-contraceptive	1.5%
All other nonusers includes male sterility of unknown origin	0.0%

Adapted from ref. *2*.

Although most women report using only one method, use of the pill and the condom to prevent pregnancy and transmission of STDs is most common in younger, women who have never been married. The portion of women who use both the pill and the condom as contraception is 15% in teenagers and 1% in women 40–44 years of age. Table 3 shows the percentage of women using more than one method of contraception by age and marital status.

The percentage of all women ages 15–44 who were sexually active and not using contraception increased from 5.4% in 1995 to 7.4% in 2002. This represents an apparent increase of 1.43 million women between 1995 and 2002, and could raise the rate of unintended pregnancy.

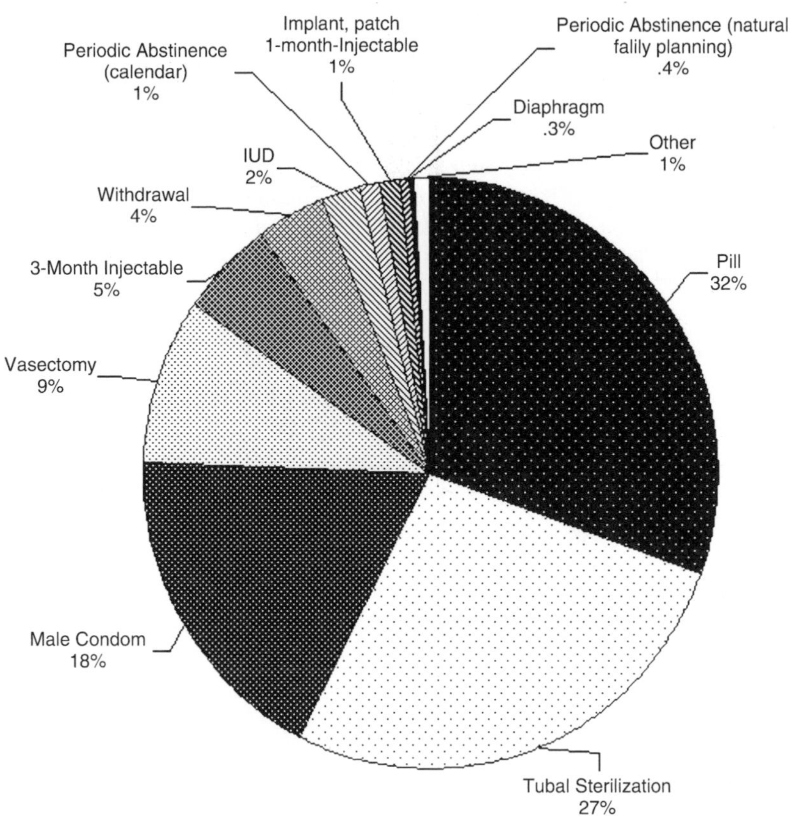

Fig. 1. Primary contraceptive methods among US women aged 15–44 years, 2002. (Adapted from ref. *2*.)

EFFECTIVENESS OF METHODS COMPARED

Perfect Versus Typical Use

- The typical use effectiveness of a particular contraceptive method is dependent on the inherent effectiveness of the method and on whether or not it is used correctly and consistently. Depending on the method, correct and consistent use may be highly or only minimally dependent on user intervention and motivation. For some methods, correct and consistent use is affected by the inherent "usability" of the method that includes how easy the method is to use correctly and by the incidence of side effects of the method.
  - Easy-to-use methods with minimal side effects are generally used more consistently than hard-to-use methods or those methods that might be easy to use but have bothersome side effects.

Table 3
Percentage of US Women Aged 15–44 Using More Than One Method of Contraception

Age	*Women using more than one method (%)*	*Contracepting women using more than one method (%)*	*Using condom and pill (%)*	*Using condom only (%)*	*Using condom at all (%)*
15–19	10.6	31.2	14.5	19.4	44.6
20–24	12.7	18.9	11.1	20.3	36.0
25–29	10.8	14.5	3.3	16.5	25.5
30–34	9.5	13.0	1.8	13.2	21.0
35–39	8.9	11.4	0.9	12.2	17.8
40–44	8.7	10.7	0.5	9.1	13.5
Marital status					
Never married	11.0	23.8	11.4[a]	19.2[a]	38.4[a]
Currently married	9.6	11.3	1.3	12.7	18.3

[a]Not cohabitating.
Columns with the percentage in each age group using condom only or condom at all show for the purpose of comparison.
Adapted from ref. 2.

 - After placement, IUDs require little or no user intervention, and their typical use effectiveness rate is almost identical to their perfect use rate.

- The perfect use effectiveness rate reflects the inherent efficacy of the method, that is, how effective the method is if used consistently and properly on each sexual act. The perfect use rates are determined either by well-done clinical studies, clinical experience, or "best guess."

The effectiveness of a contraceptive method is usually given as the percentage of couples that experience an accidental pregnancy during the first year of either perfect or typical use of the method. The perfect and typical use rates of contraceptive methods currently available in the United States are shown in Table 4. The difference between the perfect and typical use rates primarily reflects the degree to which the method is dependent on ongoing user intervention. It also may include a variety of other factors including the ease of use of the method, how easily it can be used incorrectly, and how effective the method is if not used correctly. IUDs, implants, and female sterilization are, for the most part, not subject to ongoing user intervention and as a result, have almost identical perfect use and typical use failure rates.

Table 4
Unintended Pregnancy Rates in US Women Using Various Contraceptive Methods and the Percentage Continuing Use at 1 Year

	Failure rate during the first year of use (percentage of women with unintended pregnancy)		*Continuation rate (approximate percentage still using the method at end of 1 year)*
Contraceptive method	*Typical use*	*Correct and consistent use: Perfect use: Lowest expected rate*	
No method	85	85	
Spermicides only	20–30	6–18	40
Behavior methods of family planning	25	1–9	50–75
Calendar method	25	1–9	
Ovulation	25	3	
Sympto-thermal	25	2	
Post-ovulation	25	1	
Withdrawal	19–27	4	40
Caps[a]			
Parous women	30–40	20–26	40–45
Nulliparous women	16–20	9	50–60
Sponge[a]			
Parous women	30–40	9–20	40–45
Nulliparous women	16–20	9	50–60
Diaphragm (with spermicides)	16–20	6	50–60
Condoms			
Female (Reality®)	12–22	5	50
Male	12–15	2–3	50–55
Oral contraceptives			
Progestin only	5–8	0.5	60
Combined	3–8	0.2–0.3	70
Evra patch™	3–8	0.2–0.3	70
NuvaRing®	3–8	0.2–0.3	60–70
Intrauterine devices			
CuT 380A ParaGard®	0.5–1 0.6	0.1	80
Mirena® LNG-IUS	0.1	0.1	80
Depo-Provera and depo-subQ provera 104	0.3–3	0.3	50–60
Implant: Norplant and Implanon	0.09–1.4	0.05–0.09	80
Female sterilization	0.5–0.7	0.5	100
Male sterilization	0.15–0.2	0.1	100

[a]Newly introduced caps and sponges report effectiveness rates in parous women similar to effectiveness rates in nulliparous women although studies are limited.

Ranges shown are a compilation of various studies and reports found in refs. *5–13*.

The more that a method is dependent on ongoing user intervention, the higher the differences between the perfect and typical failure rates. In study populations with highly motivated users, typical method failure will be low, approaching a perfect use rate. In studies using poorly motivated users, the failure rates are elevated. The typical failure rates are also dependent on the underlying fecundity factors of the study population including age, frequency of sexual relations, and underlying health.

The typical use failure rates include pregnancies that have occurred during improper or inconsistent use of the contraceptive method. The typical use failure rates associated with the male condom includes those couples reporting that the condom is their "chosen" method, but who may only occasionally use them. Typical use for OCs includes those women who miss pills often or even those whose prescription ran out several months ago. The typical failure rates reported in IUD studies include those women who had placement of the IUD, but later were discovered to have had an expulsion.

Perfect use is generally an estimated probability of failure based on perfect, consistent use. For each method, a set of different factors are taken into consideration and a theoretical "best guess" can be determined. For some methods, large, well-done clinical trials with very low pregnancy rates have supported these "best guess" estimates.

The continuity rate reflects the average number of couples that continue using a particular method for 1 year. As with typical use, the continuity rate is affected by ease of method use, side effects, and user motivation (*see* Table 4).

BETTER EFFICACY AFTER EXTENDED USE

The risk of method failure for a population generally declines over time for a number of reasons. Often the least compliant users either stop using the method entirely or experience a method failure during the first year of use. The most fertile couples are most likely to experience method failure during the first year. Additionally, there is a period of time for learning to use the contraceptive method that may contribute to method failure.

For each individual couple, the failure rate of a chosen method changes only slightly after the first year of use. After the learning period, unless there is a change in intercourse frequency, there is very little change in contraceptive effectiveness. With increasing age, fecundity for a woman slowly declines and this will gradually lower the risk of method failure *(3,4)*.

COSTS OF DIFFERENT METHODS

The cost of different methods of contraceptives is shown in Table 1. Some private insurances cover contraceptives and almost all cover sterilization costs. Some private insurance companies cover the cost of OCs if there is a medical indication, such as dysmenorrhea, acne, or heavy bleeding. The public sector

Table 5
Five-Year Cost of Contraception for Those At Risk for Pregnancy

1. Baseline cost for comparison
   a. No method of contraception: $14,663
2. Highly efficacious methods
   a. Copper T IUD (Paragard): $540
   b. Vasectomy: $764
   c. Implantable progestin Norplant: $850
   d. Depo Provera injections: $1290
   e. Oral contraceptives: $1784
   f. Tubal ligation: $2424
3. Less efficacious methods
   a. Male condom: $2424
   b. Withdrawal method: $3666
   c. Periodic abstinence/natural family planning: $3450
   d. Contraceptive diaphragm: $3666
   e. Vaginal spermicide: $4102
   f. Female condom: $4872
   g. Contraceptive sponge: $5700
   h. Cervical cap: $5730

Cost calculations include cost of adverse events expected from use of a method, cost of unwanted pregnancy, direct health care costs to obtain method plus direct cost of method.

Adapted from ref. 5.

generally provides some coverage for contraceptives, making the cost of certain methods very affordable for low-income users.

The cost of the method, however, represents only a small part of the overall costs associated with use or nonuse of a contraceptive method. The 5-year costs associated with various contraceptive methods are shown in Table 5. Some contraceptives lower the risk of STIs and therefore lower the associated treatment costs. The net decreases of the costs of treating STIs and the net increase of medical costs related to method side effects, however, are small compared with the net costs of an unintended pregnancy. For sexually active women, net 5-year costs are substantially lower with use of any method compared with no method.

ADVANCES IN REPRODUCTIVE HEALTH

During the past five decades, there have been significant advances in contraceptive technology. Our contraceptive options today are safer than the options of the past. All of the contraceptives on the market today are linked with numerous contraceptive as well as non-contraceptive health benefits that may improve a user's quality as well as quantity of life. Providers of reproductive health care now often address a wide range of health-related issues, including dysmenorrhea, acne, PMS, STIs, menstrual irregularities, menopausal symptoms, as well as infertility and pregnancy planning. The new methods that are entering the market and those currently undergoing clinical trials are important new options and will hopefully further advance contraceptive effectiveness, safety, and the associated benefits.

REFERENCES

1. Henshaw SK. (1998) Unintended pregnancy in the United States. Fam Plan Persp 30:24–29, 46.
2. Mosher WD, Martinez GM, Chandra A, Abma JC, Wilson SJ. (2004) Use of contraception and use of family planning services in the United States: 1998–2002. Adv Data Stat 350: Dec. 10.
3. Vessey, Lawless M, Yeates D. (1982) Efficacy of different contraceptive methods. Lancet 1:841–842.
4. Sivin I, Schmidt F. (1987) Effectiveness of IUDs: a review. Contraception 36:55–84.
5. Trussell J, Leveque JA, Koenig JD, et al. (1995) The economic value of contraception: a comparison of 15 methods. Am J Public Health 954:494–503.
6. Alan Guttmacher Institute, and Fu H, Darroch JE, Haas T, et al. (1999) Contraceptive failure rates: new estimates from the 1995 National Survey of Family Growth. Fam Plann Perspect 31:2.
7. Trussell J. (1998) Contraceptive efficacy. In: Hatcher RA, Trussell J, Stewart F, et al., eds. Contraceptive Technology, 17th edition. New York: Ardent, pp. 779–844.
8. Trussell J. (2004) The essentials of contraception: efficacy, safety, and personal considerations. In: Hatcher RA, Trussell J, Stewart F, et al., eds. Contraceptive Technology, 18th edition. New York: Ardent, pp. 211–248.
9. Schwallie PC, Assenzo JR. (1973) Contraceptive use—efficacy study utilizing medroxyprogesterone acetate administered as an intramuscular injection once every 90 days. Fert Steril 24:331–339.
10. McCann MF, Potter LS. (1994) Progestin-only oral contraception: a comprehensive review. Contraception 50(Suppl):S1–S195.
11. Wilcox AJ, Dunson D, Baird DD. (2000) The timing of the "fertile window" in the menstrual cycle: day-specific estimates from a perspective study. BMJ 321:1259–1262.
12. Areevalo M, Jennings V, Sinai I. (2002) Efficacy of a new method of family planning: the standard days method. Contraception 65:333–338.
13. Klaus H. (1995) Natural Family Planning: A Review, 2nd edition. Bethesda, MD: Natural Family Planning Center of Washington, DC.

2 Oral Contraceptives

History, Pharmacology, Metabolic Effects, Side Effects, and Health Benefits

Donna Shoupe, MD *and Daniel R. Mishell, Jr.,* MD

Contents

INTRODUCTION

Because of social, political, financial, or legal reasons, many contraceptive methods have been removed from the contraceptive armamentarium, sometimes almost as quickly as they were introduced. The original subdermal implant, a monthly intramuscular injection containing medroxyprogesterone acetate and estradiol cypionate, and a multitude of intrauterine devices have all been withdrawn from the US market after facing insurmountable problems. Over the last 45 years, however, oral contraceptives (OCs) have undergone extensive study,

From: *Current Clinical Practice: The Handbook of Contraception: A Guide for Practical Management*
Edited by: D. Shoupe and S. L. Kjos © Humana Press, Totowa, NJ

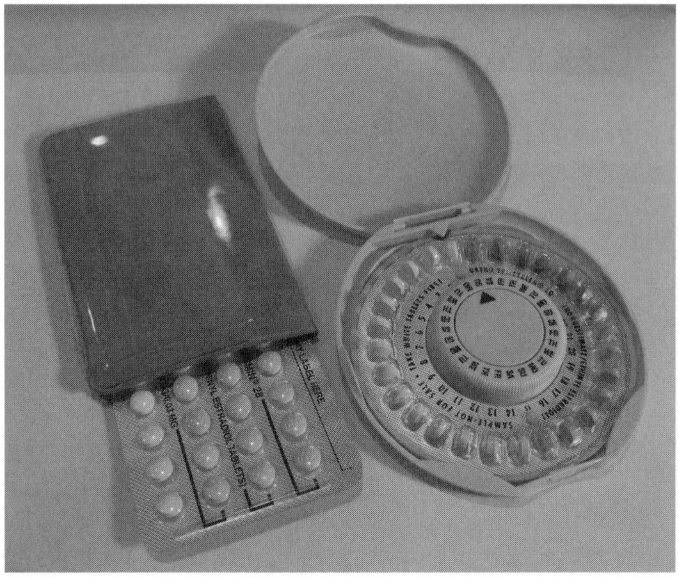

Fig. 1. Current options for oral contraception.

continual development and significant improvements. Unlike the original OCs, new low-dose OCs, as shown in Fig. 1, have few health risks when used in properly selected users and many health benefits. Currently, more than 100 million women worldwide and 18 million women in the United States rely on OCs *(1)*.

LEGAL HISTORY

The birth control pill was first introduced in 1960, but for many years its use was illegal in many states. In 1965, the Supreme Court took up the case of Estelle Griswold, executive director of the Planned Parenthood League in New Haven, CT. She and others at the Planned Parenthood Center were arrested for giving information and instruction to married couples about how to prevent pregnancies. Justice William Douglas, writing for the majority in the 7–2 opinion, cited constitutional guarantees of privacy that prevented the government from interfering in people's bedrooms. Since this landmark decision, OCs have become one of the most widely used contraceptive methods.

Connecticut Law Found Unconstitutional "Any person who uses any drug, medicinal article or instrument for the purpose of preventing conception shall be fined not less than fifty dollars or imprisoned not less than sixty days nor more than one year or be both fined and imprisoned."

Development History

- OCs are the most widely studied pharmaceutical *(2)*.
- Many misperceptions regarding OCs still exist, and many women are unaware of the significant non-contraceptive health benefits associated with OC use.

In 1951, Carl Djerrasi synthesized the first orally active progestin norethindrone from its plant source. In 1953, Cotton synthesized norethynodrel. During the process of synthesis of norethynodrel, a small amount of the estrogen, mestranol (ethinyl estradiol-3-methyl ether), was serendipitously produced as a byproduct. This discovery led to the introduction of the first OC in the United States in 1960 that contained a large amount of these compounds, namely 150 μg of mestranol and 9.85 mg of norethynodrel. During the next several decades, after scientists learned how to independently synthesize mestranol and ethinyl estradiol (EE) from the plant source, EE gradually replaced mestranol in OC formulations.

Because orally administered estrogen is thrombophilic and increases the risk of both arterial and venous thrombosis in a dose-dependent manner, an effort was made to reduce the dose of EE in OC formulations. In the United States, the estrogen dose was initially lowered from 150 μg of mestranol to 50 μg and then EE was lowered to 20 μg. Mestranol is more potent than EE per unit weight, and 50 μg of mestranol is roughly equivalent to 35 μg of EE *(3)*. The true low-dose formulations are those with less than 35 μg. A formulation with 15 μg EE is now marketed in Europe.

The dose of progestin was also reduced and newer, more potent progestins than norethynodrel were developed. Most modern OCs contain progestins derived from norethindrone or norgestrel (Table 1). These progestins chemically resemble testosterone and have a low degree of androgenic activity. The more recently introduced progestins (norgestimate, desogestrel, and gestodene) are also derivatives of testosterone but are more selective and have less androgenic activity. The anti-progestogen mefipristone was derived by manipulation of the norethinedrone molecule and tibolone is a derivative of norethynodrel (Fig. 2).

In 2001, a new oral contraceptive, Yasmin®, was introduced containing drospirenone (DRSP), a progestin structurally related to spironolactone (Table 1). This progestin exhibits progestogenic, antimineralocorticoid, and antiandrogenic activities. A transdermal method (Ortho Evra®) received regulatory approval for use in the United States in 2001. The transdermal contraceptive system was designed to release a constant rate of 150 μg of norelgestronomin (the active metabolite of norgestimate) and 20 μg of EE into the systemic circulation each day. Marketing of the contraceptive vaginal ring (NuvaRing®) that daily releases 120 μg of etonogestrel, the biologically active metabolite of desogestrel, and 15 μg of EE began in 2002.

Table 1
Family of Progestins

	Parent compounds		
Progesterone	*Testosterone*		*Spirolactone*
	Derivatives		
17α-acetoxyprogestrone	**19-nortestosterone**		**17α-spironolactone**
Pregnane derivatives	Estrane derivatives	Gonane derivatives	
Megestrol acetate	Norethindrone (OCs)	Norgestrel (OCs)	Drospirenone (OCs)
Medroxyprogesteone acetate (DMPA)	Norethindrone acetate (OCs)	Levonorgestrel (OCs)	
Chlormadinone acetate	Ethynodiol diacetate (OCs)	Desogestrel (OCs)	
Cyproterone acetate	Mefipristenone (RU-486)	Etonogestrel (implant, ring)	
	Norethynodrel	Gestodene (OCs)	
	Tibolone	Norgestimate (OCs)	
		Norelgestromin (patch)	

The parent compounds progesterone, testosterone, and spironolactone and their derivatives. Some of these derivatives are further modified to produce other derivatives. Many are currently marketed in the United States in hormonal contraceptives including OCs, the contraceptive patch, ring, implant, or DMPA injection. Gestodene, chlormadinone, and cyproterone acetate are progestin derivatives that are marketed as European OCs but not in the United States.

Adapted from ref. *3a*.

OC, oral contraceptive.

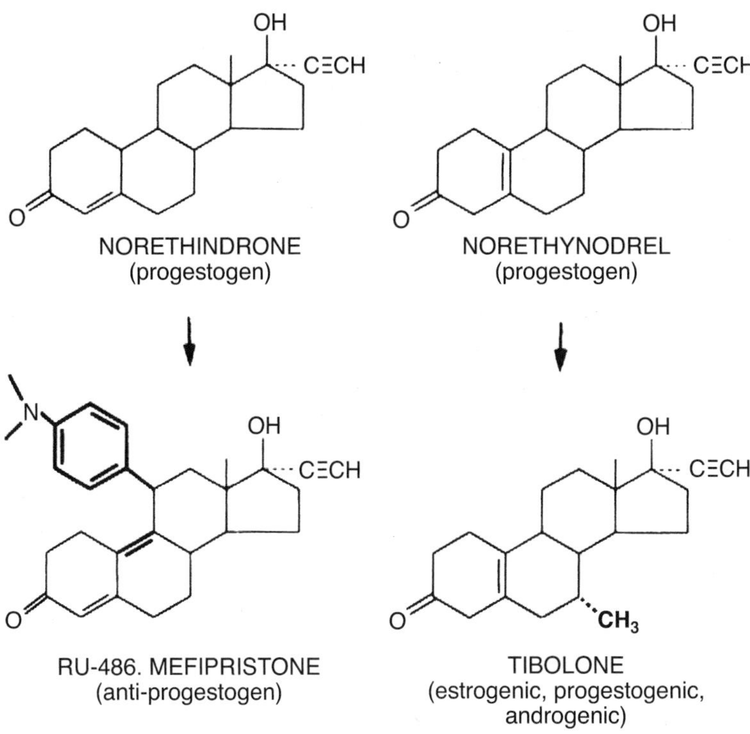

Fig. 2. Manipulation of norethindrone—a strong progestogen—results in an antihormone (RU-486). Tibolone is a derivative of the progestogen norethynodrel and displays a mixture of estrogenic, progestogenic, and androgenic properties. (From ref. *135* with permission.)

In 2003, the Food and Drug Administration (FDA) approved an extended regimen OC product (Seasonale®) containing 30 μg of EE and 150 mg of levonorgestrel (Fig. 3). Active pills are taken for 84 days followed by a 7-day pill-free interval to reduce the number of scheduled withdrawal bleeding episodes from 13 to 4 per year. Several new lower dose (20 μg EE) extended-regimen OCs, and a continuous-regimen OC (Lybrel™), are in development and should be available in the near future.

Several recently developed OCs also altered the traditional hormone-free interval. Whereas the extended regimen OC was developed to reduce the number of withdrawal menses, this new OC shortened the 7-day interval to a 4-day interval to improve bleeding profiles and decrease the incidence of ovulation and pregnancy that may occur when there is a delay in restarting the active pills in the beginning of a new cycle *(4)*. The US Food and Drug Administration has approved a new OC called Yaz® containing 20 μg ethinyl estradiol and 3 mg DRSP with a dosing regimen of 24 active pills followed by 4 days of placebo.

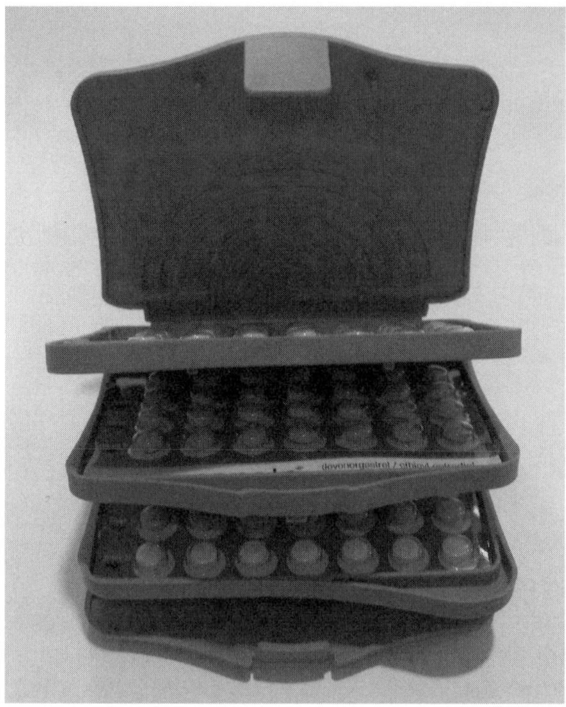

Fig. 3. Extended-cycle pill that comes with three packets.

MECHANISM OF ACTION

There are three major types of OC formulations: fixed-dose combination, combination phasic, and daily progestin-only (*see* Chapter 4). The combination estrogen–progestin formulations consistently inhibit the midcyle luteinizing hormone surge and effectively prevent ovulation. Several studies demonstrated a direct inhibitory effect on the pituitary and the hypothalamus *(5)*. The progestin-only formulations have a lower dose of progestin than the combined agents and do not consistently inhibit ovulation.

All formulations act on other areas of the reproductive tract by altering the following:

- Cervical mucus: making it viscid, thick, and scanty, thus preventing sperm penetration and inhibiting capacitation of the sperm.
- Decreasing motility of the uterus and oviduct thus inhibiting ova and sperm transport.
- Diminishing endometrial glandular production of glycogen making less energy available for the blastocyst to survive in the uterine cavity.
- Decreasing ovarian responsiveness to gonadotropin stimulation.

Because the doses of steroids in currently marked OCs are low, neither gonadotropin production nor ovarian steroidogenesis is completely suppressed. Complete absence of follicular activity, as was often noted during high-dose OC use, no longer occurs *(6)*.

The magnitude of hypothalamic–pituitary suppression is unrelated to the age of the woman or the duration of steroid use, but is related to the potency of the progestin and estrogen in the formulation. The magnitude of the hypothalamic–pituitary suppression is correlated with the incidence and severity of prolonged amenorrhea after stopping OCs. After discontinuing current low-dose formulations, return to ovulation is usually rapid. However, because the suppression is so quickly reversible, there is less room for error when using current low-dose OCs. Extending the pill-free interval for more than 7 days may result in breakthrough ovulation and pregnancy. Women should be advised that the most important pills to remember to take are the first ones of each cycle. The new low-dose OC Yaz shortens the pill-free interval to 4 days to potentially increase effectiveness with typical use.

CLINICAL EFFECTIVENESS

No significant differences in clinical effectiveness have been demonstrated for the various combination OCs currently available. With perfect use, the pregnancy rate is 0.2–0.3% at the end of 1 year with all products. However, the typical use failure rate is higher and varies between 3 and 8% depending on the population. The risk of contraception failure is highest if pills are missed at the beginning of the cycle. Because the contraceptive patch and ring have basically the same mechanism of action, their perfect and typical use failure rate is considered to be the same as combination OCs *(7)*. OCs, the contraceptive patch, and ring are very effective but are considered to be in the second tier of contraceptive effectiveness. The first tier methods, intrauterine devices, implants, and injections, have lower typical failure rates as they are not as subject to user error.

A recent study suggested that high body weight may alter the metabolism of the steroids in low-dose OCs enough to reduce their effectiveness. In a retrospective study, women weighing more than 160 lb (70.5 kg) taking OC formulations with less than 50 μg had a failure rate 2.6 times greater than women with lower body weight, and a 4.5 times greater failure rate when using formulations with less than 35 μg *(8)*. A lower contraceptive effectiveness was also reported in patch users weighing more than 198 lb *(9)*. The risks associated with using a pill with higher amounts of EE should be balanced against this possible increased failure rate when deciding on an appropriate formulation.

Progestin-only pills (POPs), often referred to as "minipills," have about 25–70% of the progestin dose contained in combination OCs. POPs, even if taken at the same time each day, are slightly less effective than combination pills. With perfect use, POPs' failure rate is 0.5%. As with combination OCs, data indicates the failure rates with POPs are higher for users who weigh more than 127.4 lb (57.8 kg; *see* Chapter 4).

ADVANTAGES OF LOW-DOSE OCS

OCs are:

- Highly effective if taken correctly.
- Relatively easy to use and require no special precautions at the time of intercourse.
- Rapidly reversible: most women become pregnant within 2–3 months after discontinuing use.
- Safe: healthy, nonsmoking, normotensive women can use OCs safely throughout their reproductive years.
- Low cost for women covered by various family planning programs (can be as low as $1.50 per month).
- OCs are associated with a long list of contraceptive and non-contraceptive health benefits that are detailed extensively in sections below. OCs are associated with:
    - Decreased menstrual blood loss, decreased menstrual cramping, control of bleeding patterns.
    - Decreased dysmenorrhea.
    - Decreased androgen-related problems and premenstrual syndrome.
    - Decreased risk of pelvic inflammatory disease (PID), ovarian cysts, and benign breast disease.
    - Decreased risk of ovarian and endometrial cancer.

DISADVANTAGES OF LOW-DOSE OCS

- The major disadvantage of OCs is that they must be taken daily.
    - Studies show that in some populations 11% discontinue pills in the first month of use, 28% discontinue by 6 months and 33–50% discontinue by 1 year *(10)*.
- OCs do not provide protection from STDs or HIV transmission (lower tract infections).
- The cost of OCs to women not on special family planning programs generally ranges from $15 to $50 per cycle. (The generic brands are generally less expensive.) The contraceptive ring and patch cost around $40 per cycle.
- The side effects of OCs include the following:
    - Breast tenderness, nausea, headache.
    - Mood changes, bloating.
- The risks of OC use include the following:
    - Venous thromboembolism (venous thrombosis and pulmonary embolism). Although OCs increase the risk of venous thromboembolism two- to four-fold, the risk is half compared with the risk associated with pregnancy (Chapter 3, Table 1).

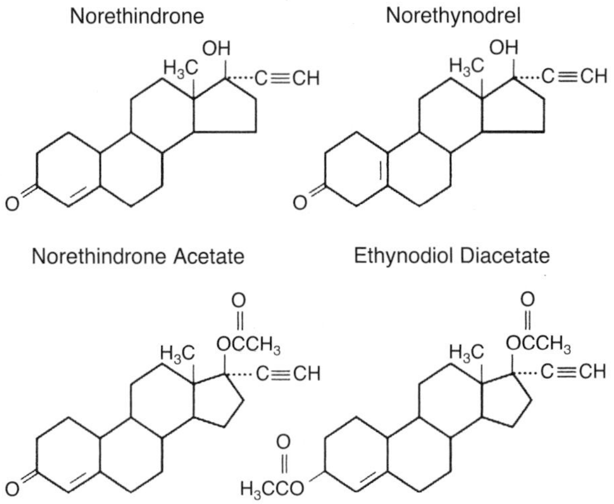

Norethindrone

Norethynodrel

Norethindrone Acetate

Ethynodiol Diacetate

Fig. 4. Chemical structure of the estrane progestins, derivatives of norethindrone, used in oral contraceptives. (© 2004 Elsevier, reprinted from ref. *136* with permission.)

- Ischemic or hemorrhagic stroke. Several studies indicate that young users of low-dose OCs who do not smoke and have no risk factors for cardiovascular disease have no increased risk.
- Myocardial infarction. Several studies show no increased risk in healthy low-dose estrogen OC users who do not smoke and do not have significant cardiovascular disease risk factors *(11,12)*.
- Breast cancer. There is conflicting information, but during use, some studies show a very small increase in the diagnosis of breast cancer in users and others show no change in risk. There is evidence that OCs do not cause breast cancer but may promote an existing lesion. The length of use does not affect risk and the risk returns to baseline after discontinuation *(13)*.

PHARMACOLOGY

All currently marketed combination OCs are composed of a synthetic estrogen plus a progestin. The progestin component provides most of the contraceptive protection while the estrogen provides cycle control and boosts the contraceptive effectiveness of the progestin.

All but one of the synthetic progestins currently marketed in the United States in hormonal contraceptives are derivatives of either 19-nortestosterone or 17α-acetoxyprogesterone (*see* Chapter 7) as shown in Table 1. The derivatives of 19-nortestosterone are either estranes or gonanes. The original OC containing norethynodrel, an estrane derivative of 19-nortestosterone, is no longer marketed, but the estrane norethindrone and its derivatives along with levonorgestrel and other gonane derivatives are used in currently marketed formulations (Fig. 4).

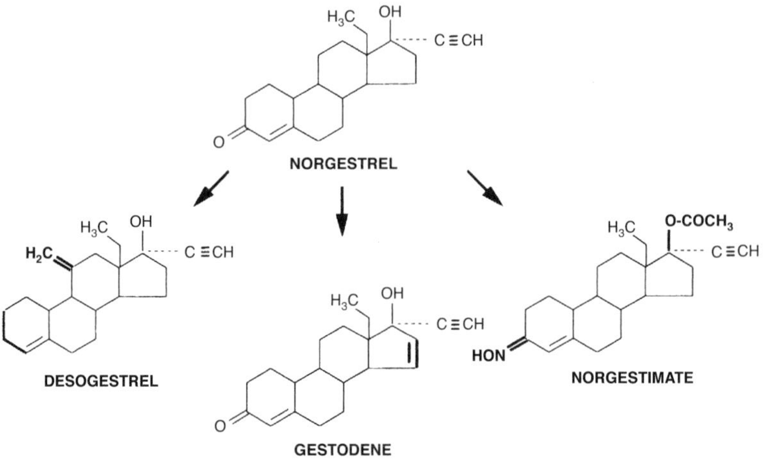

Fig. 5. Gonane progestogens derived from manipulation of the norgestrel molecule. (From ref. *135* with permission.)

The gonane derivatives have greater progestational activity per unit weight than estranes. Modifications in the chemical structure of gonane derivatives resulted in compounds that have altered biological activity. The magnitude of difference in androgenic and progestational effects produced by each progestin is called selectivity. The so-called "third-generation" progestins, norgestimate, desogestrel, and gestodene, derived from the gonane norgestrel, have high selectivity and demonstrate high progestational activity and low androgenic activity when compared with the other gonanes (Fig. 5). The OC formulations containing desogestrel, norgestimate, and gestodene are called third-generation OCs. The patch contains norelgestromin, a metabolite of norgestimate, and the ring and implant contain etonogestrel, a metabolite of desogestrel.

There has recently been introduced a new progestin, DRSP (Fig. 6), that is an entirely different progestin. It is structurally related to spironolactone and in addition to its progestogenic activity, exhibits antimineralocorticoid and antiandrogenic activities.

The newer selective progestins, including DRSP, do not counter the effects of the estrogen component as strongly as the older progestins, and are associated with higher sex hormone-binding globulin (SHBG) and other liver globulins compared with combination products with the same estrogen dose and a less selective progestin. Adjustment of the new progestin products with a lower dose of estrogen is being studied and may result in a better safety profile.

Only two estrogens are used in OCs in the United States. The so-called first-generation OCs contain 50 μg of either EE or mestranol (Fig. 7). The second-generation OCs contain 20–35 μg of EE. OCs containing one of the three newer gonane progestins and are called third-generation OCs.

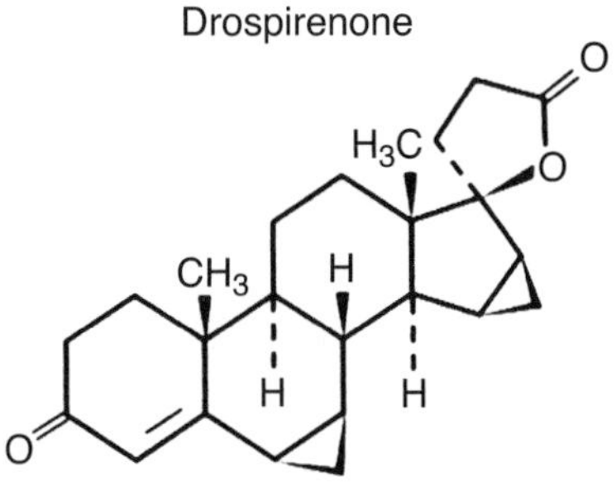

Fig. 6. Chemical structure of drospirenone. (© 2004 Elsevier, reprinted from ref. *136* with permission.)

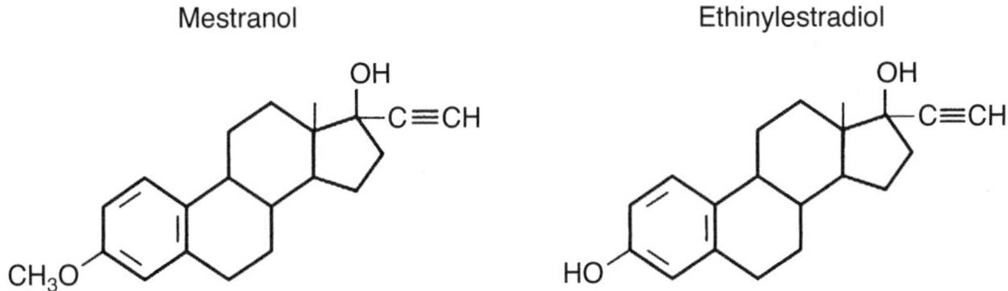

Fig. 7. Structure of the two estrogens used in combination oral contraceptives. (© 2004 Elsevier, reprinted from ref. *136* with permission.)

All the synthetic estrogens and progestins in OCs have an ethinyl group at position C17 (Fig. 8). The presence of this ethinyl group enhances the oral activity of these agents because they are not as rapidly metabolized as they pass through the intestinal mucosa and the liver through the portal system. EE has about 100 times the potency of an equivalent weight of conjugated equine estrogen or estrone sulfate for stimulating synthesis of hepatic proteins.

The two estrogens used in OCs, EE and its 3-methyl ether, mestranol, have different biological potency. Mestranol must be demethylated to EE to bind to the estrogen cytosol receptor and become biologically active. The degree of conversion of mestranol to EE varies among individuals, although overall, EE is about 1.7 times as potent as the same weight of mestranol *(14)*.

METABOLIC EFFECTS AND SIDE EFFECTS: ESTROGEN AND PROGESTIN

In addition to their contraceptive actions, OCs have many other metabolic effects (Table 2). These metabolic effects may be associated with mild or moderate side effects that often disappear over time or after switching to another formulation. The magnitude of the effects is directly related to the potency and

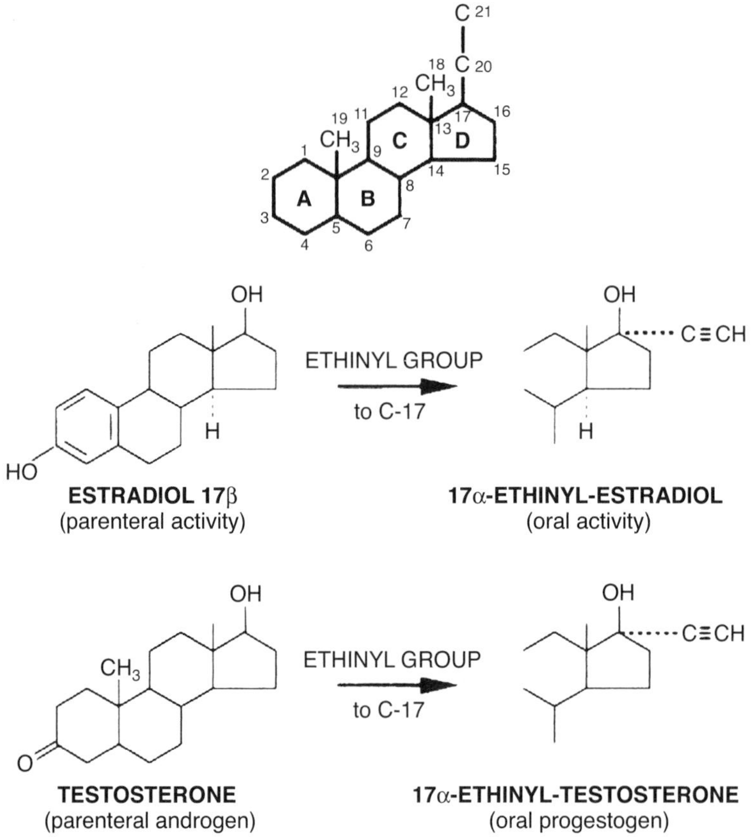

ETHINYL GROUP to C-17

ESTRADIOL 17β (parenteral activity)

17α-ETHINYL-ESTRADIOL (oral activity)

ETHINYL GROUP to C-17

TESTOSTERONE (parenteral androgen)

17α-ETHINYL-TESTOSTERONE (oral progestogen)

Fig. 8. The importance of the ethinyl group (C≡CH) on C-17 for oral activity of steroids. Introduction of the ethinyl group into the estradiol molecule resulted in the first orally active synthetic estrogen—ethinyl-estradiol. Similar manipulation of the testosterone molecule resulted in the first orally active progestogenic agent—ethinyl testosterone. The numbering system of the steroid molecule is given for reference. (From ref. *135* with permission.)

dosage of the steroids in the formulations, thus the trend toward lower-dose OCs. Fortunately, serious adverse complications are rare in healthy young women and in properly selected perimenopausal (Chapter 14) or medically complicated women (Chapter 15).

Estrogen-Related Problems

The most common estrogen-related symptoms include nausea (a central nervous system effect), breast tenderness, increased breast size, headaches, and cyclic fluid retention. The fluid retention is a result of an increased estrogen-stimulated aldosterone secretion causing decreased sodium excretion. The cyclic

Table 2
Clinical and Metabolic Effects of Contraceptive Steroids (Progestins)

	Metabolic effects	*Possible associated clinical effects*
Estrogens: ethinyl estradiol		
Hepatic proteins		
Albumin	Decrease	
Angiotensinogen	Increase	Increased blood pressure
Clotting factors	Increase	Hypercoagulability, increased DVT risk
Carrier proteins	Increase	
SHBG	Increase	Lowers circulating free testosterone and other circulating sex steroids, lowered libido
TBG	Increase	Lowers free thyroid hormones; may prompt adjustment of oral dose
CBG	Increase	
Transferrin	Increase	
Ceruloplasmin		
Glucose tolerance	Small decrease, especially with high-dose OCs	Increased insulin resistance
Plasma insulin	Slight increase	Possible increased CVD risk
Lipids		
Cholesterol	Increase	Possible increased CVD risk
Triglycerides	Increase	Possible increased CVD risk
HDL cholesterol	Increase	Possible decreased CVD risk
LDL cholesterol	Decrease	Possible decreased CVD risk
Sodium excretion	Decrease	Cyclic fluid retention, edema
Vitamins		
B complex	Decrease	Rare vitamin deficiency with older, high-dose OCs
Ascorbic acid	Decrease	
Vitamin A	Increase	
Breast	Stimulate	Breast tenderness, increase in breast size
Endometrial estrogen receptors	Increase	Endometrial stimulation, increased bleeding, endometrial hyperstimulation
Skin		
5α-reductase and other androgen receptors	Decrease	Decreased sebum (oily skin), acne, hirsutism, and other androgenic problems
Pigmentation	Increase	Increased facial pigmentation
Other	Increase	Telangiectasia
Progestins: 19-nortestosterone derivatives		
Hepatic proteins		
SHBG	Decrease	Increased free circulating testosterone and other sex steroids, increased androgen activity

(continued)

Table 2 *(Continued)*
Clinical and Metabolic Effects of Contraceptive Steroids (Progestins)

	Metabolic effects	*Possible associated clinical effects*
APC, clotting factors	Possibly oppose thrombotic effect of estrogen	
Glucose tolerance	Decrease	Possible increased CVD risk
Insulin resistance	Increase	
Cholesterol	Decrease	Possible decreased CVD risk
Trigylcerides	Decrease	Possible decreased CVD risk
HDL cholesterol	Decrease	Possible increased CVD risk
LDL cholesterol	Increase	Possible increased CVD risk
Appetite		
Nitrogen	Increase	Increased body weight, bloating
Retention	Increase	
Skin		
Androgen		
Activity	Increase	Increased sebum (oily skin), acne, hirsutism
CNS effects	Increased activity	Nervousness, fatigue, depression, tiredness, PMS symptoms
Endometrial steroid receptors	Decrease	Less menstrual bleeding, no withdrawal bleeding

Metabolic and clinical effects are related to dose, potency, and particularly estrogen and progestin, and are often minimal in current low-dose oral contraceptives.

CBG, corticosteroid-binding globulin; TBG, thyroid-binding globulin; HDL, high-density lipoprotein; LDL, low-density lipoprotein; CVD, cardiovascular disease; OC, oral contraceptive; APC, activated protein C; CNS, central nervous system; SHBG, sex hormone-binding globulin; PMS, premenstrual syndrome.

Adapted from ref. *136*.

fluid retention generally does not exceed 3–4 lb. There are minor, clinically insignificant changes in circulating vitamins. Estrogen can also cause melasma, an increased pigmentation on the malar eminences. Melasma often takes a long time to disappear and is accentuated by sunlight. The incidences of all of these estrogen-related adverse effects are much lower than those seen with use of older high-dose OCs.

Estrogen can increase the concentration of cholesterol in gallbladder bile and older formulations were associated with an increased incidence of cholelithiasis and cholecystitis. Newer, low-dose OCs appear to avoid these side effects. The results of a large British Family Planning Association study *(15)* and a case–control study *(16)* indicate that use of OCs does not increase the incidence of gallbladder disease in women, even if used for more than 8 years *(17)*.

Mood and Depression

- Low-dose OCs have not been linked with depression *(18)*, although positive and negative mood changes can occur in certain individuals with particular formulations.

In 1984, the Royal College of General Practitioners cohort study reported that the incidence of depression in OC users was positively correlated with the dose of estrogen in the formulation *(19)*. It has been postulated that the high dosages of the synthetic estrogen in OCs divert tryptophan metabolism from its minor pathway in the brain to its major pathway in the liver. The end product, serotonin, is thus decreased in the central nervous system, resulting in depression. In this study, women using OCs containing less than 50 μg of estrogen did not have an increased incidence of depression. By contrast, postmenopausal women receiving physiological doses of estrogen report an improved mood, whereas the addition of a progestin increases depression, tension, irritability, and fatigue *(20)*.

Carbohydrate Metabolism

- Low-dose OCs do not adversely alter glucose metabolism *(21–23)*.

The adverse effect of high-dose OCs on glucose metabolism is primarily related to the potency and dose of progestin. Although estrogens may act synergistically with the progestin to further impair glucose tolerance, in general, the higher the dose and potency of the progestin, the greater the magnitude of impaired glucose tolerance. However, formulations with low doses of progestins, including levonorgestrel, do not significantly alter levels of glucose, insulin, or glucagons after a glucose load in healthy women *(24)* or in those with a history of gestational diabetes *(25)*. Data from 20 years of experience of women using OCs was reported in a large cohort study. There was no increased risk of diabetes mellitus among current OC users or former OC users, even among women using OCs for 10 years or more *(26)*. Recent short-term studies of low-dose OCs also show no increase in diabetes mellitus *(27)*.

Hepatic Proteins

Synthetic estrogens in OCs stimulate increases in hepatic production of several globulins in a dose-dependent manner. The progestin component suppresses the synthesis of SHBG but has little influence on other hepatic production. Estrogen increases the production of the following hepatic proteins:

- Clotting factors: factors V, VIII, and X, and fibrinogen (enhance thrombosis) *(28)*.
  - Epidemiological studies show the increased risk of both arterial and venous thrombosis is directly related to the dose of estrogen *(29)*.
- Blood pressure factors: angiotensinogen.
  - About 0.4% of low-dose OC users became hypertensive in the Nurses Health Study *(30)*.

- SHBG: measurement of SHBG is one way to determine the relative estrogenic/androgenic balance of different OC formulations. Formulations with the greatest increases are particularly useful in treating women with symptoms of hyperandrogenism.
    - Greatest increase in SHBG levels occur following ingestion of OC formulations containing desogestrel, cyproterone acetate, and gestodene and, to a lesser degree, those with low-dose norethindrone and levonorgestrel *(31)*.
    - SHBG levels have also been linked to increases in activated protein C (APC) resistance and thrombosis. Some data suggest that increases in SHBG with OCs could be interpreted as a measure of total estrogenicity and used as a predictor of the risk of venous thromboembolism (VTE) *(32–34)*. (Further research is needed to define the best balance of new progestins with low doses of estrogen.)

Lipids

The estrogen component of OCs increases high-density lipoprotein (HDL) cholesterol, total cholesterol, and triglycerides, and decreases low-density lipoprotein (LDL) cholesterol. The progestin component has the reverse effect. Older progestin-dominant formulations had adverse effects on the lipid profiles producing decreases in HDL cholesterol and increases in LDL cholesterol levels. Because estrogen has a more potent effect on trigylcerides than progestin, the older formulations also showed significant increases in trigylcerides.

The newer, low-dose OCs still show increases in trigylceride, but generally produce little or no adverse changes in HDL or LDL cholesterol *(35,36)*. No long-term effects of these changes in lipid parameters are reported in past users.

Coagulation Parameters

OCs have multiple effects on coagulation parameters.

- OCs enhance thrombosis (through increases in fibrinogen), inhibit coagulation (protein C, protein S, and antithrombin), enhance fibrinolysis (plasminogen), and inhibit fibrinolysis (plasminogen activator-inhibitor 1).
- OCs diminish the efficacy with which APC naturally downregulates thrombin formation, designated as acquired APC resistance. Several reports indicate that the use of third-generation OCs is associated with increased acquired APC resistance compared with use of second-generation OCs *(37,38)*.
- Changes in coagulation parameters in OC users are small and have a limited clinical impact in healthy users.
- Women with inherited coagulation disorders, such as deficiency of protein C, protein S, antithrombin, or APC resistance, have several-fold increased risk of thrombosis if they use combination OCs *(39)*.
    - The annual incidence of deep venous thrombosis in women of reproductive age with an APC resistance is about 6 per 10,000 but is increased to 30 per 10,000 during use of OCs.

  - At the present, screening for these coagulation deficiencies is not recommended before initiating OCs unless a woman has a personal or strong family history of thrombotic events, although screening is certainly indicated in women with a VTE, especially if it occurs during the early use of OCs *(40)*.

Cardiovascular Events

Venous Thromboembolism

- The risk of VTE is directly related to the dose of estrogen in the OC but is lower than the rate associated with pregnancy *(42)*.
  - Inherited disorders, such as factor V Leiden mutation, protein S and C synthesis, or prothrombin mutation disorders (found in 0.5 to 5% of reproductive aged women), can dramatically increase an OC user's risk of VTE.
    - Women with a strong family or personal history of clotting problems should not use estrogen-containing OCs and should undergo screening.
- Thrombosis can occur in a variety of sites including leg or thigh veins, lung, eye, intestines, brain, or heart.

The risk of VTE is directly related to the dose of estrogen in the OC. The background rate VTE in reproductive age women in about 0.8 per 10,000 woman-years. The rate in OC users taking pills with 20 to 50 μg EE is reported to be 3 per 10,000 woman-years. Although this is about four times the background rate of reproductive-age women, it is half the rate of 6 per 10,000 woman-years associated with pregnancy *(43)*.

Controversy exists as to whether or not the OCs containing gestodene and desogestrel are associated with an increased risk of VTE or whether the increased risk (1.5 to 2.5 times the risk with levonorgestrel low-dose OCs) reported in several studies *(44–46)* may result from certain types of bias. Selection, diagnostic, and reference biases could account for the differences, but a causal relationship may exist *(47,48)*. Lower rates of myocardial infarction with third-generation products is also reported *(49)*.

It has been suggested that the phenomenon designated as acquired APC resistance (increased resistance to the anticoagulant action of APC) is more pronounced in women using third-generation versus second-generation OCs *(50)*. The fact that the third-generation progestins do not oppose the various effects of estrogen as strongly as older progestins may play a role. The newer selective progestins may not counter the thrombotic effect of the estrogen component in combined OCs as well as the older progestins *(51)*. The trend toward even lower doses of EE may be particularly beneficial for new OCs with the new progestins.

Myocardial Infarction

The cause of the increased incidence of cardiovascular disease including myocardial infarction, in users of OCs appears to be thrombosis not atherosclerosis (41).

> *A recent World Health Organization technical report states that women who do not smoke, have their blood pressure checked, and do not have hypertension or diabetes mellitus have no increased risk of myocardial infarction (MI) if they use combined OCs, regardless of their age (52). However, women with these risk factors or those with known vascular disease/vessel narrowing should not use OCs because they are at significantly increased risk.*

- The increase in MI attributable to OCs is due to estrogen-induced arterial thrombosis not atherosclerosis.
- The increased risk of MI with OC use only occurs in women with known risk factors *(53)*.
  - The risk of death attributable to OC use in low-risk women is lower than their risk of death from pregnancy, regardless of their age.
  - Large increases in the relative risk of MI or stroke (7- to 100-fold increase) are reported for OC users who smoke or have hypertension *(54)*.
  - Because of their narrowed vessels, women with underlying vascular disease are at highest risk for the estrogen-induced changes in thrombosis.
  - For many years, uncontrolled hypertension or women over age 35 who smoke cigarettes have been contraindications to the use of OCs.

Nearly all the published epidemiological studies confirm that there is no increased risk of MI among former users of OCs *(55)*. Studies with cynomolgus macaque monkeys found that, although ingestion of OCs containing high doses of norgestrel and EE resulted in lowered HDL cholesterol, these animals had a significantly smaller amount of coronary artery atherosclerosis than did a control group of female monkeys not ingesting OCs but fed the same atherogenic diet after 2 years of use *(56)*. This study suggests that the estrogen component of OCs does not promote atherosclerosis but rather has a direct protective effect on the coronary arteries.

Since the 1970s, epidemiological studies have reported significantly increased risk of MI, mainly among older OC users who had risk factors that caused arterial narrowing, such as hypertension, diabetes mellitus, or smoking *(57,58)*. A case–control study analyzed the risk of MI after OC use in women admitted to hospitals in northeastern United States between 1985 and 1999. The relative risk of MI among current OC users was not significantly increased; however, among women who smoked at least 25 cigarettes a day, current OC use increased the risk of MI 32-fold compared with nonsmokers not using OCs. However, smoking alone was an independent risk factor and increased the risk of MI about 12-fold even without use of OCs *(59)*. A more recent meta-analysis reported that current use of OCs increased this risk of MI by 2.48 *(60)*. In a rigorous meta-analysis, low-dose OCs with second- and third-generation progestogens increased the risk of cardiac and vascular arterial events; the increased risk seemed less robust for the use of third-generation OCs. The authors link much of the increased risk to baseline risk factors including hypertension, migraines, smoking, or metabolic syndrome *(61)*.

Stroke

- Recent studies of low-dose OCs show no increased risk of stroke for nonsmoking women without risk factors for cardiovascular disease *(62–64)*.
- OC users who smoke or have hypertension or migraines with aura have a threefold increased risk of stroke compared with nonusers *(65)*.

As occurred with MI, the epidemiological studies of OCs that show increased risk of stroke in OC users, indicated that the increased risk was mainly limited to older women who also smoked or were hypertensive. There appears to be no difference between second- and third-generation OCs *(66)*.

Hypertension

The OC-induced increases in angiotensin II and aldosterone may be associated with increases is systolic or diastolic blood pressure in some women. A significant increase is seen in only 1 to 3% of users. Blood pressure normalizes within 2 to 3 months after OC discontinuation.

Progestin-Related Problems

Because progestins are derivatives of testosterone, the progestin components of OCs may have androgenic side effects. With the use of low-dose progestins or new, low-androgenic progestins, these side effects are reduced. Additionally, all current combination OCs suppress endogenous testosterone production and increase SHBG that binds up free testosterone. Therefore, most combination OCs actually decrease androgenic activity and androgenic problems, including acne, hirsutism, and oily skin. Some products have a particularly good anti-androgenic action and have specific FDA approval for treatment of acne.

Other androgenic and progestogenic side effects include cyclic mood changes, increased appetite, tiredness, anxiety, and depression. Progestin's impact on lipids, glucose metabolism, hepatic proteins, skin, and CNS effects are listed in Table 2.

Androgenic Effects

- Most currently marketed OCs have a beneficial impact on acne or facial hair through multiple estrogenic actions (increases in SHBG, direct skin effects, and suppression of endogenous androgens).

Although all low-dose OCs are associated with a reduction in androgen-related problems, the gonane and estrane progestins are structurally related to testosterone and may produce certain androgenic side effects. These include nervousness, acne, weight gain, and increased sebum production. The current low-dose OCs have less androgenic side effects than the high-dose OCs of the past because of lower doses of progestins. For women with primary complaints of moderate to severe acne or other manifestations of hyperandrogenism, OCs with norgestimate, desogestrel, and DRSP are considered the formulations of choice.

REPRODUCTIVE EFFECTS OF LOW-DOSE OCS

There is a slight delay in the return of ovulation in women discontinuing use of OCs. For about 2 years after stopping, the rate of return of fertility is lower in previous OC users compared with previous barrier method users, but eventually the percentage of women in both groups becomes the same *(67)*.

Neither the rates of birth defects *(68)*, spontaneous abortion, or chromosomal abnormalities in abortuses *(69)* are increased in women conceiving during the first or second month after discontinuing OCs. If OCs are accidentally ingested during the first few months of pregnancy, a large cohort study reported no increased risk of congenital malformations among the offspring *(70)*.

NEOPLASTIC EFFECTS OF LOW-DOSE OCS

Breast Cancer

- OCs have undergone extensive study for more than 40 years in an attempt to determine the relationship between OCs and the development of breast cancer.
- The vast amount of studies show small or no changes in the relative risk of breast cancer during OC use. Following discontinuation of OCs, the risk returns to baseline.
  - It is reassuring that the risk of having had breast cancer diagnosed by age 65 is the same in past users as in never users.
- It appears that the dose or type of either steroid, as well as duration of OC use, is not related to breast cancer risk.

The results of a study by the National Institute of Child Health and Human Development are very reassuring *(71)*. This study reported that current or prior use of OCs did not affect a women's risk of diagnosis of breast cancer between the ages of 35 and 64; the relative risk (RR) estimates were 1.0 and 0.9 for current or prior OC users compared with nonusers, respectively. The risk was not increased among women who had taken OCs for long periods of time or had used formulations with high amounts of estrogen. Additionally, women with a family history of breast cancer did not have a further increased risk of breast cancer with OCs use.

It is important to also consider the findings of an international collaborative study that analyzed the data from 54 studies performed in 25 countries, involving more than 53,000 women with breast cancer and more than 100,000 control subjects. Current OCs users had a slightly increased risk of having breast cancer (RR: 1.24, confidence interval [CI]: 1.15–1.30) *(72)*. After discontinuing OCs, the risk declined steadily and by 10 years, the risk was no longer significant (RR: 1.01, CI: 0.96–1.05). The cancers diagnosed in women taking OCs in this study were less advanced clinically than those in nonusers. The authors concluded that these results could be explained by the fact that breast cancer is diagnosed earlier in OC users than in nonusers or could result from biological effects of the OCs.

- There are two factors that may explain this increased risk of breast cancer: detection bias or a promoter effect. A detection bias would occur if OCs users are more likely to have breast exams or receive mammograms and thus more likely to have their breast cancer diagnosed. Alternatively, the epidemiological findings are compatible with the hypothesis that OCs may act to promote the growth of increase the chance of diagnosis of existing cancers. Like early first-term pregnancy, OCs slightly increase the risk of breast cancer diagnosis at a young age with no appreciable effect on lifetime risk of breast cancer and no change in risk during the perimenopausal years when the disease becomes more common.

Cervical Cancer and Cervical Dysplasia

- Although it is uncertain whether OCs increase the risk of cervical cancer, act as a co-carcinogen, or have no effect, users of OCs as a group have an increased risk of cervical neoplasia and require at least annual screening of cervical cytology, especially if they have used OCs for more than 5 years.

The epidemiological data is conflicting regarding OC use and risk of invasive cervical cancer. Confounding factors may account for the different results in various studies, such as the woman's age at first sexual intercourse, exposure to human papillomavirus (HPV), number of sexual partners, cytological screening (possibly more frequent among OC users), use of barrier contraceptives or spermicides, and cigarette smoking (an independent risk factor). However, most of the studies made statistical correction for these confounding factors.

Pooled data from eight case–control studies reported that the RR of invasive cervical cancer was 0.73 for less than 5 years of OC use, 2.82 for 5–9 years of use, and 4.03 for 10 or more years of use *(73)*. In this analysis, OCs increased the risk of cervical cancer only in women infected with HPV, but not in women without HPV. In an even larger meta-analysis of 28 studies including 12,531 women with cervical cancer, 5 years of OC use was associated with an RR of 1.1. OC use for 5 to 10 years was associated with an RR of 1.6 and an RR of 2.2 after 10 years of use *(74)*.

Endometrial Cancer

- Women who use OCs for at least 1 year have an age-adjusted RR of 0.5 for the diagnosis of endometrial cancer between 40 and 55 years compared with nonusers.

Three cohort studies and 12 case–control studies examined the relationship between endometrial cancer and OCs. All but two of these studies indicated that OCs have a protective effect *(75)*. This protective effect is related to duration of use increasing from 20% reduction with 1 year of use to 40% reduction with 2 years use to about 60% reduction with 4 years of use. It appears that both high- and low-dose formulations are protective *(76)*.

Ovarian Cancer

- The RR of ovarian cancer among ever-users of OCs is around 0.64, a 36% reduction.

Of 20 reports on the use of OCs with subsequent development of ovarian cancer, 18 found a reduction in risk *(77)*. OCs were found to reduce the risk of the four main histological types of epithelial ovarian cancer (serous, endometrioid, clear cell, and mucinous) and the risk of those with low malignant potential. The decreased risk is directly related to the duration of OC use, increasing from about 40% reduction with 4 years of use to a 53% reduction with 8 years and a 60% reduction with 12 years of use.

Liver Adenoma and Cancer

Although rare, the prolonged use of high-dose OCs, particularly those containing mestranol, has been linked to an increased risk of hepatocellular adenoma. Although two British studies reported an increased risk of liver cancer among OC users, data from a large World Health Organization multicenter study found no increased risk of liver cancer associated with OC users in countries with a high prevalence rate of this neoplasm *(78)*.

Colorectal Cancer

Although a meta-analysis published in the year 2000 showed a significant reduction of risk for OC users (0.81 for the case–control studies and 0.84 for the cohort studies), a causal relationship between OCs and colorectal cancer remains to be established *(79)*. Support for the belief that estrogen causes a reduction in colon cancer is provided by multiple studies showing that postmenopausal estrogen use has also been associated with a lower risk of colon cancer.

Pituitary Adenomas

Discontinuing OCs may unmask the amenorrhea associated with a pituitary adenoma, suggesting a causal relationship. However, data from three separate studies document that the incidence of pituitary adenoma among users of OCs is not higher than that among matched nonusers *(80)*.

Malignant Melanoma

The results of many large studies of long duration indicate that OC use does not increase the risk of malignant melanoma *(81)*.

DRUG INTERACTIONS

As a result of substrate competition, synthetic sex steroids can retard the biotransformation of certain drugs, such as phenazone and meperidine. Such interference is generally not clinically significant. However, some drugs can interfere clinically with the action of OCs by inducing liver enzymes that convert the steroids to more polar, less biologically active metabolites. For this reason, drugs such as barbiturates, carbamazepine, griseofulvin, sulfonamides, antiretinal, cyclophosphamide, and rifampin *(82)* should not be given concomitantly with OCs (Chapter 3, Table 2).

The clinical data linking certain antibiotics (penicillin, ampicillin, and sulfonamides), antiepileptics (phenytoin), and barbiturates are less clear. A few anecdotal studies have appeared in the literature, but reliable evidence for a clinical inhibitory effect of these drugs on OC effectiveness, such as occurring with rifampin, is not available. The best data is on antiepileptic medications that are known to induce hepatic P450 enzymes and thus increase estrogen metabolism. Based on this data, it is recommended that women with epilepsy requiring medication should consider a 35 μg or higher formulation *(83)*, although a risk–benefit evaluation should be done.

CONTRACEPTIVE HEALTH BENEFITS

In 2003, the Centers for Disease Control and Prevention reported that there was an average of 11.8 pregnancy-related deaths per 100,000 live births during the 1990s in the United States *(84)*. By protecting the user from pregnancy, this risk is substantially reduced. The user is also protected from ectopic pregnancies (≥90% reduced risk) *(85)*, the leading cause of pregnancy-related deaths in the first trimester of pregnancy. It is estimated that OC use prevents 1–7 million abortions worldwide annually. For most healthy, nonsmoking women, the risk of using any contraceptive method is safer than using no method (Chapter 3, Table 1).

NON-CONTRACEPTIVE HEALTH BENEFITS

In addition to their effective contraceptive protection, OCs provide a wide range of other health benefits *(86)*. These benefits are not FDA-approved indications, but the clinician and users may want to consider them in their overall assessment.

- Reduction in the amount of monthly blood loss resulting from a progestin "antiestrogenic" action on the endometrium *(87)*. In an ovulatory cycle, the mean blood loss is about 35 mL, compared with 20 mL in OC users.
  - OCs are often an effective treatment for menorrhagia *(88,89)*.
  - Less iron-deficiency anemia *(90,91)*.
- Fewer menstrual irregularities: OCs are designed to produce regular withdrawal bleeding *(92)*.
  - Less frequent curettage or hysterectomy.
  - Eighty percent improvement in dysfunctional uterine bleeding *(93)*.
- Lowered risk of endometrial cancer.
  - OC use for 1 year reduces the risk by 40% *(94)* and by 80% after 10 years of use *(95)*.

    - Protection lasts for up to 20 years *(96)*.
- Lowered risk of ovarian cancer.
    - Risk is reduced by 40% *(97)* after ever-use and 80% reduced after 10 years of use *(98)*.
        - Protection lasts for up to 20 years *(99)*.
        - Protection may include women with *BRCA* mutations *(100–102)* or strong family history of ovarian cancer *(103,104)*, although some studies show that protection is limited to those that are not genetically at risk *(105)*.
        - High-dose progestin OCs may give more protection than low-progestin OCs *(106)*.
- Lowered risk of benign breast disease *(107)*.
    - Reduced risk of cysts, fibrocystic changes, fibroadenomas *(108)*.
        - Progestins inhibit the synthesis of estrogen receptors in breast tissue.
- Less dysmenorrhea (63%) *(109)*.
    - OC use can reduce absences from work or school.
- Lowered incidence of symptomatic endometriosis *(110)*.
- Less premenstrual syndrome symptoms (29%) *(111,112)*.
    - Less bloating, pain, cramping, mastalgia.
    - OCs containing DRSP reported to improve symptoms of water retention, negative affect *(113,114)*.
- Lowered rate of functional cysts *(115)*, although follicular cyst formation may not be eliminated with low-dose OCs *(116)*.
- Lowered incidence of androgen excess conditions.
    - Reduction in acne lesions *(117,118)* and hirsutism *(119,120)*.
        - All formulations associated with improvements in mild to moderate acne; only Ortho Tri-Cyclen® *(121)* and Estrostep® have FDA approval for treatment.
- Lowered risk of PID *(122)* primarily because of reductions in gonorrhea PID.
    - Upper tract infections may be prevented.
        - Thickened cervical mucus preventing the movement of sperms carrying pathogens into the uterus.
        - Less menstrual bleeding with OC use: blood in the cervix may facilitate pathogen transport.
    - There is no decreased risk of chlamydial PID *(123)* or lower tract infections, such as chlamydia or other STDs.
- Less mittelschmerz (midcycle ovulation pain).
- Reduction in symptomatic endometriosis during use *(124,125)*.
- Reduction in hot flashes and other perimenopausal symptoms *(126,127*; *see* Chapter 14).

Possible Non-Contraceptive Benefits

The following potential benefits from OCs are controversial because there are conflicting studies.

- Reduced risk of hip fracture *(128)*, increased bone mineral density *(129)*, mixed findings in a comprehensive review *(130)*.
- Lowered risk or slower growth of uterine fibroids *(131)*.
- Reduced risk of colon cancer *(132)*.
- Reduced risk or slower progression of rheumatoid arthritis *(133)* or no effect *(134)*.
- Reduced symptoms appearing during menses.
  - Seizures, asthma, porphyria.

REFERENCES

1. Blackburn RD, Cunkelman A, Zlidar VM. (2000) Oral contraceptives—an update. Popul Rep A 28:1–16, 25–32.
2. Woltersz TB. (1991) Benefits of oral contraception: thirty year's experience. In J Fertil 36:26–31.
3. Bordy SA, Turkes A. Goldzieher JW. (1989) Pharmacokinetics of three bioequivalent norethindrone/mestranol-50 micrograms and three norethindrone/ethinyl estradiol-35 micrograms OC formulations: are "low-dose" pills really lower? Contraception 40:269–284.
4. Mishell DR. (2005) Rationale for decreasing the number of days of the hormone-free interval with use of low-dose oral contraceptive formulations. Contraception 71:304–305.
5. Mishell DR Jr, Kletzky OA, Brenner PF, et al. (1977) The effect of contraceptive steroids on hypothalamic-pituitary function. Am J Obstet Gynecol 128:60–74.
6. Tayob Y, Robinson G, Adams J, et al. (1990) Ultrasound appearance of the ovaries during the pill-free interval. Br J Family Planning 16:94–96.
7. Audet MC, Moreau M, Koltun WD, et al. (2001) ORTHO EVRA/EVRA 004 Study Group. Evaluation of contraceptive efficacy and cycle control of a transdermal contraceptive patch vs and oral contraceptive: a randomized controlled trial JAMA 285:2347–2354.
8. Holt VL, Cushinig-Haugen KL, Daling JR. (2002) Body weight and risk of oral contraceptive failure risk. Obstet Gynecol 99:820–827.
9. Zacur HA, Hedon B, Mansour D, et al. (2002) Integrated summary of Ortho Evra contraceptive patch adhesion in varied climates and conditions. Fertil Steril 77:S32–S35.
10. Potter LS. (1991) Oral contraceptives compliance and its role in the effectiveness of the method. In: Cramer JA, Spilker B, eds. Patient Compliance in Medical Practice and Clinical Trials. New York: Raven Press, pp. 195–207.
11. Tanis BC, van den Bosch MA, Kemmeren JM, et al. (2001) Oral contraceptives and the risk of myocardial infarction. N Engl J Med 345:1787–1793.
12. Khader YS, Rice J, John L, Abueita O. (2003) Oral contraceptives use and the risk of myocardial infarction: a meta-analysis. Contraception 68:11–17.
13. Collaborative Group on Hormonal Factors in Breast Cancer. (1996) Breast cancer and hormonal contraceptives: Collaborative reanalysis of individual data on 53,297 women with breast cancer and 100,239 women without breast cancer from 54 epidemiological studies. Lancet 347:1713–1727.
14. Goldzieher JW, Dozier TS, de la Pena A. (1980) Plasma levels and pharmacokinetics of ethinyl estrogens in various populations. Contraception 21:17–27.
15. Vessey M, Painter R. (1994) Oral contraceptive use and benign gallbladder disease revisited. Contraception 50:167–173.
16. La Vecchia C, Negri E, D'avanzo B, Parazzini F, Gentile A, Franceschi S. (1992) Oral contraceptives and noncontraceptive oestrogens in the risk of gallstone disease requiring surgery. J Epidemiol Community Health 46:234–236.
17. Strom BL, Tamragouri RN, Morse ML, et al. (1986) Oral contraceptives and other risk factors for gallbladder disease. Clin Pharmacol Ther 39:335–341.

18. Rosenberg MJ, Meyers A, Roy V. (1999) Efficacy, cycle control, and side effects of low and lower dose oral contraceptives: a randomized trial of 20 micrograms and 35 micrograms estrogen preparations. Contraception 60:321, 329.
19. Kay CR. (1984) The Royal College of General Practitioners' Oral Contraception study: some recent observations. Clin Obstet Gynaecol 11:759–786.
20. Holst J, Backstrom T, Hammarback S, von Schoultz B. (1989) Progestogen addition during oestrogen replacement therapy-effects on vasomotor symptoms and mood. Maturitas 121:13–20.
21. Troisi RJ, Cowie CC, Harris MI. (2000) Oral Contraceptive use and glucose metabolism in a national sample of women in the United States. Am J Obstet Gynecol 183:389–395.
22. Kim C, Siscovick DS, Sidney S, et al. (2002) Oral contraceptive use and association with glucose, insulin, and diabetes in young adult women: the CARDIA Study. Coronary Artery Risk Development in Young Adults. Diabetes Care 25:1027–1032.
23. Kjos SL, Peters RK, Xiang A, Thomas D, Schaefer U, Buchanan TA. (1998) Contraception and the risk of type 2 diabetes mellitus in Latina women with prior gestational diabetes mellitus. JAMA 280:533–538.
24. Van der Vange N, Blankenstein MA, Kloosterhoer JH, et al. (1990) Effects of seven low-dose combined oral contraceptives on sex hormone binding globulin, corticosteroid binding globulin, total and free testosterone. Contraception 41:345–352.
25. Kung AW, Ma JT, Wong VC, et al. (1987) Glucose and lipid metabolism with triphasic oral contraceptives in women with history of gestational diabetes. Contraception 325:257–269.
26. Hannaford PC, Kay CR. (1989) Oral contraceptives and diabetes mellitus. Br Med J 299:1315–1316.
27. Rimm EB, Manson JE, Stampfer MJ, et al. (1992) Oral contraceptive use and the risk of type 2 (non-insulin-dependent) diabetes in a large prospective study of women. Diabetologia 35:967–962.
28. MeadeTW. (1982) Oral contraceptives, clotting factors, and thrombosis. Am J Obstet Gynecol 142:758–761.
29. Gerstman BB, Piper JM, Tomita DK, et al. (1991) Oral contraceptives estrogen dose and the risk of deep venous thromoembolic disease. Am J Epidemioil 133:32–37.
30. Chasen-Taber L, Willett WC, Manson GE, et al. (1996) Prospective study of oral contraceptives and hypertension among women in the United States. Circulation 94:483–489.
31. Van der Vange N, Blankenstein MA, Kloosterboer JH, et al. (1990) Effects of seven low-dose combined oral contraceptives on sex hormone binding globusin, corticosteroid binding globulin, total and free testosterone. Contraception 41:345.
32. Odlind V, Milsom I, Persson I, Victor A. (2002) Can changes in sex hormone binding globuoin predict the risk of venous Thromboembolism with combined oral contraceptive pills. Acta Obstet Gynecol Scand 81:482–490.
33. van Vliet H AAM, Frolich M, Christella M, et al. (2005) Association between sex hormone-binding globulin levels and activated protein C resistance in explaining the risk of thrombosis in users of oral contraceptives containing different progestogens. Human Reproduction 20:563–568.
34. van Rooijen M, Silveira A, Hamsten A, Bremme K. (2004) Sex hormone-binding globulin-A surrogate marker for the prothrombotic effects of combined oral contracetptives. Am J Obstet Gynecol 190:332–327.
35. Speroff L, DeCherney A, the Advisory Board for the New Progestins. (1993) Evaluation of a new generation of oral contraceptives. Obstet Gynecol 81:1034.
36. Notelovitz M, Feldman EB, Gillespy M, et al. (1989) Lipid and lipoprotein changes in women taking low-dose, triphasic oral contraceptives: a controlled, comparative, 12-month clinical trial. Am J Obstet Gynecol 160:1269.
37. Rosing J, Middeldorp S, Curvers J, et al. (1999) Low-dose oral contraceptives and acquired resistance to activated protein C: a randomized cross-over study. Lancet 354:2036–2040.

38. Rosing J, Tans G. (1999) Effects of oral contraceptives on hemostasis and thrombosis. Am J Obstet Gynecol 180:S375–S382.
39. Vanderbroucke JP, Koster T, Briet E, et al. (1994) Increased risk of venous thrombosis in oral-contraceptive users who are carriers of factor V Leiden mutation. Lancet 344:1453.
40. Bloemenkamp KWM, Rosendaal FR, Helmerhorst FM, Vandenbroucke JP. (2000) Higher risk of venous thrombosis during early use of oral contraceptives in women with inherited clotting defects. Arch Intern Med 169:49–52.
41. Stampfer MJ, Willett WC, Colditz GA, Speizer FE, Hennekens CH. (1990) Past use of oral contraceptives and cardiovascular disease: a meta-analysis in the context of the Nurses' Health Study. Am J Obstet Gynecol 163:285–291.
42. Schwingl PJ, Shelton J. (1997) Modeled estimates of myocardial infarction and venous thromboembolic disease in users of second and third generation oral contraceptives. Contraception 55:125–129.
43. Lidegaard O, Edstrom B, Kreiner S. (2002) Oral contraceptives and venous thromboembolism: A five-year national case-control study. Contraception 65:187–196.
44. Jick H, Jick SS, Gurewich V, Myers MW, Vasilakis C. (1995) Risk of idiopathic cardiovascular death and nonfatal venous thrmoboembolism in women using oral contraceptives with differing progestogen components. Lancet 346:1589–1593.
45. World Health Organization Collaborative Study of Cardiovascular Disease and Steroid Hormone Contraception. (1995) Venous thromboembolic disease and combined oral contraceptives. Lancet 346:1575–1582.
46. Spitzer WO, Lewis MA, Heinemann LAJ, et al. (1996) Third-generation oral contraceptives and risk of venous thromboembolic disorders: An international case-control study. Br Med J 312:83–88.
47. Lewis MA, Heinemann LA, MacRae KD, Bruppacher R, Spitzer WO. (1996) The increased risk of venous thromboembolism and the use of third generation progestagens: role of bias in observational research. The Transnational Research Group on Oral Contraceptives and the Health of Young Women. Contraception. 1996 54:5–13.
48. Shelton T. (2002) Dutch GPs warned against new contraceptive pill. BMJ 324:869.
49. Lewis AL, Spitzer WO, Heinemann LAJ, MacRae KD, Bruppacher R, Thorogood M on behalf of Transnational Research Group on Oral Contraceptives and the Health of Young Women. (1996) Third generation oral contraceptives and risk of myocardial infarction: an international case-control study. BMJ 312:88–90.
50. Rosing J, Middeldorp S, Curvers J, et al. (1999) Low-dose oral contraceptives and acquired resistance to activated protein C: a randomized cross-over study. Lancet 354:2036–2040.
51. Kemmeren JM, Algra A, Meijers JC, et al. (2004) Effect of second- and third-generation oral contraceptives on the protein C system in the absence or presence of the factor V Leiden mutation: a randomized trial. Blood 103:927–933.
52. World Health Organization. (1998) Cardiovascular disease and steroid hormone contraception, report of a WHO scientific group. WHO Technical Report Series no. 877, Geneva, Switzerland.
53. Tanis BC, van den Bosch MA, Kemmeren JM, et al. (2001) Oral contraceptives and the risk of myocardial infarction. N Engl J Med 345:1787–1793.
54. Pettiti DB. (2003) Combination estrogen-progestin oral contraceptives. N Engl J Med 349:1443–1450.
55. Stampfer MJ, Willett WC, Colditz GA, Speizer FE, Hennekens CH. (1988) A prospective study of past use of oral contraceptive agents and risk of cardiovascular diseases. N Engl J Med 319:1313–1317.
56. Adams MR, Clarkson TB, Korinik DR, et al. (1987) Contraceptive steroids and coronary artery atherosclerosis in cynomolgus macaques. Dertil Steril 47:1010.

57. Mann JL, Doll R, Thorogood M, et al. (1986) Risk ractors for myocardial infarction in young women. Br J Prev Soc Med 30:94.
58. Croft P, Hannaford PC. (1989) Risk factors for acute myocardial infarction in women. Br Med J 298:165–168.
59. Rosenberg L, Palmer JR, Rao RS, et al. (2001) Low-dose oral contraceptives use and the risk of myocardial infarction. Arch Intern Med 161:1065–1070.
60. Khader YS, Rice J, John L, Abueita O. (2003) Oral contraceptives use and the risk of myocardial infarction: a meta-analysis. Contraception 68:11–17.
61. Baillargeon J-P, McClish DK, Essah PA, Nestler JE. (2005) Association between the current use of low-dose oral contraceptives and cardiovascular arterial disease: a meta-analysis. J Clin Endocrinol Metab 90:3863–3870.
62. Pettiti DB, Sidney S, Bernstein A, et al. (1996) Stroke in users of low-dose oral contraceptives. N Engl J Med 335:8–15.
63. Lidegaard O, Kreiner S. (2002) Contraceptives and cerebral thrombosis: a five-year national case-control study. Contraception. 65:197–205.
64. Siritho S, Thrift AG, McNeil JJ, You RX, Davis SM, Donnan GA. (2003) Melbourne Risk Factor Study (MERFS) Group. Risk of ischemic stroke among users of the oral contraceptive pill: The Melbourne Risk Factor Study (MERFS) Group. Stroke 34:1575–1580.
65. Chang CL, Donaghy M, Poulter N. (1999) Migraine and stroke in young women: case-control study. The World Health Organization Collaborative Study of Cardiovascular Disease and Steroid Hormone Contraception. BMJ 318:13–18
66. Kemmeren JM, Tanis BC, van den Bosch MA, et al. (2002) Risk of Aterial Thrombosis in Relation to Oral Contraceptives (RATIO) study: oral contraceptives and the risk of ischemic stroke. Stroke 33:1202–1208.
67. Vessey MP, Wright NH, McPherson K, et al. (1978) Fertility after stopping different methods of contraception. Br Med J 1:265–267.
68. Rothman KJ, Louik C. (1978) Oral contraceptives and birth defects. N Engl J Med 299:522–524.
69. Jacobsen C. (1974) Cytogenic Study of Immediate Post Contraceptive Abortion. Washington, DC: US Government Printing Office.
70. Harlap S, Shiono PH, Ramcharan S. (1985) Congenital abnormalities in the offspring of women who used oral and other contraceptives around the time of conception. In J Fertil 30:39.
71. Marchbanks PA, McDonald JA, Wilson HG, et al. (2002) Oral contraceptives and the risk of breast cancer. N Engl J Med 342:2025–2032.
72. Collaborative Group on Hormonal Factors in Breast Cancer. (1996) Breast cancer and hormonal contraceptives: further results. Contraception 54:1S–106S.
73. Moreno V, Bosch FX, Munbor N, et al. (2002) Effect of oral contraceptives on risk of cervical cancer in women with human papillomavirus infection: the IARC multicentric case-control study. Lancet 359:10–85.
74. Smith JS, Green J, Berrington de Gonzalez A, et al. (2003) Cervical cancer and use of hormonal contraceptives: a systematic review. Lancet 361:1159–1167.
75. The Cancer and Hormone Study of the Centers for Disease Control and the National Institute of Child Health and Human Development. (1987) Combination oral contraceptives use and risk of endometrial cancer. JAMA 257:796–800.
76. Voigt LF, Deng Q, Weiss NS. (1994) Recency, duration, and progestin content of oral contraceptives in relation to the incidence of endometrial cancer. Cancer Causes Control 3:227–233.
77. Hankinson SE, Colditz GA, Hunter DJ, Spencer TL, Rosner B, Stampfer MJ. (1992) A quantitative assessment of oral contraceptive use and risk of ovarian cancer. Obstet Gynecol 80:708–714.

78. World Health Organization. Collaborative Study of Neoplasia and Steroid Contraceptives. (1989) Combined oral contraceptives and liver cancer. Int J Cancer 43:254–259.
79. Fernandez E, La Vecchia C, Balducci A, et al. (2001) Oral contraceptives and colorectal cancer risk: a meta-analysis. Br J of Cancer 84:722–727.
80. Pituitary Adenoma Study Group. (1983) Pituitary adenomas and oral contraceptives: a multicenter case-control study. Fertil Steril 39:753–760.
81. Hannaford PC, Villard-Macintosh L, Vessey MP, Kay CR. (1991) Oral contraceptives and malignant melanoma. Br J Cancer 63:430–433.
82. Back DJ, Breckenridge AM, Crawford FE, et al. (1980) The effects of rifampicin on the pharmacokinetics of ethinylestradiol in women. Contraception 21:135–143.
83. Mattson RH, Rebar RW. (1993) Contraceptive methods for women with neurologic disorders. Am J Obstet Gynecol 168:2027–2032.
84. Chang J, Elam-Evans LD, Berg CJ, et al. (2003) Pregnancy related mortality surveillance—United States, 1991–1999. MMWR Surveill Summ 52:1–8.
85. Marchbanks PA, Annegers JF, Coulam CB, Strathy JH, Kurland LT. (1988) Risk factors for ectopic pregnancy. A population-based study. JAMA 259:1823–1827.
86. Mishell DR Jr. (1982) Noncontraceptive health benefits of oral steroidal contraceptives. Am J Obstet Gynecol 142:809–816.
87. Runnebaum B, Grunwald K, Rabe T. (1992) The efficacy and tolerability or norgestimate/ethinyl estradiol; results of an open, multicenter study of 59,701 women. Am J Obstet Gynecol 166:1963–1968.
88. Fraser IS, McCarron G. (1991) Randomized trial of 2 hormonal and 2 prostaglandin inhibiting agents in women with a complaint of menorrhagia. Aust N Z J Obstet Gynaecol 31:66–70.
89. Iyer V, Farquhar C, Jepson R. (2000) Oral contraceptive pills for heavy menstrual bleeding. Cochrane Database Syst Rev (2):CD000154.
90. Larsson G, Milsom I, Linstedt G, Rybo G. (1992) The influence of a low-dose combined oral contraceptive on menstrual blood loss and iron status. Contraception 46:327–334.
91. Task Force for Epidemiological Research on Reproductive Health, United Nations Development Programme/United Nations Population Fund/World Health Organization/World Bank Special Programme of Research, Development and Research Training in Human Reproduction, World Health Organization. (1998) Effects of contraceptives on hemoglobin and ferritin. Contraception 58:262–273.
92. Royal College of General Practitioners. (1974) Oral Contraceptives and Health: An Interim Report from the Oral Contraceptive Study of the Royal College of General Practitioners. New York: Pitman Medical Publishing.
93. Davis A, Godwin A, Lippman J, Olson W, Kafrissen M. (2000) Triphasic norgestimate ethinyl estradiol for treating dysfunctional uterine bleeding. Obstet Gynecol 96:913–920.
94. The Cancer and Steroid Hormone Study of the Centers for Disease Control and the National Institute of Child Health and Human Development. (1987) Combination oral contraceptive use and the risk of endometrial cancer. JAMA 257:796–800.
95. Vessey MP, Painter R. (1995) Endometrial and ovarian cancer and oral contraceptives—findings in a large cohort study. Br J Cancer 71:1340–1342.
96. Schlesselman JJ. (1997) Risk of endometrial cancer in relation to use of combined oral contraceptives. A practioner's guide to meta-analysis. Hum Reprod 12:1851–1863.
97. Vessey MP, Painter R. (1995) Endometrial and ovarian cancer and oral contraceptives—findings in a large cohort study. Br J Cancer 71:1340–1342.
98. Rosenberg, L, Palmer JR, Zauber AG, Warshauer ME, et al. (1994) A case-control study of oral contracetpvie use and invasive epithelial ovarian cancer. Am J Epidemiol 139:654–661.
99. Ness RB, Grisso JA, Klapper J, et al. (2000) risk of ovarian cancer in relation to estrogen and progestin dose and use characteristics of oral contraceptives. SHARE Study Group. Steroid Hormones and reproductions. Am J Epidemiol 152:233–241.

100. Narod SA, Risch H, Moslehi R, et al. (1998) Oral contraceptives and the risk of hereditary ovarian cancer. Hereditary Ovarian Cancer Clinical Study Group. N Eng J Med 339:424–428.
101. Modan B, Hartge P, Hirsh-Yechezkel G, et al. (2001) Parity, oral contraceptives, and the risk of ovarian cancer among carriers and noncarriers of a BRCA1 or BRCA2 mutation. N Engl J Med 345:235–240.
102. Jensen JT, Speroff L. (2000) Health benefits of oral contraceptives. Obstet Ghynecol Clin North Am 27:705–721.
103. Gross TP, Schlesselman JJ. (2002) The estimated effect of oral contraceptives on ovarian cancer risk. J Natl Cancer Inst 94:32–38.
104. Walker GR, Schlesselman JJ, Ness RB. (2002) Family history of cancer, oral contraceptive use, and ovarian cancer risk. Am J Obstet Gynecol 186:8–14.
105. Narod SA, Dube MP, Klijn J, et al. (2002) Oral contraceptives and the risk of breast cancer in BRCA1 and BRCA2 mutation carriers. J Nat Cancer Inst 94:1773–1779.
106. Schildkraut JM, Calingaert B, Marchbanks PA, Moorman PG, Rodriguez GC. (2002) Impact of progestin and estrogen potency in oral contraceptives on ovarian cancer risk. J Natl Cancer Inst 94:32–38.
107. Ory H, Cole IP, MacMahon B, et al. (1976) Oral contraceptives and reduced incidence of benign breast disease. N Engl J Med 294:419–422.
108. Brinton LA, Vessey MP, Flavel R, Yeates D. (1981) Risk factors for benign breast disease. Am J Epidemiol 113:203–214.
109. Milsom I, Sundell G, Andersch B. (1990) The influence of different combined oral contraceptives on the prevalence and severity of dysmenorrheal. Contraception 42:497–506.
110. Sangi-Haghpeykar H, Poindexter AN 3rd. (1995) Epidemiology of endometriosis among parous women. Obstet Gynecol 85:983–992.
111. Royal College of General Practitioners. (1974) Oral Contraceptives and Health: An Interim Report from the Oral Contraceptive Study of the Royal College of General Practitioners. New York: Pitman Medical Publishing.
112. Shargil AA. (1985) Hormone replacement therapy in perimenopausal women with a triphasic contracetpvie compound: a three year prospective study. In J Fertil 30:15;18–28.
113. Borenstein J, Yu HT, Wade S, Chiou CF, Rapkin A. (2003) Effect of an oral contraceptive containing ethinyl estradiol and drospirenone on premenstrual symptomatology and health-related quality of life. J reprod Med 48:79–85.
114. Parsey KS, Pong A. (2000) An open-label, multicenter study to evaluate Yasmin, a low-dose combination oral contraceptive containing drospirenone, a new progestogen. Contraception 61:105–111.
115. Lanes AF, Birmann B, Walter AM, Singer S. (1992) Oral contraceptive type and functional ovarian cysts. Am J Obstet Gynecol 166:956–961.
116. Chiaffarino F, Parazzini F, La Vecchia C, Ricci, Crosignani PG. (1998) Oral contraceptive use and benign gynecologic conditions. A review. Contraception 57:11–18.
117. Redmond GP, Olson WH, Lippman JS, et al. (1997) Norgestimate and ethinyl estradiol in the treament of acne vulgaris: a randomized, placebo-controlled trial. Obstet Gynecol 89:615–622.
118. Jemec GB, Linneberg A, Nielsen NH, et al. (2002) Have oral contraceptives reduced the prevalence of acne? A population-based study of acne vulgaris, tobacco smoking and oral contraceptives. Dermatology 204:179–184.
119. Dewis P, Petsos P, Newman M, Anderson DC. (1958) The treatment of hirsutism with a combination of desogestrel and ethinyl oestradiol. Clin Endocrinol (Oxf) 22:29–36.
120. Lobo RA. (1988) The androgenicity of progestational agents. Int J Fertil 33:6–12.
121. Lucky AW, Henderson TA, Olson WH, et al. (1997) Effectiveness of norgestimate and ethinyl estradiol in treating moderate acne vulgaris. J Am Acad Dermatol 37:746–754.
122. Panser LA, Phipps WR. (1991) Type of oral contraceptive in relation to acute, initial episodes of pelvic inflammatory disease. Contraception 43:91–99.

123. Washington AE, Gove S, Schachter J, Sweet Rl. (1985) Oral contraceptives, Chlamydia trachomatis infection, and pelvic inflammatory disease. A word of caution about protection. JAMA 253:2246–2250.
124. Sangi-Haghpeykar H, Poindexter AN 3rd. (1995) Epidemiology of endomjetriosis among parous women. Obstet Gynecol 85:983–992.
125. Parrazzini F, Ferraroni M, Bocciolone L, Tozzi L, Rubessa S, La Vecchia C. (1994) Contraceptive methods and risk of pelvic endometriosis. Contraception 49:47–55.
126. Shargil AA. (1985) Hormone replacement therapy in perimenopausal women with a triphasic contraceptive compound: a three-year prospective study. Int J Fertil 30:15, 18–20.
127. Casper RF, Dodin S, Reid RL, Study Investigators. (1997) The effect of 20 μg of ethinyl estradiol/1 mg norethindrone acetate (Minestrin™), a low-dose oral contraceptive on vaginal bleeding patterns, hot flashes, and quality of life in symptomatic perimenopausal women. Menopause 4:139–147.
128. Seeman E, Szmukler Gi, Formica C, Tsalamandris C, Mestrovicd R. (1992) Osteroporosis in anorexia nervosa; the influence of peak bone densithy, bone loss, oral contraceptive use and exercise. J Bone Miner Res 7:1467–1474.
129. Pasco JA, Kotowica MA, Henry MJ, Panahi S, Seeman E, Nicholson GC. (2000) Oral contraceptives and bone mineral density: A population-based study. Am J Obstet Gynecol 182:265–269.
130. Kuohung W, Borgatta L, Stubblefield P. (2000) Low-dose oral contraceptives and bone mineral density: an evidence-based analysis. Contraception 61:77–82.
131. Chiaffarino F, Parazzini F, La Vecchia C, Marsico S, Surace M, Ricci E. (1999) Use of oral contraceptives and uteirne fibroids: results from a case-control study. Br J Obstet Gynaecol 106:857–860.
132. Fernandez E, La Vecchia C, Balducci A, Chatenoud L, Franceschi S, Negri E. (2001) Oral contraceptives and colorectal cancer risk: a meta-analysis. Br J Cancer 84:722–727.
133. Spector TD, Hochberg MC. (1990) The protective effect of the oral contraceptive pill on rheumatoid arthritis; an overview of the analytic epidemiological studies using meta-analysis. J Clin Epidemiol 43:1221–1230.
134. Pladevali-Vila M, Delclos Gl, Varas C, Guyer H, Brugues-Tarradellas J, Anglada-Arisa A. (1996) Controversy of oral contraceptives and risk of rheumatoid arthritis; meta-analysis of conflicting studies and review of conflicting meta-analyses with special emphasis on analysis of heterogeneity. Am J Epidemiol 144:1–14.
135. Henzl M. (1993) Evolution of steroids and their contraceptive and therapeutic use. In: Shoupe DS, Haseltine FP, eds. Contraception. New York: Springer-Verlag, pp. 1–16.
136. Mishell DR. (2004) Contraception. In: Strauss J, Barbieri R, eds. Yen and Jaffe's Reproductive Endocrinology, 5th Edition. New York: Elsevier, pp. 904.

3 Oral Contraceptives

Patient Screening and Counseling, Pill Selection, and Managing Side Effects

Donna Shoupe, MD

CONTENTS

INTRODUCTION

> *It is recommended to use of the lowest dose OC that is effective, particularly a low-dose estrogen pill.*

Concerns regarding the estrogen-related adverse effects with use of combination oral contraceptives (OCs) have led to a progressive reduction in the estrogen dose since their introduction in the 1960s. Prompting these concerns were the numerous epidemiological studies linking estrogen in OCs to breast cancer *(1)* and cardiovascular complications, including an increase in thromboembolic events and myocardial infarction *(2)*. By the early 1990s, low-dose OCs containing 20–35 μg of ethinyl estradiol (EE) were the most commonly used formulations, and products with more than 50 μg of EE were no longer being marketed. Epidemiological studies reported improved safety profiles of these lower dose formulations *(3–7)* (Fig. 1).

From: *Current Clinical Practice: The Handbook of Contraception: A Guide for Practical Management*
Edited by: D. Shoupe and S. L. Kjos © Humana Press, Totowa, NJ

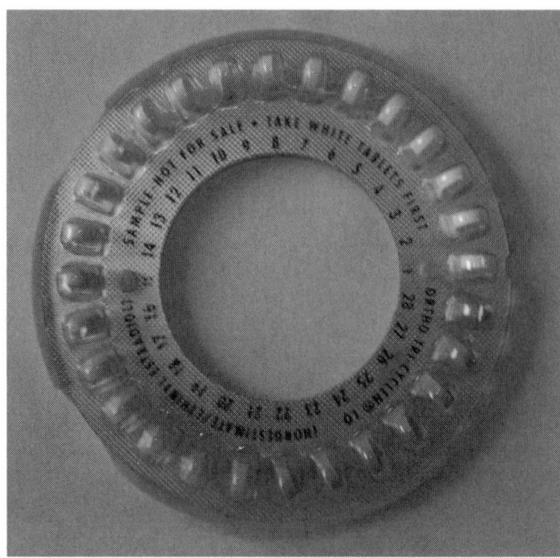

Fig. 1. Current pill packet.

By 1998, about 8% of the OC prescriptions in the United States were for 20 μg OCs and their use has steadily increased since then. Many health care providers and women chose the 20 μg OCs because of projected improvements in safety parameters owing to the lower estrogen dose and decreased incidence of estrogen-related side effects *(8)*. However, to date, randomized controlled trials have been inadequate to detect possible differences in contraceptive safety or efficacy of the 20 μg compared with the 35 μg OCs *(9)*. Some recently introduced 20 μg OCs have altered the duration of the active and pill-free interval and used newly synthesized progestins to improve bleeding profiles and efficacy *(10)*.

PATIENT EDUCATIONAL POINTS

The new package inserts supplied with OCs are easy to read and provide useful information to patients. The insert includes the general counseling information as listed below. As part of their counseling, health care providers may want to direct users to read the patient package insert.

- Many side effects associated with OCs are mild and subside within the first 3 months of use. These side effects include breast tenderness, bleeding between periods, cyclic fluid retention, headaches, nausea, and difficulty wearing contact lenses.
- OCs provide important non-contraceptive benefits including less dysmenorrhea, less menstrual blood loss and anemia, fewer pelvic infections (pelvic inflammatory disease [PID]/upper tract infections), and fewer cancers of the ovaries and endometrium.

Table 1
Estimated Risk of Birth-Related Deaths Plus Method-Related Deaths in Women Using Different Birth Control Methods

Method	*15–19*	*20–24*	*25–29*	*30–34*	*35–39*	*40–44*
None (deaths are birth-related)	7.0	7.4	9.1	14.8	25.7	28.2
Oral contraceptives (nonsmoker; method-related deaths)	0.3	0.5	0.9	1.9	13.8	31.6
Oral contraceptives (smoker; method-related deaths)	2.2	3.4	6.6	13.5	51.1	117.2
Intra-uterine device (method-related deaths)	0.8	0.8	1.0	1.0	1.4	1.4
Condom (deaths are birth-related)	1.1	1.6	0.7	0.2	0.3	0.4
Diaphragm/spermicide (deaths are birth-related)	1.9	1.2	1.2	1.3	2.2	2.8
Periodic abstinence (deaths are birth-related)	2.5	1.6	1.6	1.7	2.9	3.6

Annual number of birth- or method-related deaths per 100,000 nonsterile, sexually active women. Adapted from ref. *12a*.

- OCs are designed to prevent pregnancy and do not protect against HIV infections or other STDs (lower tract infections).
- Women who use OCs should not smoke.
  - Cigarette smoking dramatically increases the risk of serious adverse cardiovascular events from OC use. The risk increases with age and with heavy smoking (≥15 cigarettes per day) and is quite marked in women over 35 years of age.
  - The risk of death from any birth control method is less than the risk of childbirth in nonsmoking women under the age of 40 (Table 1).
- There are conflicting results on the relationship between breast cancer and OC use. Overall, most experts believe that OCs have little to no effect on the overall risk of a woman developing breast cancer.
  - In 1990, a large collaborative group reanalyzed most of the worldwide data and reported that estrogen dose, progestin type/dose, or duration do not increase the risk of breast cancer. However, there is a slight increase in the relative risk in current OC user and for women who stopped using OCs within the past 1–4 years. The risk returns to normal 10 years after stopping use *(11)*.
  - An important, well-done study reported that OC users and former users aged 35–65 have no difference in breast cancer risk than nonusers. The relative risk did not increase with longer use or higher doses of estrogen *(12)*.

- Patients should notify their health care provider if they notice any unusual physical disturbances while taking the pill. Taking rifampin, anticonvulsants, certain antibiotics, or St. John's Wort may decrease OC effectiveness.
- When starting OCs, the physical examination may be delayed to another time if a patient requests it and the health care provider believes that it is appropriate to postpone it. Examinations once per year are recommended.

PATIENT SELECTION AND SCREENING

Although OCs are safe in healthy, normotensive women, there are important contraindications to their use, and it is important to identify certain risk factors. Additionally, OCs are associated with many non-contraceptive benefits (*see* Chapter 2) and the identification of conditions that may be improved with OC use is also important.

- Pertinent gynecological issues.
  - Menstrual cycle irregularities, heavy bleeding, anemia.
  - Leiomyomata uterus, previous surgery.
  - Polycystic ovary syndrome, recurrent ovarian cysts.
  - Dysmenorrhea, pelvic pain.
  - Sexual history, exposure to HIV (consider condom protection).
  - Current and future childbearing plans.
  - Androgen excess, acne, hirsutism, alopecia.
  - Premenstrual syndrome (PMS)/premenstrual dysphoric disorder (PMDD).
- Demographics.
  - Age, gravity, parity, marital status, occupation.
- Medications (Table 2).
  - Good data stating that certain drugs accelerate the biotransformation of steroids in OCs and concomitant use may make OCs less effective.
    - Rifampin *(13)*, sulfonamides, cyclophosphamide, barbiturates, certain antiepileptics (Dilantin®), butazolindin.
    - St John's Wort.
  - Data less convincing for certain antibiotics (penicillin, ampicillin), fluconazole.
    - Low-dose, long-term antibiotic use for acne appears to be compatible with OC use *(14)*.
  - Product labeling suggests that women taking potassium-sparing diuretics, angiotensin-converting enzyme inhibitors, angiotensin-II receptor antagonists, chronic daily use of nonsteroidal anti-inflammatory drugs should consult their health care provider to check if a drospirenone (DRSP)-containing OC is right for them. Under these conditions, serum potassium levels should be checked during the first month. Clinical studies have reported minimal incidences of problems in women on these medications who also take a DRSP-containing OC.

Table 2
Oral Contraceptives and Other Drug Interactions

Drugs that may decrease the effectiveness of OCs, may result in breakthrough spotting, or may interfere with the drug's blood level or therapeutic action.

Medications that may interfere with OC action:

Over-the-counter medications: St. John's Wort *(26)* may reduce effectiveness of OCs.

Anti-convulsants: Many anti-convulsants induce cytochrome P-450 activity and can have significant effects on OC hormone levels. Likewise, estrogen may stimulate clearance of anti-convulsants and lessen their effectiveness.

Barbituates
Carbamazepine (Tegretol®)
Felbamate
Phenobarbital
Phenytoin (Dilantin®)
Primidone (Mysoline®)
Topiramate (Topamax®)
Felbamate (Felbatol®)
Oxcarbazine
Vigabatrin

Anti-fungal medications: May adversely affect OC effectiveness.

Griseofulvin

Anti-HIV protease inhibitors: May adversely affect OC effectiveness.

Anti-TB medications: May adversely affect OC effectiveness.

Rifampin *(27)*

Certain antibiotics: Data is not consistent and many clinicians do not recommend back-up method while on short-term therapy of the antibiotics listed below. Some studies report that certain antibiotics may adversely affect OC effectiveness, whereas others show no effect. *Note:* long-term anti-acne treatment usually does not interfere with OC use *(28)*.

Ampicillin
Neomycin
Nitrofurantoin
Amoxicillin
Metronidazole
Penicillin
Chloramphenicol
Tetracycline
Sulfonamide
Quinolones

Oral contraceptives may interfere with the action of certain medications

Fluoroquinolones: Serum levels of fluoroquinolones are lower in OC users *(29)*.

Moxifloxacin
Trovafloxacin

(continued)

Table 2 *(Continued)*
Oral Contraceptives and Other Drug Interactions

Thyroid medication: Increases in sex hormone-binding globulin may impact thyroid function testing results and may alter required dosage of medication.

Diazepam (Valium®), cholordiazepoxide (Librium®), and cyclic antidepressants: OCs may increase their effect but generally they can be used safely together.

Asthma medication: OCs may increase their effect.
Theophylline

Potassium-sparing drugs: Women who use ACE inhibitors, potassium-sparing diuretics, heparin, angiotensin-II receptor inhibitors, aldosterone antagonists, or daily NSAIDs should be monitored for potassium before and during use of DRSP containing OCs. Multiple studies demonstrate safety of DRSP-containing pills in for patients on these medications.

OC, oral contraceptive; ACE, angiotensin-converting enzyme; NSAID, nonsteroidal anti-inflammatory drug; DRSP, drospirenone.

- Allergies.
- Family history.
    - Thrombosis/thrombophlebitis/inherited clotting disorders.
    - Breast cancer: studies indicate that OC use in women with a family history of breast cancer does not appear to alter their overall risk *(15)*.
- Social history.
    - Smoking.
    - Sexual history.
- Concurrent problems, medical illnesses.
    - History of thrombosis/thrombophlebitis, pulmonary embolism, or known clotting disorder.
    - Known cardiovascular disease.
    - Significant risk factors for cardiovascular disease.
        - Hypertension, diabetes, lipid abnormalities.
        - Chronic disease associated with vascular disease (e.g., lupus).
        - Obesity.
    - Migraine headaches.
    - Liver disease.
- Physical examination.
    - Vital signs: blood pressure measurement and weight (these may have profound effects on safety or efficacy of OCs).
    - Breast and pelvic examination, cervical cytology (pelvic exam may be postponed if the provider believes it is appropriate).
- Laboratory assays.

  - Cervical tests for STDs as indicated (rarely necessary if mutually monogamous).
  - Screening for anemia, diabetes, clotting abnormalities, or abnormal lipids as clinically indicated.

CONTRAINDICATIONS TO USE

OCs are safe for the majority of women of reproductive age, however, there are absolute contraindications. The following recommendations are based on 2004 World Health Organization (WHO) medical eligibility criteria.

> *It is important to screen a potential user for possible existing cardiovascular disease or clotting abnormalities including evaluation of her blood pressure, smoking status, and risk factors for vascular disease.*

Absolute Contraindications to Low-Dose OC Use

- Valvular heart diseases with thrombogenic complications.
  - Pulmonary hypertension, subacute bacterial endocarditis, or atrial fibrillation.
- Known or suspected vascular disease.
  - Cerebrovascular or coronary artery disease, history of stroke.
  - Myocardial infarction, known atherosclerosis.
  - Diabetes with vascular disease including retinopathy or nephropathy.
  - Diabetes for more than 20 years.
- Hypertension.
  - WHO medical criteria classify controlled, adequately evaluated hypertension as category 3; the risks generally outweigh the benefits.
- Multiple risk factors for atherosclerosis (older age, diabetes, obesity, hypertension, smoking, statin use, hyperlipidemia).
- Personal history of thrombosis or high risk for thrombosis.
  - Thromboembolism, thrombophlebitis, deep vein thrombosis.
  - Polycythemia vera.
  - Known or suspected inherited clotting disorder (factor V Leiden, protein S, protein C, prothrombin, or antithrombin deficiency).
- Cigarette smoking in women older than 35.
- Cancer of the breast (past or present).
  - Any current estrogen-dependent neoplasia.
- Known or suspected pregnancy.
- Migraine headaches with localizing neurological signs, including scotomata at any age.
  - Migraine without aura over age 35.
  - Worsening migraines during use of OC.

- Acute or chronic liver disease.
  - Active viral hepatitis, abnormal liver functions, severe cirrhosis.
  - Benign hepatic adenomas/liver carcinoma.
- Prolonged immobilization, major surgery.
- Hypersensitivity to any component of the pill.

Risks Generally Outweigh Benefits

- History of OC-induced cholestatic jaundice or current symptomatic gall bladder disease treated medically.
- Mild compensated cirrhosis.
- Postpartum less than 21 days or less than 6 months if primarily breastfeeding.
- Cigarette smoking of less than 15 cigarettes per day in women 35 years or older.
- History of hypertension (including pregnancy-induced) in which blood pressure cannot be monitored or moderately elevated; systolic blood pressure 140–159 mmHg or diastolic blood pressure 90–99 mmHg.
- Hypertriglyceridemia (>350 mg/dL), known hyperlipidemias (screening not necessary).
- Migraine without aura over 35 years of age.
- Previous breast cancer but no evidence of current disease for 5 years.
- Certain antibiotics (rifampin) or anticonvulsants (barbiturates, phenytoin, carbamezapine, primidone, topiramate, oxcarbazepine).

Benefits Generally Outweigh Risks: Consider Use of OCs After Evaluation of Risks and Benefits and Develop an Appropriate Monitoring Plan

- Unexplained (suspicious) vaginal bleeding before evaluation.
- Undiagnosed breast mass.
- Varicose veins.
- Migraine headaches without localizing neurological signs or aura more than 35 years.
  - Non-migranous headaches mild or severe during use.
- Cigarette smoking by women younger than age 35.
- Age over 40.
- Prolactin-secreting pituitary microadenoma.
- Valvular heart disease uncomplicated.
- Unexplained amenorrhea after evaluation.
- Diabetes (insulin- and non-insulin-dependent) with no vascular disease in women.
  - Under 35 years of age and less than 20 years duration of diabetes.
- Surgery without prolonged immobilization.
- Known hyperlipidemias (except as listed above) with no other risk factors for cardiovascular disease.
- On antiretinoviral therapy (consult WHO website).

- On Griseofulvin.
- Obesity: body mass index 30 kg/m^2 or more.
- Non-migrainous mild or severe headache.
- Cervical cancer awaiting treatment.
- Cervical intraepithelial neoplasia.
- Sickle cell disease *(16)* or trait.
- Symptomatic gall bladder disease treated with cholecytectomy or asymptomatic.
- Gall bladder disease or history of pregnancy induced cholestatic jaundice.
- History of pregnancy-induced hypertension (in which current blood pressure is measured and normal).
- Family history in first-degree relative of deep vein thrombosis/polmonary embolism.
- Superficial thrombophlebitis.

Conditions Where OC Use Is Generally Safe

- Benign breast disease.
- Family history of breast cancer.
- Immediately after first or second trimester pregnancy, ectopic pregnancy, septic abortion, molar pregnancy, or malignant trophoblastic disease.
- Minor surgery without immobilization.
- Epilepsy.
- Varicose veins.
- Depressive disorders.
- Unexplained vaginal bleeding after evaluation.
  - Menorrhagia, metorrhagia.
- Endometriosis.
- Ovarian cysts.
- Uterine fibroids.
- Past history of PID, STDs, or current PID.
  - Purulent cervicitis, chlamydial infection, or gonorrhea.
  - Current vaginitis.
- HIV-infected, AIDS.
- Malaria.
- Pelvic or non-pelvic tuberculosis.
- Thyroid disease: goiter, hypo-, or hyperthyroid.
- Carrier, non-active viral hepatitis.
- Thalassemia.
- Iron deficiency anemia.
- Antibiotics (except griseofulvin, rifampin).
- Endometrial cancer.
- Ovarian cancer.
- Schistosomiasis.
- History of gestational diabetes.
- Carrier, non-active viral hepatitis.

COUNSELING TIPS

- There are two common methods for initiating OC use.
  - "First-day start" has the advantage that no back-up method is needed.
    - First-day start means starting OCs on the first day of normal menstrual bleeding.
  - "Sunday start" has the advantage that withdrawal bleeding will occur mid-week and not on the weekends (desired by some users), but 7 days' back-up method (or abstinence) is recommended.
    - Sunday start means starting the first Sunday after menses begins.
    - Helpful to give examples: "If you happen to start your menses on Monday, you would start pills 6 days later, or if you started on Saturday, that means you'd be starting the next day."
- Abnormal bleeding or spotting may be expected for 1–2 months after starting a new OC.
- Minor side effects, such as breast tenderness, nausea, and headache, are likely to decrease after several cycles.
  - Side effects may be minimized if the pill is taken the same time every day or if taken with a meal.
- OCs provide no protection from STDs (lower tract infections) and users at risk for STD or HIV exposure should use a condom back-up.
- Missing pills during second or third week of pill packet (or a non-placebo pill during fourth week of pill packet).
  - Missing one pill: take two pills as soon as possible; no backup needed.
  - Missing two pills (2 days in a row): take two pills as soon as possible and then two more the following day. Use back-up protection until the next pill cycle.
  - Missing more than two pills: discard current pack and begin a new cycle on the following Sunday, use a back-up method until 7 days into the next cycle (consider emergency contraception if intercourse occurred within the past 5 days).
- Missing pills during first week of pill packet.
  - Missing one pill in first week of a new cycle: take tablet as soon as remembered and the next one at the correct time. Use barrier back-up method for 7 days (consider emergency contraception if intercourse occurred within the past 5 days).
  - Missing two or more pills: take two pills as soon as possible and then two more the following day. Use back-up protection until the next pill cycle (consider emergency contraception if intercourse occurred within past 5 days).
- A 3- to 6-month follow-up visit may be useful to check for problems and to check blood pressure, although the majority of users do not need frequent visits *(17)*.
- There is no need to take a "rest" from pills; there is no evidence that there is any benefit and it may result in an unintended pregnancy.
- A short or scanty period (a drop of blood) counts as withdrawal bleeding as long as it occurs during the pill-free/placebo pill interval.

    - If one period is missed and no pills in that cycle have been missed, pregnancy is unlikely.
        - If any pills were missed in that cycle or if there is concern, a pregnancy test is advised.
    - If no withdrawal bleeding occurs for two cycles, a pregnancy test should be done and if negative, switch to more estrogenic OC.
- OCs are a good choice for women who want future fertility.
    - Rates of anovulation are not higher in ever-users than in never-users (i.e., being on pills for a long time does not increase the risk of irregular periods/ anovulation after stopping pills).
    - Many of the non-contraceptive benefits associated with OCs may protect fertility (e.g., OCs users have lowered rates of PID and often benefit from control of endometriosis and fibroid growth).
    - It is optimal that OCs are stopped 2 months before desired time of pregnancy so that more accurate dating of the pregnancy is possible. Prenatal vitamins with folate should be started.
        - After stopping OCs and the final withdrawal bleeding has occurred, a back-up barrier method may be desired. There is often a 1- to 2-week delay in the return of ovulation following discontinuation of OCs. This means that ovulation will generally occur about 3–4 weeks after the last active pill. During the first pill-free month, it is difficult to know for certain when ovulation will occur. If pregnancy occurs during the first month, an ultrasound can be used to accurately determine gestational age because dating from last menstrual period is typically inaccurate.
            - The second cycle after stopping OCs is an optimal time to start trying to get pregnant.
    - If regular menses have not returned by 4–6 months after stopping OCs, a diagnostic evaluation should be performed.

TIMING OF INITIATION

- Adolescents: after three regular menstrual cycles.
- Post-abortion: initiate immediately.
- Post-ectopic pregnancy: initiate immediately.
- Postpartum: initiate at 3–4 weeks postpartum if not breastfeeding (*see* Chapter 14).
    - Fully breastfeeding: a progestin-only method is preferred because combination OCs can decrease milk production.
    - Partially breastfeeding: a combination OC can be used at 6 months postpartum.
- Perimenopausal: use of 20 μg OC for cycle control or symptoms, especially if contraception is needed (*see* Chapter 14).
- Switching from intrauterine device (IUD): start immediately, consider back-up barrier for 1 week (*see* Chapter 9).
- Switching from implants: start immediately after removal.

- Switching from injectable progestin: start on day of next injection due date or on first Sunday before (*see* Chapter 7).
- Switching OCs or changing from patch or ring: start new pack on first day of next cycle or alternatively start new pack on any day of previous cycle. Replace new pill for old pill (discontinue old OC or other method) and continue new pack normally.
- Switching from barrier: stop barrier method on initiation of first pill if using first day start method or after first week of OC use if using Sunday-start method.

WARNING SIGNS

Users should contact their physician/health care provider if they have any of the following:

- No withdrawal bleeding (not even a blood spot during pill-free interval) for 2 months—rule out pregnancy.
- Severe leg pain—rule out blood clot.
- Abdominal pain—rule out pregnancy, ectopic pregnancy, upper tract infection, blood clot (mesentery, pelvic vessel).
- Chest pain, shortness of breath—rule out pulmonary embolism, myocardial infarction.
- Blurred vision, speech problem, visual problem—rule out stroke, blood clot in eye, hypertension.
- Severe or increased frequency of headache (warning sign of stroke)—rule out hypertension, stroke.
- Weakness, numbness, or pain in extremity—rule out blood clot, stroke.

OPTIONS

*Low-Dose OCs (*See *Tables 3 and 4)*

There are four different estrogen (EE) doses currently available in low-dose OCs: 35, 30, 25, and 20 μg. A 15-μg EE dose is available in Europe.

Pills are classified as monophasic (traditional cycle), monophasic with extended cycle or continuous use, monophasic with shortened hormone-free interval, biphasic, biphasic with shortened hormone-free interval, triphasic (with phasic progestin), triphasic with phasic estrogen, and triphasic with phasic estrogen and progestin.

High-Dose OCs (Table 5)

There are currently eight different 50-μg OCs marketed in the United States. The use of high-dose OCs is usually limited to special cases (e.g., women on antiepileptic medications).

CHOOSING AN OC FORMULATION

The guidelines shown below may be helpful in choosing the best OC formulation. It is generally recommended to use the lowest effective dose. As women

Table 3
Combination Oral Contraceptives

Product	*Estrogen*	*Progestin*	*Days with active pills*	*Manufacturer*
Monophasic 20 μg				
Alesse®	20 μg EE	0.1 mg	21 (+ 7 inert)	Wyeth
Aviane®		LNG	21 (+ 7 inert)	Barr
Lutera®			21 (+ 7 inert)	Watson
Lessina® 28			21 (+ 7 inert)	Barr
Lessina 21			21	
Levlite®			21 (+ 7 inert)	Berlex
Loestrin® 1/20			21	Barr
Loestrin Fe 1/20			21 (+ 7 iron)	Barr
Junel 1/20			21	Barr
Junel Fe1/20			21 (+ 7 iron)	Barr
Microgestin®			21	Watson
Microgestin Fe®	20 μg EE	1 mg NEA	21 (+ 7 with 75 mg iron)	Watson
Biphasic 20 μg with shortened hormone-free interval				
Kariva®				Barr
Mircette®	20 μg EE/10 EE	0.15 mg DSG	21 + 5 EE (+ 2 inert)	Organon
Monophasic 20 μg with shortened hormone-free interval				
Yaz®	20 μg EE	3 mg DSPG	24 (+ 4 inert)	Berlex
Loestrin® 24 Fe	20 μg EE	1 mg NEA	24 (+ 4 iron)	Warner Chilcott
Triphasic 25 μg				
Cyclessa®				Organon
Velivet®	25 μg EE	0.1 mg/ 0.125 mg/ 0.15 mg DSG	7 + 7 + 7 (+ 7 inert)	Barr
Ortho Tri-Cyclen-Lo®	25 μg EE	0.18 mg/ 0.215 mg/ 0.25 mg NGM	7 + 7 + 7 (+ 7 inert)	Ortho-McNeil
Monophasic 30 μg				
Levlen®				Berlex
Levora®				Watson
Portia®				Barr
Nordette®	30 μg EE	0.15 mg LNG	21 (+ 7 inert)	King
Desogen®				Organon
Ortho-Cept®				Ortho-McNeil
Apri®	30 μg EE	0.15 mg DSG	21 (+ 7 inert)	Barr

(continued)

Table 3
Combination Oral Contraceptives

Product	*Estrogen*	*Progestin*	*Days with active pills*	*Manufacturer*
Cryselle®				Barr
Lo/Ovral®				Wyeth
Low-Ogestrel®	30 μg EE	0.3 mg NOR	21 (+ 7 inert)	Watson
Loestrin 1.5/30	30 μg EE	1.5 mg NEA	21	Barr
Loestrin Fe 1.5/30			21 (+ 7 iron)	Barr
Microgestin Fe 1.5/30			21 (+ 7 iron)	Watson
Junel 1.5/30			21	Barr
Junel Fe 1.5/30			21 (+ 7 iron)	Barr
Yasmin®	30 μg EE	3 mg DRSP	21 (+ 7 inert)	Berlex

EE, ethinyl estradiol; NEA, norethindrone acetate; NOR, norgestrel; NE, norethindrone; LNG, levonorgestrel; DRSP, drospirenone; NGM, norgestimate; DSG, desogestrel.

age, there are different issues that affect proper selection of an OC formulation. Because of the higher potency of EE (about 1.8 times as potent as mestranol), OCs containing 35 μg EE are similar to the 50-μg OCs containing mestranol.

> *The OCs containing 20 and 25 μg EE should be considered the low-dose OC options.*

New-Start Healthy Patients

1. **Adolescents (Chapter 14):** 20, 25, (or 30) μg EE OCs. Going with the lowest dose 20 μg EE OCs in adolescents may be associated with a lack of bleeding control, a leading cause of discontinuation. In this population, starting with a 25 or 30 μg EE OC may be associated with better bleeding control and ultimately better compliance. However, the biphasic or monophasic 20-μg OCs with shortened pill-free intervals are associated with improved bleeding control and may be a good option to consider.
   a. OCs are often used in young girls not at risk for pregnancy because of the many non-contraceptive benefits:
      i. Dysmenorrhea, bleeding control. All OC brands show benefit; 25 and 30 μg OCs may have better bleeding control than traditional 20-μg OCs with a 7-day pill-free interval. Reviews have shown that OCs with levonorgestrel have good bleeding control *(18)*.
      ii. Acne, androgenic problems. All OCs brands show benefit. If symptoms are severe or continue to be a problem while on an OC, switch OC with formulation containing a low androgenic progestin (norgestimate,

Table 4
Combination Oral Contraceptives

Product	Estrogen	Progestin	Days with active pills	Manufacturer
Triphasic 20–35 μg				
Estrostep® 21	20/30/35 μg EE	1 mg NEA	5 + 7 + 9	Warner Chilcott
Estrostep Fe	20/30/35 μg EE	1 mg NEA	5 + 7 + 9 (+ 7 iron)	Warner Chilcott
Monophasic 30 μg with extended cycle				
Seasonale®	30 μg EE	0.15 mg LNG	84 (+ 7 inert)	Barr
Triphasic 30–40 μg with phasic progestin				
Trivora®				Watson
Triphasil®				Wyeth
Tri-Levlen®				Berlex
Enpresse®	30/40/30 μg EE	0.05/0.75/ 0.125 mg LNG	6 + 5 + 10 (+ 7 inert)	Barr
Monophasic 35 μg				
MonoNessa®				Watson
Ortho-Cyclen®				Ortho-McNeil
Previfem®				Teva
Sprintec®	35 μg EE	0.25 mg NGM	21	Barr
Ovcon®	35 μg EE	0.4 mg NE	21 + (7 inert)	Warner Chilcott
Brevicon®	35 μg EE	0.5 mg NE	21 + (7 inert)	Watson
Modicon®				Ortho-McNeil
Necon® 0.5/35				Watson
Nortrel® 0.5/35	35 μg EE	0.5 mg NE	21 + (7 inert)	Barr
Necon 1/35				Watson
Norinyl® 1 + 35				Watson
Nortrel 1/35	35 μg EE			Barr
Ortho-Novum® 1/35		1 mg NE	21 + (7 inert)	Ortho-McNeil
Demulen®				Pfizer
Zovia®	35 μg EE	1 mg ED	21 + (7 inert)	Watson
Triphasic 35 μg				
Ortho Tri-Cyclen®				Ortho-McNeil
Tri-Previfem®				Teva
TriNessa®				Watson

(continued)

Table 4
Combination Oral Contraceptives

Product	*Estrogen*	*Progestin*	*Days with active pills*	*Manufacturer*
Tri-Sprintec®	35 µg EE	0.18/0.215/ 0.25 mg NGM	7 + 7 + 7 (+ 7 inert)	Barr
Ortho-Novum 7/7/7				Ortho-McNeil
Nortel 7/7/7				Barr
Necon 7/7/7	35 µg EE	0.5/0.75/ 1 mg NE	7 + 7 + 7 (+ 7 inert)	Watson
Aranelle®				Barr
Tri-Norinyl®	35 µg EE	0.5/1/ 0.5 mg NE	7 + 9 + 5 (+ 7 inert)	Watson
Biphasic 35 µg				
Necon 10/11				Watson
Ortho-Novum 10/11	35 µg EE	0.5/1 mg NE	10 + 11 (+ 7 inert)	Ortho-McNeil

EE, ethinyl estradiol; NEA, norethindrone acetate; NOR, norgestrel; NE, norethindrone; LNG, levonorgestrel; DRSP, drospirenone; NGM, norgestimate; DSG, desogestrel.

Table 5
Combination Oral Contraceptives

Product	*Estrogen*	*Progestin*	*Days with active pills*	*Manufacturer*
Monophasic 50 µg				
Ovral®				Wyeth
Ogestrel® 0.5/50	50 mg EE	0.5 mg NOR	21 (+ 7 inert)	Watson
Demulen® 1/50				Pfizer
Zovia® 1/50	50 mg EE	1 mg ED	21 (+ 7 inert)	Watson
Ovcon® 50	50 mg EE	1 mg NE	21 (+ 7 inert)	Warner Chilcott
Neocon® 1/50				Watson
Norinyl® 1 + 50	50 mg MES			Watson
Ortho-Novum® 1/50		1 mg NE	21 (+ 7 inert)	Ortho-McNeil

EE, ethinyl estradiol; LNG, levonorgestrel; NEA, norethindrone acetate; MES, mestranol DRSP, drospirenone; NE, norethindrone; NOR, norgestrel; NGM, norgestimate; DSG, desogestrel; ED, ethynodiol diacetate.

desogestrel [DSG], or DRSP) Ortho Tri-Cyclen® is approved by the Food and Drug Administration (FDA) to treat acne vulgaris.

iii. Users with at risk of STD or HIV exposure need additional protection and should use condoms and OCs.

2. **Early reproductive (18–29 years) first choice:** 20, 25, (or 30) μg EE OCs. Young women may have increased bleeding problems on 20-μg OCs with a traditional 7-day pill-free interval and use of a 20 μg EE monophasic or biphasic OC with a shortened pill-free interval; a 25 μg EE OC may result in better bleeding control (Table 3). Use of a levonorgestrel-containing pill is associated with good bleeding control.
   a. Dysmenorrhea, bleeding control: all OC brands show benefit; 25- and 30-μg OCs better than some of the 20-μg OCs. Reviews have shown levonorgestrel-containing OCs to have good bleeding control *(14)*.
   b. PMS, PMDD, or fluid retention: all OCs may show benefit. The progestin DRSP is a derivative of spironolactone and has some diuretic effect. Selection of an OC with DRSP is a good choice for users with significant complaints of PMS, PMDD, or fluid retention.
   c. Acne, androgenic problems: all OCs show benefit. Consider low-androgenic progestin OCs (norgestimate, DSG, or DRSP) if severe or if non-responsive to other OCs. Ortho Tri-Cyclen is FDA-approved to treat acne vulgaris.
3. **Late reproductive (30–35 years) first choice:** 20–25 μg EE OCs (Table 3).
   a. Menorrhagia (heavy menses): all OCs show benefit. If menorrhagia is a problem while on an OC, switch to OC with levonorgestrel or one with lower EE dose. Switching to pill with higher progestin to estrogen ratio results in less endometrial stimulation and may result in less menstrual bleeding.
   b. Bleeding problems: all OCs show benefit. If midcycle bleeding and spotting is a problem while on OC, consider switching to an OC with stronger progestin, such as one with levonorgestrel, or consider switching to a higher EE dose OC. Estrogen increases endometrial growth and may improve bleeding control. In some instances, switching to a lower EE dose OC may be effective because it lowers endometrial stimulation, which results in less endometrial tissue and less bleeding.
   c. Fibroids or endometriosis: all OCs may show benefit. Consider a stronger progestin OC, such as one with levonorgestrel, or OC with as low a dose of EE as possible.
   d. Significant menstrual related problems: consider a low-dose 21-day extended-cycle or continuous OC.
   e. Obesity: for heavier women (>160 lb), consideration of 30- to 35-μg pill *(19)*, extended-use OC *(20)*, or vaginal ring (or Depo-subQ provera®, IUD, barriers). Using more than 35-μg OCs may increase the risk of venous thromboembolisms and a risk–benefit ratio should be considered. As a user gets older, risk of thrombosis may increase and fecundity decreases, therefore, using a low EE dose OC may be considered. Women over 35 with long-standing obesity are good candidates for progestin only methods, barriers, IUDs, or tubal sterilization.

4. **Perimenopausal or women over 35 years old (Chapter 14)** who are healthy, non-hypertensive, nonsmokers: first choice is 20 or 25 μg OCs. Women in this age group with longstanding obesity, hypertension, cigarette smoking, known or suspected vascular disease, or diabetes may consider progestin-only methods, barriers, IUDs, or tubal sterilization.
   a. Perimenopausal symptoms (headaches, hot flushes) during pill-free interval: consider switching to OC with shortened pill-free interval (Mircette®, Kariva®) with EE 20 μg/150 μg DSG for 21 days, 5 days of 10 μg EE, and only 2 days hormone-free (placebo pills) interval; or the new 20-μg OC containing 3 mg DRSP with a 4-day hormone-free interval (Yaz®). (*Note:* product labeling states DSG-containing OCs have elevated risk of venous thromboembolism compared with other low-dose OCs. New 20-μg [lower dose] EE OC pills Yaz or Loestrin® 24 Fe are good options.)

MANAGING PROBLEMS

The amount and potency of either the particular estrogen or progestin component in an OC and the balance between the particular estrogen and progestin is associated with hormonal side effects as listed in Table 6. Management of these problems generally involves changing to an OC with a different estrogen to progestin balance.

- Consider switching to another OC if current OC is associated with:
  - Breakthrough bleeding, heavy menses: irregular, bothersome, or heavy bleeding that continues after 2 months of use, consider OC with levonorgestrel or lower EE to progestin ratio pill.
  - Amenorrhea for two cycles: after negative pregnancy test, switch to OC with higher EE to progestin ratio (switch either to an OC with a low progestin impact, i.e., OCs with norgestimate [Ortho Tri-Cyclen-Lo®], or DRSP [Yasmin®], or DSG [Cyclessa®, Velivet®] or switch to OC with higher dose EE).
  - Acne is exacerbated on OC: switch to OC with norgestimate, DSG, or DRSP. Ortho Tri-Cyclen is FDA-approved to treat acne vulgaris.
  - Minor estrogen-related side effects that continue after 2 months: switch to OC with lower EE dose, consider 20 μg EE OC.
    - Nausea or vomiting: switch to OC with 20 μg EE or consider taking OCs with dinner.
    - Breast tenderness: switch to OC with lower EE (consider 20 μg EE OC *[21]*).
  - Headaches: stop OCs immediately if there are concomitant localizing signs, auras (flashing lights), blurred vision, weakness, or numbness or if the user is experiencing a worsening of migraines (could be a warning sign of impending stroke—plan for appropriate follow-up).

Table 6
Hormonal Side Effects of Oral Contraceptives

Estrogen excess	*Estrogen deficiency*	*Progestin excess*	*Progestin deficiency*
Breast tenderness, increase in breast size	Early midcycle spotting	Shortened menses	Late breakthrough bleeding and spotting
Heavy menstrual flow and clots	Decreased amount of menstrual flow	Acne, oily skin, hirsutism	Heavy menstrual flow and clots
Dysmenorrhea	No withdrawal bleeding	No withdrawal bleeding	Delayed onset of menses
Uterine cramps		Increased appetite	Dysmenorrhea
Nausea, vomiting		Irritability	
Cyclic weight gain		Nervousness	
Chloasma		Cholestatic jaundice	
Lactation suppression		Mood swings	
Vascular headaches			
Irritability			
Decreased libido			

Adapted from and quoted in ref. *31*.

- Check blood pressure.
- If blood pressure normal, headaches are simple, and there are none of the symptoms above, consider switching to 20 μg EE OC or progestin-only method.

◦ Decreased libido: there is a dose-dependent suppression of endogenous testosterone production by OCs *(22)*. Additionally, estrogen-dominant pills increase sex hormone-binding globulin that binds up endogenous androgens: switching to OC with 20 μg EE or to a progestin-only OC may result in more normal free testosterone levels and less negative impact on libido.
◦ Melasma: switch to progestin-only OC or consider one with 20 μg EE.
◦ Mood swings: switch to 20- to 25-μg OC; consider OC with a different progestin from current OC; consider DRSP, norgestimate, or DSG, consider extended-cycle or continuous OC.
◦ Weight gain: currently available low-dose OCs are generally not associated with a weight gain *(23–25)*, consider switching to 20–25 μg EE OC. If fluid retention is a problem, use an OC containing DRSP.

REFERENCES

1. Collaborative Group on Hormonal Factors in Breast Cancer. (1996) Breast cancer and hormonal contraceptives: collaborative reanalysis of individual data on 53,297 women with breast cancer and 100,239 women without breast cancer from 54 epidemiologic studies. Lancet 347:1713–1727.
2. Anonymous. Oral contraceptives and cardiovascular risk. (2000) Drug Ther Bull 38:1–5.
3. Rosenberg L, Palmer JR, Rao RS, et al. (2001) Low-dose oral contraceptives use and the risk of myocardial infarction. Arch Intern Med 161:1065–1070.
4. Pettit DB, Sidney S, Bernstein A, et al. (1996) Stroke in users of low-dose oral contraceptives. N Engl J Med 335:8–15.
5. Siritho S, Thrift AG, McNeil JJ, et al. (2003) Risk of ischemic stroke among users of the oral contraceptive pill: the Melbourne Risk Factor Study (MERFS) Group. Stroke 34:1575–1580.
6. Kemmeren JM, Tanis BC, van den Bosch MA, et al. (2002) Risk of Aterial Thrombosis in Relation to Oral Contraceptives (RATIO) study: oral contraceptives and the risk of ischemic stroke. Stroke 33:1202–1208.
7. Lidegaard O, Kreiner S. (2002) Contraceptives and cerebral thrombosis: a five-year national case-control study. Contraception 65:197–205.
8. Rosenberg MJ, Meyers A, Roy V. (1999) Efficacy, cycle control, and side effects of low- and lower-dose oral contraceptives: a randomized trial of 20 μg and 35 μg estrogen preparations. Contraception 60:321–329.
9. Gallo M, Nanda K, Grimes D, Schutz K. (2005) Twenty micrograms vs >20 μg estrogen oral contraceptives for contraception: systematic review of randomized controlled trials. Contraception 71:162–169.
10. Mishell DR Jr. (2005) Rationale for decreasing the number of days of the hormone-free interval with use of low-dose oral contraceptive formulations. Contraception 71:304–305.
11. Collaborative Group on Hormonal Factors in Breast Cancer. (1996) Collaborative Group on Hormonal Factors in Breast Cancer and hormonal contraceptives: collaborative breast cancer reanalysis of individual data on 53,297 women and 100,239 women without breast cancer from 54 epidemiologic studies. Contraception 54:S100–S106.
12. Marchbanks PA, McDonald JA, Wilson HG, et al. (2002) Oral contraceptives and the risk of breast cancer. N Engl J Med 346:2025–2032.

12a. Ory HW. (1983) Making choices: evaluating the health risks and benefits of birth control methods. Int Fam Plan Perspect 15:57–63.

13. Back DJ, Breckenridge AM, Crawford FE, et al. (1980) The effects of rifampicin on the pharmacokinetics of ethinyl estradiol in women. Contraception 21:135–143.
14. Murphy AA, Zacur HA, Charache P, Burkmand RT. (1991) Ehe effect of Tetracycline on levels of oral contraceptives. Am J Obstet Gynecol 164:28–33.
15. Marchbanks PA, McDonald JA, Wilson HG, et al. (2002) Oral contraceptives and the risk of breast cancer. N Engl J Med 346:2025–2032.
16. World Health Orgnization. Medical eligibility criteria. Available from: http://www.who.int/reproductive-health/publications/mec/mec.pdf. Accessed: March 2006.
17. Grimes DA. (1993) Editorial: over the counter oral contraceptives- a immodest proposal? Am J Public Health 83:1092–1103.
18. Rosenberg MJ, Long SC. (1992) Oral contraceptives and cycle control: a critical review of the literature. Adv Contracep (Suppl)1:35–40.
19. Zieman M, Nelson AL. (2002) Contraceptive efficacy and body weight. Female Patient 27:36–38.
20. Anderson FD, Hait H. (2003) The seasonale-301 Study Group. A multicenter, randomized study of an extended cycle oral contraceptive. Contraception 68:89–96.

21. Rosenberg MJ, Meyers A, Roy V. (1999) Efficacy, cycle control, and side effects of low- and lower-dose oral contraceptives: a randomized trial of 20 micrograms and 35 micrograms estrogen preparations. Contraception 60:321–329.
22. Graham CA, Ramos R, Bancroft J, Maglaya C, Farley TMM. (1995) The effects of steroidal contraceptives on the well-being and sexuality of women: A double-blind, placebo-controlled, two-centre study of combined and progestogen-only methods. Contraception 52:363–369.
23. Rosenberg M. (1998) Weight change with oral contraceptive use and during the menstrual cycle. Results of daily measurements. Contraception 58:345–349.
24. Lloyd T, Lin HM, Matthews AE, Bentley CM, Legro RS. (2002) Oral contraceptive use by teenage women does not affect body composition. Obstet Gynecol 100:235–239.
25. Rosenberg M. (1998) Weight change with oral contraceptives use and during the menstrual cycle. Results from daily measurement. Contraception 58:345–349.
26. Henney JE/ From the Food and Drug Administration. (2000) Risk of drug interactions with St. John's wort. JAMA 283:1679.
27. Back DJ, Breckenridge AM, Crawford FE, et al. (1980) The effect of rifampin on the pharmacokinetics of ethinyl estradiol in women. Contraception 21:235–239.
28. Helms SE, Bredle DL, Zajic J, et al. (1997) Oral contraceptive failure rates and oral antibiotics. J Am Acad Dermatol 36:705–710.
29. Amsden GW, Mohamed MA, Menhinick AM. (2001) Effect of hormonal contraceptives on the pharmacokinetics of trovafloxacin in women. Clin Drug Invest 21:281–286.
30. Sanfilippo JS. (1991) Adolescents and oral contraceptives. Intl J Fertil 36:65–79.
31. Bailey P, Sanfilippo JS. (1993) Contraception in the adolescent. In: Shoupe DS, Haseltine FS, eds. Contraception. New York: Springer-Verlag, pp. 93–111.

4 Progestin-Only Oral Contraceptives

Donna Shoupe, MD

CONTENTS

INTRODUCTION

Progestin-only pills (POPs) are often referred to as mini-pills. POPs contain about 35–75% of the progestin dose contained in combination oral contraceptives (OCs) but they are taken continuously without a pill-free interval. Their effectiveness is generally similar to combination OCs. It is critical that POPs be taken at the same time every day; failure to do this may explain the higher typical-use failure rates reported in some studies. They are associated with more breakthrough spotting and bleeding but fewer serious side effects. Although not as well-studied as combination OCs, POPs are thought to have many of the same non-contraceptive health benefits.

MECHANISM OF ACTION

To a limited degree, POPs suppress the midcyle peak of luteinizing and follicle-stimulating hormone, and are only able to suppress ovulation in about half of the cycles during use. POPs have multiple other actions that prevent pregnancy including the following:

From: *Current Clinical Practice: The Handbook of Contraception: A Guide for Practical Management*
Edited by: D. Shoupe and S. L. Kjos © Humana Press, Totowa, NJ

- Produce "hostile" cervical mucus—making it viscid, thick, and scanty, thus preventing sperm penetration. Some reports indicate that the cervical mucus becomes so impermeable to sperm that a back-up contraception method is not needed until three consecutive pills are missed *(1)*.
- Reduce cilia motion in the fallopian tube and decrease motility of the uterus and oviduct, thus inhibiting ova and sperm transport.
- Reducing the size and number of endometrial glands, thus inhibiting implantation.

CLINICAL EFFECTIVENESS

With perfect use, the pregnancy rate for POP users is only slightly higher than that seen with perfect use of combination OCs (0.5% versus 0.2–0.3%). For typical use, the effectiveness rate is generally around 92–95%, although different studies report significant variations. These variations likely result from differences in a study population's ability to adhere to the strict criteria of taking the POP at the same time each day. In a study of 358 obviously very compliant women using POPs, the pearl index was 0.2 per 100 woman-years *(2)*. Other clinical studies report failure rates as high as 13% *(1)*. Having a back-up method for cycles in which pills are missed or ensuring easy access to emergency contraception is recommended, especially for the first 6 months of use.

Women with lower fecundity, such as breastfeeding women or women over 40 years of age, are ideal candidates for POPs. A nearly 100% effectiveness rate was reported in as study of postpartum lactating women *(3)*.

Recent studies have showed that women with the highest body weight have the highest failure rates, although the differences are small.

ADVANTAGES OF POPs

POPs are a good option for many women for whom estrogen is contraindicated. POPs are generally safer and not linked to many of the serious side effects of combination OCs, such as thrombophlebitis and pulmonary embolism *(1,4)*. POPs are a good option in women over age 35 who smoke.

- POPs are rapidly reversible.
- Decreased risk of ectopic pregnancy (although as many as 10% of pregnancies that do occur may be ectopic) *(5)*.
- Easy to use because the user takes the same pill every day with no break.
- More sexual freedom because taking the POP does not interfere with sexual relationships.
- Less menstrual blood flow.
- Less menstrual cramping.

Although not well-studied, the non-contraceptive health benefits of POPs may include:

- Decreased menstrual blood loss.
  - Lowered risk of anemia.
- Decreased dysmenorrhea.
- Decreased cyclic mood changes or other premenstrual syndrome problems.
- Lowered risk of benign breast disease.
- Protection from endometrial cancer.
- Decreased pain from endometriosis.
- Decreased pelvic inflammatory disease (from thickened, impenetrable cervical mucus).

DISADVANTAGES OF POPs

Unlike combination OCs, POPs must be taken at the same time each day with no pill-free interval. The following disadvantages and risks are associated with the use of POPs:

- Functional ovarian cysts are slightly more common in POP users compared with users of combination OCs.
- Pregnancies (method failures) that occur are more likely to be ectopic pregnancies (this a concern in heavier patients in which method failure may be higher).
- All progestin-only methods are associated with irregular bleeding *(6)*.
  - Breakthrough bleeding/spotting may account for 10–25% of POP users discontinuing use during the first year.
  - POPs have a higher number of spotting/bleeding days than combination OCs.
- Minor side effects include:
  - Headache, breast tenderness, and nausea.
  - Androgenic side effects, such as acne or hirsutism.
- Weight gain has been a concern but is generally not a significant problem in POP users (very low dose of progestin in POPs).
- There is no protection from sexually transmitted infections (STI) or HIV.
- Critical necessity to take the pill at the same time everyday.
- Contraceptive efficacy may be decreased substantially by other medications that induce liver enzymes.
- Less information available than for combination OCs.
  - There is limited data from large-scale population studies available and limited data to establish a risk–benefit profile.

CONTRAINDICATIONS TO USE

POPs are safe for the majority of women of reproductive age, although there are certain absolute contraindications. The number of absolute contraindications is much smaller than the list for combination OCs.

- Pregnancy or suspected pregnancy.
- Current or history of breast cancer.
- Undiagnosed genital bleeding.
- Acute liver disease.
  - Hepatic adenomas/carcinoma.
- Hypersensitivity to any component of the pill.

A relative contraindication would be current coronary artery disease or cerebrovascular disease. As discussed in Chapter 15, use of POPs in women with cardiovascular disease must be individualized. A risk–benefit analysis, informed decision, and proper follow-up are advised.

EVALUATIONS, PATIENT SELECTION, AND COUNSELING

When evaluating a potential POP user, the following may be considered. These are very similar to the issues covered when evaluating a potential combination OC user.

- Current gynecological issues:
  - Sexual history, risk of STI exposure.
  - Present and future fertility plans.
  - Bleeding problems, fibroids, endometriosis.
- Demographics.
  - Age, smoking status.
- Current problems, medical illnesses.
  - Medications taken.
- Physical and pelvic examination.
  - Blood pressure, weight.
- Laboratory assays.
  - Pap test.
  - Cervical tests for sexually transmitted diseases as indicated (rarely necessary for a patient in a mutually monogamous relationship).
  - Screening for anemia or abnormal lipids as indicated.

Good Candidates

The following are generally suitable candidates for POP use:

- Many women for whom estrogen is contraindicated because POPs have little or no effect on clotting factors.
- Many women over 35 or 40 years of age who are not candidates or are poor candidates for combination OCs.
  - Smokers.
  - Multiple cardiovascular disease risk factors (Chapter 15).
    - Obese with risk factors.

  - Migraines.
  - Sickle cell disease *(7)*.
- Breastfeeding women (POPs have little or no effect on production of breast milk).
- Women who experience problems with combination OCs including:
  - Headaches.
  - Decreased libido.
  - Breast tenderness.
  - Nausea or gastrointestinal upset.
- Women on sodium valproate and benzodiazepines (they do not reduce POP contraceptive effectiveness).

Poor Candidates

- Women on enzyme-inducing drugs, such as phenytoin, barbiturates, or carbamazepine, because there is a significant risk of reduced contraceptive effectiveness and caution advised (includes rifampicin, phenytoin, primidone, topiramate, oxcarbazepine, and griseofulvin).
- Adolescents or adults who are unable or unwilling to be rigidly compliant.
- Obese (160 lb) women (pill may be less effective, although a risk–benefit analysis is advised); older patients have lower fecundity and this may be taken into consideration.

COUNSELING TIPS

- POPs must be taken at the same time everyday (ideally within 1 hour, but within 3 hours is acceptable).
  - Never miss any days.
  - On initiation, the very first pill is taken on the first day of normal menses (or in some cases after a negative pregnancy test, when appropriate).
- Abnormal, unpredictable bleeding may be expected.
  - Bleeding patterns may improve over time.
- Minor side effects, such as nausea or mood changes may decrease after several cycles.
  - Premenstrual syndrome symptoms may improve or worsen.
- Have a back-up method available for missed pill days or abstain from sexual intercourse for specific time period as detailed below.
- If a pill is missed or if taken late, have a back-up method available or abstain from sex for the period of time as detailed below.
  - If a pill is missed, it should be taken as soon as possible and a back-up method should be used until 7 days of uninterrupted POP use has been completed.
  - If a pill is taken more than 3 hours late, a back-up method should be used for 2 days.
  - If two pills are missed, back-up contraception should be used for one cycle.

Table 1
Progestin-Only Pills

Progestin	*Product*	*Progestin content*	*Active pills per cycle*	*Manufacturer*
Levonorgestrel	Ovrette®	Levonorgestrel 0.075 mg	28	Wyeth
Norethindrone	Micronor®	Norethindrone 0.35 mg	28	Janssen-Cilag
	Camila®		28	Barr
	Errin®		28	Barr
	Nor-QD®		28	Watson
	Jolivette®		28	Watson
	Nora-BE®		28	Watson
	Ortho-Micronor®		28	Ortho-McNeil

- Information or access to emergency contraception may be useful to some users.
- POPs offer no protection from STIs or HIV but may provide some protection from pelvic inflammatory disease (upper tract infections).
  - Adding the use of condoms advisable if a patient at risk of exposure to STIs or HIV.
- Some women may ovulate during POP use.
  - Women with regular menstrual cycles during POP use may be at slightly higher risk for method failure. If these women suddenly miss a menstrual period, they should get a pregnancy test and appropriate follow-up.

WARNING SIGNS

POP users should return to their clinic or contact their health care provider for any of the following:

- Pelvic/lower abdominal pain: rule out ectopic pregnancy (ectopic pregnancy is rare, but if patient has a positive pregnancy test, an ectopic must be ruled out).
- Heavy, continuous bleeding: rule out anemia.
- A sudden skipped period or onset of amenorrhea, especially after a pattern of regular bleeding cycles: rule out pregnancy.
- Jaundice, light stools.
- The same warning signs are appropriate for POPs as combination OCs, although many of the serious side effects are not common.

OPTIONS AVAILABLE

There are seven POPs containing 0.35 mg of norethindrone and one pill containing 0.075 mg norgestrel on the market (Table 1). All POPs are taken every day at the same time of day with no pill-free days. The cost of mini-pills is generally slightly higher than combined OCs regardless of the coverage.

REFERENCES

1. McCann MF, Potter LS. (1994) Progestin-only contraception: a comprehensive review. Contraception 50:S1–S195.
2. Broome M, Fotherby K. (1990) Clinical experience with the progestin-only pill. Contraception 42:489–495.
3. Moggia AV, Harria GS, Dunson TR, et al. (1991) A comparative study of a progestin-only oral contraceptive versus non-hormonal methods in lactating women in Buenos Aires, Argentina. Contraception 44:31–43.
4. Vessey MP, Lawless M, Yeates D, McPherson K. (1985) Progestin-only oral contraception: findings in a large prospective study with special reference to effectiveness. Br J Fam Plann 10:117–121.
5. Speroff L, Darney PD. (2001) A Clinical Guide for Contraception, 3rd ed. Philadelphia: Lippincott Williams & Wilkins.
6. D'Arcangues C. (2000) Management of vaginal bleeding irregularities induced by progestin-only contraceptives. Hum Reprod 15:24–29.
7. Bailey P, Sanfilippo JS. (1993) Contraception in the adolescent. In: Shoupe DS, Haseltine FP, eds, Contraception. New York: Springer-Verlag, pp. 93–111.

5 Contraceptive Patch

Donna Shoupe, MD

CONTENTS

INTRODUCTION

After its introduction in 2002, the transdermal contraceptive patch became one of the fastest growing birth control options in the United States (Fig. 1). Like combination oral contraceptives (OCs), the contraceptive patch is effective and rapidly reversible. The patch was designed to mimic the hormonal action of a 35-μg OC and carries many of the same advantages and disadvantages. It is expected that the patch will have many of the same contraceptive and non-contraceptive benefits associated with OCs. The biggest advantage of the patch is its once-a-week administration. The most common side effects are application site reaction, breast discomfort, nausea, and headaches *(1)*. Recently, the package insert has been changed to include a statement that patch users are exposed to about 60% more estrogen than those using a typical oral contraceptive pill containing estrogen.

From: *Current Clinical Practice: The Handbook of Contraception: A Guide for Practical Management*
Edited by: D. Shoupe and S. L. Kjos © Humana Press, Totowa, NJ

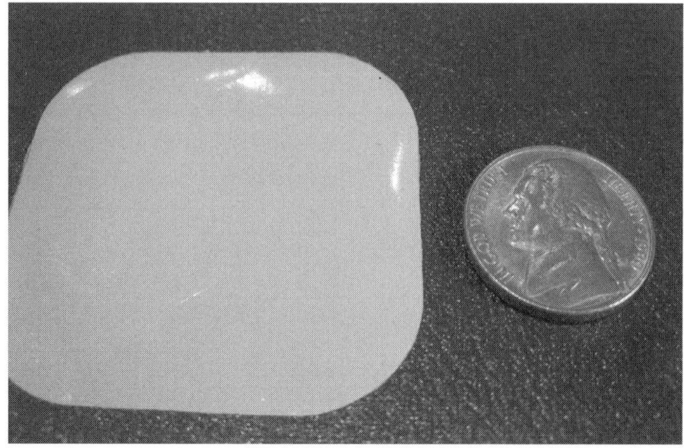

Fig. 1. Contraceptive patch shown with a nickel for size comparison.

PHARMACODYNAMICS

The contraceptive patch contains 6 mg norelgestromin and 0.75 mg ethinyl estradiol (EE) and was designed to release 150 μg of norelgestromin and 20 μg of EE through the skin into the blood stream per 24 hours. Norelgestromin is the primary active metabolite produced following oral administration of norgestimate. Following application, norelgestromin and EE rapidly appear in the circulation and reach steady-state levels at 48 hours (0.3–1.53 ng/mL and 11–137 pg/mL, respectively). These levels are within or higher than the therapeutic reference ranges established for OrthoCyclen® (0.6–1.2 ng/mL and 25–75 pg/mL, respectively). Therapeutic levels of norelgestromin and EE are maintained for the 7 days of routine patch wear and during 2 extra days of extended wear.

The half-life of norelgestromin is 28 hours and the half-life of EE is 17 hours. Absorption and serum levels are not significantly affected by exposure of the user to saunas, whirlpools, treadmills, or cold water baths.

Transdermally administered norelgestromin does not reverse the stimulatory action of EE on sex hormone-binding globulin (SHBG), resulting in significant increases in SHBG following patch administration *(2)* and other hepatic proteins (Chapters 2 and 3). Increased levels of SHBG bind endogeous androgens resulting in lower levels of free testosterone following patch application.

METABOLISM

Transdermally administered hormones avoid the first-pass metabolism through the gastrointestinal tract as seen with oral administration. Circulating norelgestromin is eventually metabolized to norgestrel as well as other metabolites. Circulating EE is metabolized to various hydroxylated metabolites and their sulfate and glucuronide conjugates and elimination by renal and fecal pathways.

MECHANISM OF ACTION

The mechanism of action of the contraceptive patch is the same as combination OCs; that is, the patch inhibits the midcyle gonadotropin surge and effectively prevents ovulation *(3)*. Although inhibition of ovulation is the primary mechanism of action, combination OCs and the contraceptive patch also act on other parts of the reproductive tract in the following ways:

- Cervical mucus: making it viscid, thick, and scanty, thus preventing sperm penetration, inhibits capacitation of the sperm.
- Decreasing motility of the uterus and oviduct, thus inhibiting ova and sperm transport.
- Diminishing endometrial glandular production of glycogen, making less energy available for the blastocyst to survive in the uterine cavity.
- Decrease in ovarian responsiveness to gonadotropin stimulation.

CLINICAL EFFECTIVENESS

Like OCs, the patch is effective if used properly. The percentage of women experiencing an unintended pregnancy during the first year of perfect and typical use of the contraceptive patch is considered to be similar to OC use (0.2–0.3% and 3–8%, respectively). In large clinical trials in North America, Europe, and South Africa, the failure rate of the contraceptive patch was approximately 1%. The patch appears to be less effective in women weighing more than 198 lb *(4)*.

ADVANTAGES OF THE PATCH

- The biggest advantage of the patch is its once-a-week dosing that is very convenient for many users.
  - High rates of perfect use in some studies (92% in patch users compared with 77.2% in OC users *[5]*).
  - Good compliance in all age groups but particularly good in adolescents in whom OC compliance is poor *(6)*.
- Rapidly reversible.
- Verifiable, visible patch.
- Norelgestromin is a derivative of norgestimate, a progestin with minimal androgencity *(7)*.
- Because patches have the same mechanism of action, they are expected to have the same non-contraceptive benefits that are associated with OCs (Chapter 2) including:
  - Bleeding control.
  - Less cyclic mood changes, premenstrual syndrome.

- Less dysmenorrhea.
- Decrease in androgen-related problems, such as acne.
- Decreased risk of endometrial and ovarian cancer.

DISADVANTAGES OF THE PATCH

- The patch is noticeable; privacy may be a concern.
- It is necessary to replace the patch weekly.
- About 1–2% of patches detach and need to be replaced.
- There are no generic equivalents and cost may be a concern.
- Room temperature storage necessary.
- Provides no protection against STDs and HIV (concurrent condom use advised for women with risk of exposure).
- 20% Incidence of minor skin irritation, local rash, or redness.
  - Residual adhesive may be left on skin.
  - About 2% of users in clinical trials discontinued use because of skin irritation from the patch.
- Common side effects are breast discomfort, nausea, headache, and dysmenorrhea.
- Health risks fall into the same categories as those seen with OCs.
  - Blood clots, thrombophlebitis, pulmonary embolism.
    - It is not known whether the patch is associated with higher risk of clotting problems than currently available OCs, but the issue has been raised.
  - Increased risk of stroke and myocardial infarction in high-risk populations, such as smokers over 35 years of age or women with vascular disease.

SIDE EFFECTS

The most frequent side effects leading to discontinuation in users participating in the clinical trials included:

- Application site reaction.
- Breast symptoms.
- Headache.
- Emotional liability.
- Nausea and/or vomiting.
- Dysmenorrhea.

Serious Side Effects

Similar contraindications for use of OCs applies to the patch. For many years, uncontrolled hypertension or women over age 35 who smoke cigarettes have been contraindications to the use of OCs. A recent World Health Organization Technical Report states that women who do not smoke, who have their blood pressure checked, and who do not have hypertension or diabetes mellitus have no increased risk of myocardial infarction if they use combined OCs, regardless of their age *(8)*. However, women with these risk factors or those with known vascular disease/vessel narrowing should not use OCs or the patch because they are at significantly increased risk *(9)*.

An increased risk of the following are associated with OC use and apply to the contraceptive patch (Chapters 2 and 3). With use of OCs, the increased risk of these conditions is particularly of concern in women over 35 who smoke, or in women with cardiovascular disease, obesity, hypertension, diabetes, or the specific risk factors listed under the Contraindications heading and in Chapter 3. Close evaluation of the risk of clotting incidences in patch users in the United States has been ongoing since media articles reported on several cases.

- Thrombophlebitis and venous thrombosis with or without embolism.
- Arterial thromboembolism.
- Pulmonary embolism.
- Myocardial infarction.
- Cerebral hemorrhage, cerebral thrombosis.
- Gallbladder disease.
- Hepatic adenomas or benign liver tumors.
- Mesenteric or retinal thrombosis.

Reproductive Effects

As with OCs, there is a slight delay (usually only a few weeks) in the return of ovulation in women discontinuing use of the patch.

Breast Cancer Risk

The risk is assumed to be similar to the risk in OC users (Chapter 2). The vast amount of studies show small or no changes in the relative risk of breast cancer with OC use. It appears that the dose or type of either steroid, as well as duration of OC use, is not related to breast cancer risk.

CONTRAINDICATIONS

OCs and patches are considered to be safe for the majority of women of reproductive age, although there are certain absolute contraindications that are listed in detail in Chapter 3.

- Significant risk factors for thrombosis or cardiovascular disease.
  - Over age 35 with cigarette smoking, significat hyperlipidemia, migraine headaches, diabetes, systemic disease, obesity, or hypertension.
  - Thrombophlebitis or thromboembolic disorders (current or past), known thrombogenic mutations.
- Valvular heart diseases (other than asymptomatic mitral valve prolapse).
- Cerebrovascular or coronary artery disease.
  - Systemic disease that affects the vascular system.

    - Lupus erythematosus.
    - Diabetes with vascular involvement, retinopathy, or nephropathy.
- Hypertension.
- Surgery or prolonged immobilization.
- Cancer of the breast (past or present).
- Known or suspected pregnancy.
- Migraine headaches with localizing signs or worsening headaches during use.
- Undiagnosed genital bleeding.
- Acute or chronic hepatocellur disease with abnormal liver function, hepatic adenomas/carcinoma.
- Known hypertriglyceridemia (between 350 and 600 mg/dL).
- OC-related jaundice.
- Hypersensitivity to any component of the product.

Relative Contraindications

Consider other methods after an appropriate risk–benefit analysis for the following conditions:

- Sickle cell disease/trait.
- Cigarette smoking (>15 cigarettes/day) by women younger than age 35.
- Migraine headaches.
- Weight more than 198 lb (effectiveness may be a problem).

Use when appropriate and follow as needed in women with the following:

- Gallbladder disease.
- Depression.
- Prolactin-secreting pituitary macroadenoma.
- History of cholestatic jaundice of pregnancy.

DRUG INTERACTIONS

Some drugs can interfere clinically with the action of OCs by inducing liver enzymes that convert the steroids to more polar, less biologically active metabolites. For this reason, drugs such as barbiturates, sulfonamides, griseofulvin, phenylbutazone, phenytoin, carbamazepine, cyclophosphamide, and rifampin *(10)* should not be given concomitantly with OCs and patches. Herbal products containing St. John's Wort may induce hepatic (cytochrome P450) enzymes and may reduce effectiveness and result in breakthrough bleeding (Chapter 3).

COUNSELING AND PATIENT SELECTION

Evaluation of a potential patch user is similar to evaluation of a potential OC user and includes the following:

- Current gynecological issues:
  - Menstrual cycle irregularities, anemia.
  - Exposure to STD.
  - Dysmenorrhea, premenstrual syndrome.
  - Androgen excess, acne, hirsutism, polycystic ovarian syndrome.
  - Endometriosis, fibroids.
  - Recurrent ovarian cysts.
  - Current and future childbearing plans.
  - Past experience with use of OCs.
- Demographics:
  - Age, marital status, occupation.
- Medications.
- Allergies.
- Surgeries.
- Smoking history.
- Family history, especially thrombosis or cardiovascular disease.
- Medical problems:
  - Known clotting irregularities, thromboembolic disease.
  - Known cardiovascular disease or risk factors.
  - Hypertension.
  - Obesity.
  - Diabetes.
- Physical examination:
  - Vital signs and weight (elevated blood pressure and long-standing obesity may have a significant impact on safety; additionally, current weight may have significant impact on efficacy).
  - Breast and pelvic examination with cervical cytology are recommended at baseline and yearly.
- Laboratory assays if indicated:
  - Cervical tests for STDs as indicated (not necessary for women in mutually monogamous relationships).
  - Screening for anemia, insulin resistance, or abnormal lipids if indicated.

INSTRUCTIONS TO USE

- If user chooses a first-day start (applying the patch within 24 hours of the start of a period), no back-up contraceptive is needed.
  - If a patch is not applied within 24 hours of menses, or if choosing a Sunday start, 1 week of a back-up contraception method, such as condom, spermicide, or diaphragm, should be used. (Alternatively, a new user can abstain from sexual contact for 1 week.)

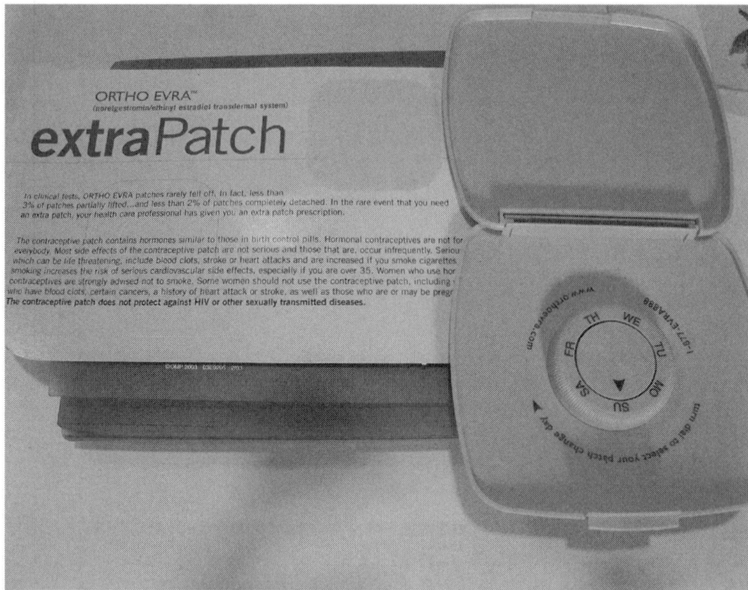

Fig. 2. Case for storage of second- and third-week patches, shown with information on the extra patch that is included as a spare.

- The patch is applied to dry, healthy skin in one of four areas (buttocks, abdomen, upper torso excluding breasts, or outside upper arm; detailed instruction available at website) *(11)*.
  - Half the protective liner is peeled away and the sticky surface is applied to the skin. The other half of the liner is removed and the patch is pressed firmly with the palm of the hand for 10 seconds.
  - Apply patch to dry, nonirritated skin (do not apply right after bath or shower as skin may have microscopic wetness that can lead to increased skin irritation).
  - Make sure patch is firmly placed making sure that all the edges are sticking and that the patch remains smooth after application.
  - Check the patch every day to make sure it is in place.
  - Extra patches are available in case a patch comes off (Fig. 2).
- If a patch is partially or completely detached for less than 24 hours, reapply the same patch or replacement patch immediately; no back-up contraception necessary.
- If a patch is detached for more than 24 hours or user is unsure on how long it has been detached, the user should start a new cycle immediately by applying a new patch and establishing a new patch change day. Back-up contraception, such as condoms, spermicides, or diaphragm must be used for 1 week of the new cycle.
  - Do not use supplemental adhesives or wraps to hold the patch in place.
  - Any residual adhesive can be removed with baby oil.

- A new patch is used weekly for 3 weeks followed by 1 week off.
  - Remove the old patch and apply a new patch to a different area of the skin.
- Withdrawal bleeding should occur during the patch-free fourth week.
  - Abnormal bleeding/spotting may occur for 1–3 months after starting use of the patch.

Timing of Initiation

- Adolescents: after three regular menstrual cycles.
- Switching from OCs: start patch on first day of withdrawal bleeding but no later than 4–5 days after last active pill.
- Switching from DMPA: start patch on any day before the day that the next injection is due.
  - Starting the patch on the first Sunday before the day that the next injection is due is common.
- Switching from intrauterine device: start on day of intrauterine device withdrawal and use back-up method for 7 days, unless removal is on first day of menses,
- Switching from implant: start immediately on day of removal.
- Postabortion: initiate immediately (if not started within 5 days, follow instructions for new starter and use back-up method in meantime).
- Postpartum non-breastfeeding: initiate at 1 month postpartum.
  - Fully breastfeeding: a progestin-only pill is preferred because combination OCs and patch may decrease milk production.
  - Partially breastfeeding: a combination OC or patch can be used after 6 months postpartum.
- Perimenopausal: low-dose OCs or patch for cycle control and symptom relief (Chapter 14).

Warning Signals

Patients should be instructed to contact their physician/health care provider if they have any of the following:

- No withdrawal bleeding or spotting for 2 months (spotting counts as withdrawl bleeding as long as it occurs in the pill-free interval): pregnancy must be ruled out.
- Severe leg pain: rule out blood clot.
- Abdominal pain: rule out pregnancy, ectopic pregnancy, infection, or blood clot.
- Sharp chest pain, shortness of breath, coughing of blood: possible pulmonary embolism.
- Crushing chest pain or tightness in the chest: indicating possible heart attack.
- Blurred vision, speech problem, visual problem: possible blood clot or stroke.
- Numbness or weakness of arm or leg: possible blood clot or stoke.
- Severe or increased frequency of headache: discontinue method because this may be a warning of potential stroke.

- Jaundice or yellowing of the skin or eyeballs, dark-colored urine, or light-colored bowel movements: indicates liver disease.

POOR CANDIDATES FOR THE PATCH

- Women on enzyme-inducing drugs, such as phenytoin, barbiturates, or carbamazepine because there is a significant risk of reduced contraceptive effectiveness with OCs and presumably with patch use.
  - When using Griseofulvin and rifampin, caution advised.
- Disorganized, poor compliance likely.
- Multiple skin allergies, skin conditions.
- Weight more than 198 lb.

COUNSELING TIPS

- The patch can be applied to one of four areas of the body: the buttocks, abdomen, upper torso (front and back excluding the breasts), or upper outer arm.
- Every new patch is applied on the same day of the week, known as the patch change day.
  - It is important that new patches are placed in a new location each time.
  - The patch change day can be identified on the dial in the storage case (Fig. 2).
- No creams, lotions, powders, makeup, or other products should be applied to the skin where the patch will be placed.
- OCs offer no protection from STDs (no protection from lower tract transmission and infection).
- Minor side effects, such as breakthrough spotting or bleeding, breast tenderness, nausea, and headache may decrease after several cycles.
- If a user misses timely placement of patch at the start of a patch cycle: apply the first patch of new cycle. This is now the new patch change day. Back-up contraception should be used for 1 week.
  - If a user misses new patch placement in the middle of the patch cycle: for up to 48 hours late, apply the new patch immediately. The next patch should be applied as usual. No back-up protection needed. (Patch has 2-day grace period in steroid release.)
  - If a user is more than 48 hours late to place new patch: start of new cycle; this is now the new patch change day; back-up contraception needed for 1 week.
  - If a user forgets to remove a patch at the end of a patch cycle: user should remove the patch and start the next cycle on the usual patch change day.
    - There should never be more than 7 patch-free days. If there have been more than 7 patch-free days, back-up contraception is needed for 7 days.
- If the user wishes the change the patch change day, she should complete her current cycle and remove the third patch on the correct day. During the patch-free week, she should apply the new patch on the "selected" day, before the

normal date, and this becomes the new patch change day. In no case should there by more than 7 consecutive patch-free days.

- Lack of withdrawal bleeding for one cycle: user may continue using patch if she has adhered to the prescribed schedule.
  - If user has missed two consecutive periods (no bleeding or spotting), pregnancy should be ruled out.

PRODUCT

The contraceptive transdermal patch is a thin, flexible, beige-colored, 20-cm^2 (1.75 sq. in.), two-layered, matrix-type patch with a clear plastic backing that is removed before application (Fig. 1). The backing layer consists of an outer low-density pigmented polyester layer and an inner polyester layer. On the outside of the backing layer is a heat-stamped "ORTHO EVRA™ 150/20". This layer provides structural support and protects the inner layer from the environment. The inner layer contains the active medication and also a polysobulylene/polybutene adhesive. There is a clear polyester film backing that protects the adhesive layer during storage and is removed just before placement.

REFERENCES

1. Audet MC, Moreau M, Koltun WE, et al. for the ORTHO EVRA/EVRA 004 study Group. (2001) Evaluation of contraceptive efficacy and cycle control of a trandermal contraceptive patch vs an oral contraceptive: a randomized controlled trial. JAMA 285:2347–2354.
2. White T, Jain JK, Stanczyk FZ. (2005) Effect of oral versus transdermal contraceptives on androgenic markers. Am J Obstet Gynecol 192:2055–2059.
3. Mishell DR Jr, Kletzky OA, Brenner PF, et al. (1978) The effect of contraceptive steroids on hypothalamic-pituitary function. Am J Obstet Gynecol 130:817–821.
4. Burkman RT. (2002) The transdermal contraceptive patch: a new approach to hormonal contraception. Int J Fertil Womens Med 47:69–76.
5. Potter L, Oakley D, de Leon-Wong E, Canamar R. (1996) Measuring compliance among oral contraceptive users. Fam Plann Perspect 28:154–158.
6. Archer DF, Cullins V, Creasy GW, Fisher AC. (2004) The impact of improved compliance with a weekly contraceptive transdermal system (Ortho Evra™) on contraceptive efficacy. Contraception 69:189–195.
7. Anderson FD. (1992) Selectivity and minimal androgenicity of norgestimate in monophasic and triphasic oral contraceptives. Acta Obstet Gynecol Scan 156:15–21.
8. World Health Organization. (1998) Cardiovascular disease and steroid hormone contraception, report of a WHO Scientific Group. WHO Technical Report Series no. 877, Geneva, Switzerland.
9. Pettit DB, Sidney S, Bernstein A, et al. (1996) Stroke in users of low-dose oral contraceptives. N Engl J Med 335:8–15.
10. Back DJ, Breckenridge AM, Crawford FE, et al. (1980) The effects of rifampicin on the phrmacokinetics of ethinylestradiol in women. Contraception 21:135–143.
11. Ortho-McNeil Pharmaceutical. Ortho Evra. Available from: www.orthoevra.com. Accessed: March 2006.

6 Contraceptive Ring

Susan A. Ballagh, MD

CONTENTS

INTRODUCTION

In development for more than 20 years, the first vaginal ring contraceptive (NuvaRing®) was approved by the Food and Drug Administration in 2001 and marketed in 2002. Like oral contraceptive (OC) pills, the ring is safe, effective, and rapidly reversible *(1)*. It offers the lowest estrogen dose of any estrogen–progestin contraceptive product marketed in the United States. It is worn for 21 days then removed and discarded. Bleeding ensues and 7 days later a new ring is inserted to start the next cycle. The advantages and side effects are similar to OCs. Ring users are expected to experience similar non-contraceptive health benefits as pill users. The biggest advantage of ring use is its once-a-month insertion and removal. Ring users do not have the burden of taking a pill every day and yet they retain complete control of initiating and discontinuing use of the method.

PRODUCT DESCRIPTION

The vaginal ring is designed to release 15 μg of ethinyl estradiol (EE) and 120 μg of etonogestrel daily over a 24-hour period. Hormone release remains steady

From: *Current Clinical Practice: The Handbook of Contraception: A Guide for Practical Management*
Edited by: D. Shoupe and S. L. Kjos © Humana Press, Totowa, NJ

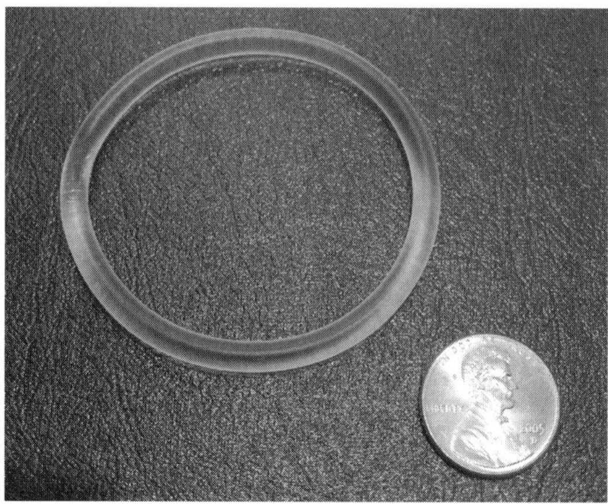

Fig. 1. Contraceptive vaginal ring shown with a penny for a size comparison.

even if use is extended up to 28 days. Unlike OCs, there are no daily fluctuations. Etonogestrel, also called 3-keto-desogestrel, is the active metabolite of desogestrel, a progestin found in several OCs. Instead of giving a pro-drug as with oral mestranol or desogestrel products, the vaginal ring releases the active estrogen and progestin compounds directly into the pelvic bloodstream.

The ring measures 54 mm in diameter, two sizes smaller (or 11 mm smaller) than the smallest ring of a diaphragm-fitting kit. It is half as thick as menopausal vaginal rings with a cross-sectional diameter of 4 mm (Fig. 1). The ring is made of a polymer called ethylene vinyl acetate or Evatane®. This plastic is used to make blood bags, ocular inserts, and the progesterone intrauterine device. Most of the ring is composed of a translucent polymer/hormone mixture coated with a thin, 0.1 mm outer layer composed of polymer alone. The outer layer meters hormone release over time.

The absorption of hormone through the vagina is rapid, reaching therapeutic hormone levels of EE and etonogestrel during the first day of use. The half-life of both steroids is 20 and 22 hours for EE and etonogestrel, respectively *(2)*. The incidence of nausea in ring users is the same as in OC users *(3)*. Bioavailability of etonogestrel and EE is 100 and 56%, respectively *(4)*. Placement of the ring is limited only by comfort issues because hormone release occurs anywhere in the vagina. The user need not fit or verify placement as long as the ring rests inside comfortably. Most women do not feel the ring because it lies on top of the pelvic floor muscles. When she sits or stands the ring occupies a nearly horizontal position.

Serum hormone levels remain therapeutic for at least 7 days beyond the 21 days of labeled use (Fig. 2). No extra contraceptive precautions are recommended for women who extend wear for up to 1 week beyond the labeled duration of action. Even then, some hormone is still released until removed.

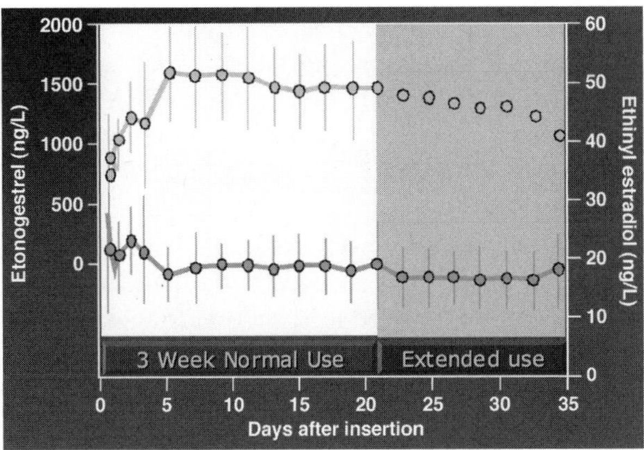

Fig. 2. Serum hormone levels remain therapeutic for at least 7 days beyond the 21 days of normal use.

METABOLISM

Both EE and etonogestrel are primarily metabolized by the liver P450 isoenzyme 3A4. The aromatic ring of EE is hydroxylated and/or methylated forming a number of water-soluble metabolites that circulate free or conjugated to sulfates or glucuronide. The estrogen metabolites have little estrogenic potency and are ultimately eliminated in urine and feces. When a single OC tablet with 30 μg of EE and 150 μg of desogestrel is ingested, the major plasma compound present during the first 24 hours is etonogestrel (3-keto-desogestrel *[5]*). Sixty percent of desogestrel radioactivity is excreted in the urine and 35% in feces. Etonogestrel is conjugated with sulfonic and glucuronic acid for excretion. Predominant etonogestrel metabolites are compounds hydroxylated at C5, C6, and the C13-ethyl moiety.

Women with impaired liver or kidney function may have difficulty metabolizing or eliminating sex steroids. Women who develop jaundice should discontinue any hormonal contraceptive including the ring. The liver is stimulated to produce globulins in proportion to the serum EE levels whether the EE is given orally or vaginally *(6)*. Sex hormone-binding globulin *(7)* and clotting factors *(8)* increase during ring use as seen with oral products. Lipid changes are minimal after 6 months of contraceptive ring use. Total cholesterol and high-density lipoprotein remain the same. There are increases in triglycerides and decreases in lipoprotein(a) similar to changes seen with use of an OC containing levonorgestrel and EE *(9)*.

MECHANISM OF ACTION

Combination hormonal contraceptives act by inhibiting ovulation in more than 97% of cycles *(10)*. Data with the ring shows that follicles of up to 13 mm in size shrink rapidly and do not progress to ovulation when the ring is administered *(11)*. Despite this fact, because individual variation is marked, hormone-free intervals more than 7 days are not recommended. A back-up birth control method is recommended for the first 7 days when initiating use more than 5 days after a natural menses or following a hormone-free interval longer than 7 days (*see* product package insert).

Other minor mechanisms of OC steroids include cervical mucus alteration *(12)*, altered uterotubal peristalsis, reduced endometrial glycogen production, reduced glycodelin secretion, and reduced endometrial gland proliferation *(13)*. It is reasonable to assume that the contraceptive ring also acts through these mechanisms. It has not been used as an emergency contraceptive and does not afford protection against acquisition of sexually transmitted infections (STIs).

CLINICAL EFFECTIVENESS

Between 1 and 2% of women using the ring for 1 year (13 cycles) experienced a pregnancy during clinical trials (Pearl index 1.2, 95% confidence interval: 0.7–1.8) *(1)*. Less than 1% of women who used the ring properly became pregnant. There was no variation in efficacy by weight when divided into deciles. Study participants in the highest decile weighing 167 lb or more were as likely to experience a pregnancy (1.2%) as other women. No pregnancies were noted in the 74 women weighing from 189 to 272 lb *(14)*.

Efficacy in "actual use" was evaluated in 130 high-risk young women randomized to use the ring for 3 months and then an OC for 3 months or vice versa. Four subjects experienced pregnancy during ring use compared with nine while assigned to the OC *(15)*. OC efficacy is estimated to be 92% in actual use compared with more than 99% with perfect use. Two-thirds of women starting pills are still using pills at 1 year *(16)*. Continuation rates in a clinical trial of the vaginal ring were similar with 70% of women completing 1 year of use *(17)*.

Unscheduled bleeding plagues hormonal contraceptive users reducing acceptability and resulting in discontinuation. A Cochrane review pointed to 20 μg oral products as being particularly prone to poor cycle control among oral options. The cycle control of the ring is superior to that of a higher dose (30 μg) OC (Fig. 3) *(3)*. Additionally, the incidence of expected bleeding during the ring-free interval is reassuring at 98.8% *(18)*.

ADVANTAGES OF THE CONTRACEPTIVE RING

- Once-a-month dosing.
- Discreet, verified only by a clinician or intimate partner.
- Rapidly reversible.
- Highly effective, even in overweight women *(11)*.
- Lowest estrogen dose of any combination hormonal contraceptive.

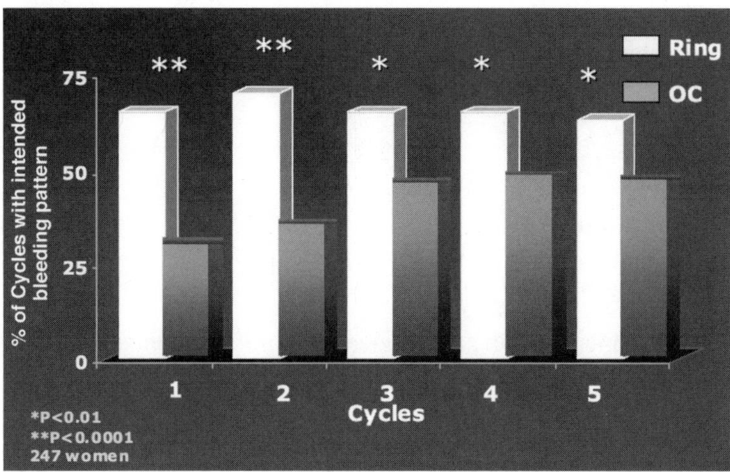

Fig. 3. Bleeding pattern. Contraceptive ring compared with 30 μg/150 μg LNG OCs. (Adapted from ref. *45*.)

- Excellent control of unscheduled breakthrough bleeding and spotting from the start.
- Simple to insert and remove (patient-controlled).
- No package to store.
- One-week reserve for women who forget to remove ring on day 21.
- Can be removed for up to 3 hours per day.
- Reduces dysmenorrhea *(19)*.
- Encourages vaginal colonization of hydrogen peroxide-producing lactobacillus *(20)*.
- The same non-contraceptive benefits expected as with combination OCs (Chapter 2).
  - Reduced monthly bleeding.
  - Reduced acne or other androgen-related problems.
  - Decreased risk of endometrial and ovarian cancer.
  - Decreased risk of pelvic inflammatory disease.

DISADVANTAGES OF THE CONTRACEPTIVE RING

- No generic equivalents.
- No protection against STIs or HIV transmission.
- Volume of normal vaginal secretions increased *(18)*.
- May slip or dislodge with straining or intercourse.
- Cannot be used by certain women with severe vaginal prolapse.
- Unfamiliar technology for drug delivery requires more counseling.

SIDE EFFECTS

The ring is associated with similar side effects as low-dose OCs, except for the 2.6% who experienced device-related events like ring expulsion, foreign body sensation, or coital problems *(21)*. The most frequent side effects reported by women using the ring in clinical trials *(1)* were:

- Headache (5.8%).
- Vaginitis (5.6%).
- Leukorrhea (4.8%).
- Nausea (3.2%).
- Emotional lability (2.8%).
- Breast tenderness (2.6%).
- Dysmenorrhea (2.6%).

There were no increases in pathological vaginitis or changes in cytology with ring use *(22)*.

Cardiovascular Disease Risk

The same contraindications for use of combination OCs apply to the ring. Women with uncontrolled hypertension *(23)* or women over age 35 who smoke cigarettes should not use them. A recent World Health Organization Technical Report *(24)* states that women who do not smoke, have normal blood pressure, and no cardiovascular risk factors such as obesity or diabetes show no increased risk of stroke *(25)*. With use of low-dose OCs, the increased risk of myocardial infarction or stroke is primarily seen in women over 35 who smoke, or in those women with risk factors such as obesity, diabetes, or hypertension (*see* Chapters 2 and 3).

Risk of thromboembolism is associated with OC use and applies to the contraceptive ring as well:

- Thrombophlebitis and venous thrombosis with or without embolism.
- Arterial thromboembolism.
- Pulmonary thromboembolism.
- Retinal or mesenteric thrombosis.

Other serious adverse events noted with OCs include:

- Hypertension (a drug-related idiosyncratic reaction).
- Gallbladder disease.
- Hepatic adenomas or benign liver tumors.

Reproductive Effects

As with combination OCs *(25)*, there may be a slight delay in the return of ovulation in women discontinuing use of the ring. Although anecdotal reports suggest a higher incidence of multiple ovulation in the first cycles after OC discontinuation, an increase in the risk of dizygotic twins has not been well substantiated *(26)*. Pregnancies conceived before normal cycles resume should be carefully dated—with a first trimester ultrasound if possible. There are no teratogenic effects apparent for pregnancies conceived during use of combination OCs or if OCs are used during the first trimester *(27)*.

Breast Cancer Risk

The risk of developing breast cancer is assumed to be similar to OCs (Chapter 2). The vast amount of studies shows small or no changes in the relative risk of breast cancer with OC use *(28)*. No dose effect is noted. Among women with hereditary breast cancer, ever-users do not show any increased risk with OC use compared with non-users *(29)*.

Contraindications

OC, rings, and patches are safe for the majority of women of reproductive age. Certain absolute contraindications apply to all combination hormonal contraceptives (Chapter 3):

- Valvular heart disease (other than asymptomatic mitral valve prolapse).
- Cerebrovascular or coronary artery disease.
  - Systemic disease that affects the vascular system.
    - Lupus erythematosus.
    - Diabetes with vascular disease including:
      - Retinopathy or nephropathy.
- Severe or uncontrolled hypertension.
  - Hypertension in women over 35 is a relative contraindication.
- Thrombophlebitis or thromboembolic disorders current or past.
- Major surgery with prolonged immobilization.
- Cigarette smoking in women older than 35.
- Cancer of the breast (past or present).
- Cancer of the endometrium or any other estrogen-dependent neoplasia.
- Known or suspected pregnancy.
- Migraine headaches that worsen with use have localizing signs.
- Undiagnosed genital bleeding.
- Acute or chronic hepatocellur disease with abnormal liver function.
- Hepatic adenomas/carcinoma.
- Known hypertriglyceridemia (between 350 and 600 mg/dL).
- Cholestatic jaundice of pregnancy or hormone-related jaundice.
- Hypersensitivity of any component of the product.

Use with caution and follow women appropriately who:

- Smoke cigarettes heavily (>15 cigarettes/day) regardless of age.
- Have common migraine headaches.
- Have prolactin-secreting pituitary macroadenoma.
- Are depressed.

- Have undiagnosed amenorrhea.
- Have sickle cell disease.
- Have well-controlled hypertension in women under age 35.
- Have gallbladder disease.

DRUG INTERACTIONS

Ring drug delivery is not altered by simultaneous tampon use. Fourteen healthy women used four tampons per day for 3 days while wearing the contraceptive ring without altering serum levels of EE or etonogestrel *(30)*. Nonoxynol-9 co-administration had no effect on serum levels either *(31)*. Concomitant use of miconazole vaginal suppositories actually resulted in a slight increase in serum hormone levels *(32)*. All these products can be used without compromising the efficacy of the contraceptive ring.

Some drugs can interfere clinically with the action of combination OCs by inducing liver enzymes that convert the steroids to more polar, less biologically active metabolites. For this reason, drugs such as barbiturates, sulfonamides, griseofulvin, phenylbutazone, phenytoin, carbamazepine, cyclophosphamide, felbamate, and rifampin *(33)* or herbal products containing St. John's Wort *(34)* given concomitantly may reduce the ring efficacy. High-dose oral products containing 50 μg EE (not mestranol) may be a better choice for women on these medications, although a risk–benefit analysis should be done. The estimated reduction in EE and progestin with anticonvulsants is at least 40% *(35,36)*.

COUNSELING AND PATIENT SELECTION

To evaluate patients for combined hormonal contraception, a thorough history that checks for absolute contraindications and a blood pressure check are all that is necessary to begin use given the remarkable safety of these products *(37)*. Weight is optional but important to obtain, if possible, given widespread concern about weight gain among users and non-users alike. Randomized, placebo-controlled studies do not suggest significant weight change in placebo versus OC users over 1 year *(38)*. It is common to suggest a follow-up visit within 3 months to encourage compliance and method continuation, but there is no clear data to support the actual impact of that practice *(39)*.

Many women prefer to receive health care and contraception simultaneously. Other gynecological issues are usually addressed simultaneously including:

- Current gynecological issues.
  - Menstrual cycle irregularities, anemia.
  - Exposure to STIs.
  - Dysmenorrhea, premenstrual syndrome.
  - Androgen excess, acne, hirsutism.
  - Endometriosis, fibroids, recurrent ovarian cysts.

- Current and future childbearing plans.
- Past experience with hormonal contraception.

- Demographics:
  - Age, marital status.
- Concurrent problems:
  - Illnesses.
  - Medications.
  - Allergies.
  - Surgeries.
  - Smoking.
  - Family history, especially of thrombophlebitis.
  - Medical problems or significant risk factors.
    - Cardiovascular disease, hypertension, diabetes.
    - Clotting abnormalities, thromboembolic disease.
- Physical examination.
  - Vital signs and weight.
  - Breast and pelvic examination.
    - Cervical cytology.
- Laboratory assays.
  - Pap test in sexually active women over 20 years old.
  - Cervical tests for STDs as indicated (strongly recommended if new partner since last examination).
  - Screening for anemia, insulin resistance, or abnormal lipids if indicated.

Instructions To Use

- New users may choose to place the ring within 5 days of the onset of normal menses without back-up contraception.
- A new ring is used for 3 weeks then discarded.
- Withdrawal bleeding occurs during the ring-free week in 99% of cycles *(19)*.

Timing of Initiation

- Adolescents: after three regular menstrual cycles.
- Switching from OCs: start ring at any time during the 28-day cycle. Wear ring for 21 days then remove.
- Switching from intrauterine device: remove intrauterine device during menses and begin ring within 5 days of the onset of menses.
- Switching from DMPA or depo-subQ provera 104™ start ring on any day up to the injection due date.
- Postabortion: initiate immediately (if not started within 5 days, user should use a back-up method or abstain during the first week of ring use).
- Postpartum non-breastfeeding: initiate at 2–4 weeks postpartum.

- Fully breastfeeding: a progestin-only or non-hormonal contraceptive is traditionally preferred because estrogen-containing hormonal products may decrease milk production *(40)*, although the evidence for this is based on women in resource-poor setting, not in a US population *(41)*.
- Partially breastfeeding: any low-dose combination hormonal contraceptive can be considered. The ring, with the lowest estrogen dose available, is an excellent option.
- Perimenopausal: the ring provides for cycle control and symptom relief.

Warning Signals

Patients should be instructed to contact their physician/health care provider if they have any of the following:

- No withdrawal bleeding for 2 months (mild spotting counts as withdrawal bleeding): pregnancy must be ruled out.
- Numbness or weakness of arm or leg (indicating possible stoke) *(42)*.
- Jaundice or yellowing of the skin or eyeballs, dark-colored urine, or light-colored bowel movement (indicating liver disease).
- A: abdominal pain.
  C: chest pain that is sharp or crushing or tightness in the chest (possible heart attack); shortness of breath or coughing blood (possible embolism).
  H: headache that increases in frequency or severity.
  E: eye problems, such as blurred vision or scotomata.
  S: speech problems (possible stroke) or severe leg pain (possible DVT).

Poor Candidates

- Women on enzyme-inducing drugs such as phenytoin, barbiturates, griseofulvin, rifampin, or carbamazepine because there is a significant risk of reduced contraceptive effectiveness with the ring *(43)*.
- Women with total procedentia.
- Women unable to touch their vagina because of musculoskeletal or other problems.

Counseling Tips

- The ring does not protect against STIs.
- Minor side effects, such as breakthrough spotting or bleeding or headache, may decrease after several cycles.
- If the user forgets to remove the ring on the correct day, the user should remove it as soon as she remembers. If it is within 28 days of insertion she should discard the ring and place a new one 7 days later. If it was worn more than 28 days, she should insert the new ring immediately, skipping the ring-free interval that month. If it was worn for more than 35 days, use back-up for 7 days.
- Women who are oriented to the calendar may use the ring for 25 days per month then remove it *(44)*.
- Expect increased normal vaginal secretions while using the ring *(18)*.

SUMMARY

The contraceptive ring delivers a combined estrogen and progestin contraceptive via a once-a-month delivery system. It has similar efficacy to oral or transdermal delivery, yet offers the lowest dose of estrogen. The ring is user-controlled and is easy to insert and remove from the vagina. It affords privacy and simplicity with once-monthly insertion and no package to store. It increases healthy secretions in the vagina without increasing vaginal infections or pathogens. The steady release of hormone over the 28-day extended life of the product affords greater contraceptive protection in high-risk young women compared with controls. Simultaneously tampon, spermicide, and antimycotic use do not reduce serum steroid delivery by the ring.

REFERENCES

1. Dieben TO, Roumen FJME, Apter D. (2002) Efficacy cycle control and user acceptability of a novel combined contraceptive vaginal ring. Obstet Gynecol 100:585–593.
2. Timmer CJ, Apter D, Voortman G. (1990) Pharmacokinetics of 3-keto-desogestrel and ethinylestradiol released from different types of contraceptive vaginal rings. Contraception 42:629–642.
3. Oddsson K, Leifels-Fischer B, Weil-Masson D, et al. (2005) Superior cycle control with a contraceptive vaginal ring compared with an oral contraceptive containing 30 microg ethinyl estradiol and 150 microg levonorgestrel: a randomized trial. Hum Reprod 20:557–562.
4. Timmer CJ, Mulders TM. (2000) Pharmacokinetics of etonogestrel and ethinylestradiol released from a combined contraceptive vaginal ring. Clin Pharmacokinet 39:233–242.
5. Verhoeven CH, Gloudeman PH, Peeters PA, et al. (2001) Excretion and metabolism of desogestrel in healthy postmenopausal women. J Steroid Biochem Mol Biol 78:471–480.
6. Goebelsmann U, Mashchak CA, Mishell DR Jr. (1985) Comparison of hepatic impact of oral and vaginal administration of ethinyl estradiol. Am J Obstet Gynecol 151:868–877.
7. van Rooijen M, Silveira A, Hamsten A, Bremme K. (2004) Sex hormone-binding globulin—a surrogate marker for the prothrombotic effects of combined oral contraceptives. Am J Obstet Gynecol 190:332–337.
8. Magnusdottir EM, Bjarnadottir RI, Onundarson PT, et al. (2004) The contraceptive vaginal ring (NuvaRing) and hemostatis: a comparative study. Contraception 69:461–467.
9. Tuppurainen M, Klimscheffskij R, Venhola M, Dieben TO. (2004) The combined contraceptive vaginal ring (NuvaRing) and lipid metabolism: a comparative study. Contraception 69:389–394.
10. Coney P, DelConte A. (1999) The effects on ovarian activity of a monophasic oral contraceptive with 100 microg levonorgestrel and 20 microg ethinyl estradiol. Am J Obstet Gynecol 181:53–58.
11. Killick S. (2002) Complete and robust ovulation inhibition with NuvaRing. Eur J Contracept Reprod Health Care 7(Suppl 2):13–18.
12. Hamilton CJ, Hoogland HJ. (1989) Longitudinal ultrasonographic study of the ovarian suppressive activity of a low-dose triphasic oral contraceptive during correct and incorrect pill intake. Am J Obstet Gynecol 161:1159–1162.
13. Durand M, Seppala M, Cravioto Mdel C, et al. (2005) Late follicular phase administration of levonorgestrel as an emergency contraceptive changes the secretory pattern of glycodelin in serum and endometrium during the luteal phase of the menstrual cycle. Contraception 71:451–457.
14. Westhoff C. (2005) Higher body weight does not affect nuvaring's efficacy. Obstet Gynecol 105:56S.

15. Stewart F. (2005) Vaginal contraceptive rings: a new alternative for hormonal contraception with important advantages. Obstet Gynecol 105(Suppl 4):58S.
16. Hatcher RA, Trussel J, Stewart F, et al. (2005) Technology, 18th Edition. New York: Irvington, p. 792.
17. Roumen FJ, Apter D, Mulders TM, Dieben TO. (2001) Efficacy, tolerability and acceptability of a novel contraceptive vaginal ring releasing etonogestrel and ethinyl oestradiol. Hum Reprod 16:469–475.
18. Vree M. (2002) Lower hormone dosage with improved cycle control. Eur J Contracept Reprod Health Care 7:25–30.
19. Novak A. (2001) From the 17th World Congress on Fertility and Sterility, International Federation of Fertility Society. Nov. 25–30, Melbourne, Australia.
20. Veres S, Miller L, Burington B. (2004) A comparison between the vaginal ring and oral contraceptives. Obstet Gynecol 104:555–563.
21. Roumen F. (2002) Contraceptive efficacy and tolerability with a novel combined contraceptive vaginal ring, NuvaRing. Eur J Contracept Reprod Health Care 7:19–24.
22. Davies, GC, Feng LX, Newton JR, Dieben TO, Coelingh-Bennink HJ. (1992) The effects of a combined contraceptive vaginal ring releasing ethinyloestradiol and 3-ketodesogestrel on vaginal flora. Contraception 45:511–518.
23. Curtis KM, Chrisman C, Peterson HB. (2002) Contraception for women in selected circumstances. WHO Program for Mapping Best Practices in Reproductive Health. Obstet Gynecol 99:1100–1112.
24. World Health Organization (WHO). (2000) Improving Access to Quality Care in Family Planning: Medical Eligibility Criteria for Contraceptive Use, 2nd ed. Geneva, Switzerland: WHO.
25. Pinkerton GD, Carey HM. (1976) Post-pill anovulation. Med J Aust 1:220–222.
26. Eriksson AW, Bresser M, Kostense PJ. (year) Are changes in twinning rates caused by oral contraceptives? Institute of Human Genetics and Department of Medical Statistics, Medical Faculty, Free University, Amsterdam, The Netherlands.
27. Raman-Wilms L, Tseng AL, Wighardt S, Einarson TR, Koren G. (1995) Fetal genital effects of first-trimester sex hormone exposure: a meta-analysis. Obstet Gynecol 85:141–149.
28. Marchbanks PA, McDonald JA, Wilson HG, et al. (2002) Oral contraceptives and the risk of breast cancer. N Engl J Med 346:2025–2032.
29. Milne RL, Knight JA, John EM, et al. (2005) Oral contraceptive use and risk of early-onset breast cancer in carriers and noncarriers of BRCA1 and BRCA2 mutations. Cancer Epidemiol Biomarkers Prev 14:350–356.
30. Verhoeven CH, Dieben TO. (2004) The combined contraceptive vaginal ring, NuvaRing, and tampon co-usage. Contraception 69:197–199.
31. Haring T, Mulders TM. (2003) The combined contraceptive ring NuvaRing and spermicide co-medication. Contraception 67:271–272.
32. Verhoeven CH, van den Heuvel MW, Mulders TM, Dieben TO. (2004) The contraceptive vaginal ring, NuvaRing, and antimycotic co-medication. Contraception 69:129–132.
33. Back DJ, Breckenridge AM, Orme ML. (1983) Drug interactions with oral contraceptive steroids. IPPF Medical Bulletin 17:1–2.
34. Pfrunder A, Schiesser M, Gerber S, Haschke M, Bitzer J, Drewe J. (2003) Interaction of St John's wort with low-dose oral contraceptive therapy: a randomized controlled trial. Br J Clin Pharmacol 56:683–690.
35. Saano V, Glue P, Banfield CR, et al. (1995) Effects of felbamate on the pharmacokinetics of a low-dose combination oral contraceptive. Clin Pharmacol Ther 58:523–531.
36. Fattore C, Cipolla G, Gatti G, et al. (1999) Induction of ethinylestradiol and levonorgestrel metabolism by oxcarbazepine in healthy women. Epilepsia 40:783–787.

37. World Health Organization (WHO). (2004) What examinations or tests should be done routinely before providing a method of contraception? www.who.int/reproductive-health/publications/mec/index.htm. Accessed: March 2006.
38. Gallo MF, Grimes DA, Schulz KF, Helmerhorst FM. (2004) Combination estrogen–progestin contraceptives and body weight: systematic review of randomized controlled trials. Obstet Gynecol 103:359–373.
39. World Health Organization (WHO). (2003) What follow-up is appropriate for combined oral contraceptive, progestogen-only pill, implant and IUD users? www.who.int/reproductive-health/publications/mec/index.htm. Accessed: March 2006.
40. Tankeyoon M, Dusitsin N, Chalapati S, et al. (1984) Effects of hormonal contraceptives on milk volume and infant growth. WHO Special Programme of Research, Development and Research Training in Human Reproduction Task force on oral contraceptives. Contraception 30:505–522.
41. Truitt ST, Fraser AB, Grimes DA, Gallo MF, Schultz KF. (2003) Hormonal contraception during lactation, systematic review of randomized controlled trials. Contraception 68:233–238.
42. Pettiti DB, Sidney S, Bernstein A, et al. (1996) Stroke in users of low-dose oral contraceptives. N Engl J Med 335:18.
43. Back DJ, Breckenridge AM, Orme ML. (1983) Drug interactions with oral contraceptive steroids. IPPF Medical Bulletin 17:1–2.
44. Ballagh SA, Babb TA, Kovalevsky G, Archer DA. (2003) Contraceptive ring compliance: "as labeled" versus calendar based use. Fertil Steril 80(Suppl 3):S54.
45. Bjarnadottir RI, Tuppurainen M, Kilick SR. (2002) Comparison of cycle control with a combined contraceptive vaginal ring and oral levonorgestrel/ethinylestradiol. Am J Obstet Gynecol 186:389–395.

7 Long-Acting Progestin Injectables

Comparison of Depo-Provera® With Depo-SubQ Provera 104™

Ronna Jurow, MD *and Donna Shoupe,* MD

Contents

INTRODUCTION

Depo-Provera® (depot medroxyprogesterone acetate [DMPA]) is an extremely effective contraceptive agent. Since its introduction into the market in the 1960s, DMPA has been used for a variety of gynecological conditions including endometriosis and abnormal menstrual bleeding. For many years, DMPA was also commonly used "off-label" as a contraceptive agent, especially in women who were not candidates for oral contraceptive (OC) pills. In 1992, the Food and Drug Administration (FDA) approved the marketing of DMPA as a contraceptive agent.

From: *Current Clinical Practice: The Handbook of Contraception: A Guide for Practical Management*
Edited by: D. Shoupe and S. L. Kjos © Humana Press, Totowa, NJ

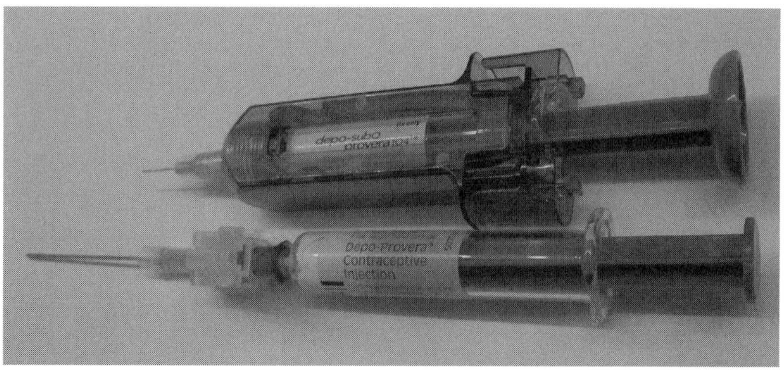

Fig. 1. Side-by-side comparison of Depo-Provera with the newer depo-subQ provera 104 showing the smaller gage needle used for the subcutaneous injection.

In December 2004, depo-subQ provera 104™, (depo-subQ), a newly formulated medroxyprogesterone acetate, was approved by the FDA as a new contraceptive option. Subsequently, depo-subQ received approval from the FDA as a treatment of endometriosis-related pain. Depo-subQ is given subcutaneously and uses a much smaller needle than DMPA (Fig. 1).

The package insert for both DMPA and depo-subQ includes a "black box" warning concerning possible bone loss. Both formulations should be used as a long-term birth control method (that is, longer than 2 years) only if other birth control methods are inadequate.

HISTORY

Unlike most of the progestins currently used in OC pills, medroxyprogesterone acetate (MPA) is a derivative of progesterone rather than testosterone. MPA is a 17-acetoxyprogesterone compound and is the only progestin of this type (i.e., a progesterone derivative) used for contraception (Fig. 2).

MPA does not have androgenic activity and was initially used in OCs more than 30 years ago. Regulatory approval of contraceptive agents containing MPA was halted when it was reported that ingestion of MPA by beagle dogs was associated with the development of mammary cancer. DMPA remained on the market only as a treatment for endometriosis. It was later discovered that beagle dogs, unlike humans, metabolize MPA to estrogen. After worldwide epidemiological studies showed no increase in breast cancer risk in DMPA users, DMPA received regulatory approval as a contraceptive method in 1992.

PHARMACODYNAMICS

MPA can be detected in the systemic circulation within 30 minutes after intramuscular injection *(1)*. Although there is some variation of serum MPA

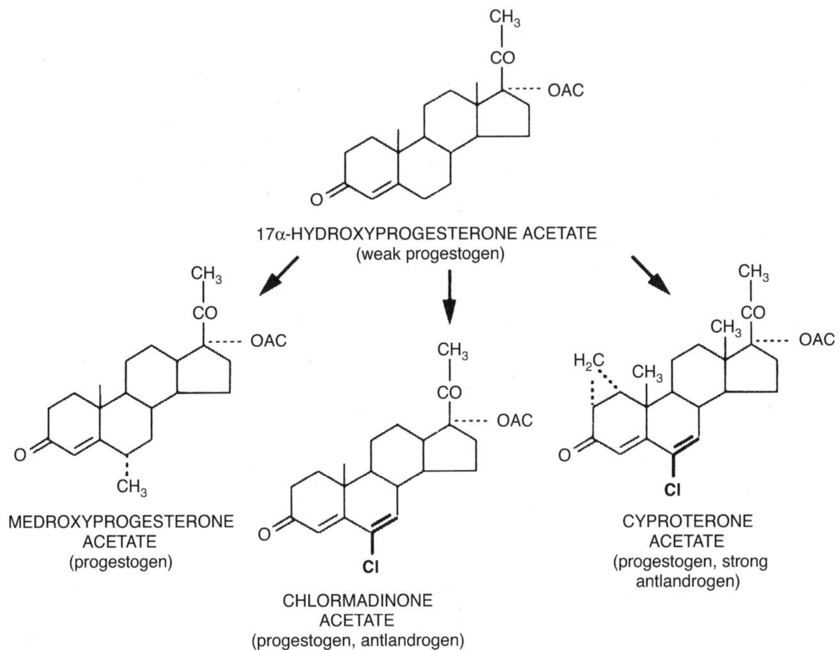

Fig. 2. Derivatives of 17α-hydroxyprogesterone acetate (17-acetoxyprogesterone) include medroxyprogesterone acetate, chlormadinone acetate, and cyproterone acetate. Manipulation of the steroid structure results in significant changes in progestational and anti-androgen activity. (From ref. *44* with permission.)

levels among individuals, serum levels of MPA rise steadily and reach effective blood levels (>0.5 ng/mL) within 24 hours after injection. Levels of MPA remain at effective levels for at least 3 months and are detectable in the circulation (>0.2 ng/mL) in some users as late as 7–9 months. MPA serum levels in many users remain at effective levels for as long as 4–6 months. The long duration of action results from its slow absorption from the injection site. The principal metabolite of MPA that has been identified is a 6α-methyl-6β,17α,21-trihydroxy-4-pregnene-3,20-dione-17-acetate that is excreted in the urine.

Estradiol levels vary considerably, but remain below 100 pg/mL during the first 4 months after injection. In one study, estradiol levels drawn on the scheduled day of a repeat DMPA injection varied between 15 and 100 pg/mL (mean, approximately 42 pg/mL) *(2)*.

MECHANISM OF ACTION

MPA is a 17-acetoxy-6-methyl progestin that has progestogenic activity in the human *(3)*. There are three mechanisms of action that make injectable MPA (iMPA) one of the most effective reversible methods of contraception currently available.

- Ovulation: suppression of the hypothalamus and inhibition of ovulation is the major mechanism of action *(2)*.
- Cervical mucus: making it viscous, thick, and scanty, thus preventing sperm penetration; sperm are unlikely to reach the oviduct and fertilize an egg.
- Endometrium: becomes thin and atrophic *(4)*.
  - Endometrium does not secrete sufficient glycogen to provide nutrition for a blastocyst entering the endometrial cavity.

Suppression of estradiol concentrations and a possible direct action of depo-subQ on lesions of endometriosis (causing thinning and atrophy) are likely to be responsible for the therapeutic effect on endometrial-associated pain.

CLINICAL EFFECTIVENESS

iMPA is an extremely effective contraceptive.

In a large World Health Organization clinical trial, the 1-year pregnancy rate with use of DMPA was only 0.1% and the 2-year cumulative rate was only 0.4% *(5)*. Following perfect use, pregnancy failure rate is 0.3%, whereas typical use failure rate is 3%. Adjusting the dose for weight is not necessary. When depo-subQ was administered for contraception, no pregnancies were detected among 2042 women using depo-subQ for up to 1 year.

- Following perfect use, pregnancy failure rate is 0.3%.
- Typical use failure rate is 3%.
- Adjusting the dose for weight is not necessary.

For the treatment of endometriosis, depo-subQ given every 3 months was statistically equivalent to leuprolide given every 3 months across all endometriosis-associated pain categories (i.e., pelvic pain, pelvic tenderness, painful periods, painful intercourse, and hardening/thickening of tissues) in an 18-month study.

ADVANTAGES OF LONG-ACTING PROGESTIN INJECTABLES

DMPA and depo-subQ have many advantages including:

- Dosing once every 3 months.
  - Depo-subQ given subcutaneously rather than intramuscularly.
- Highly effective method.
- Private.
- May be used in breastfeeding women 6 weeks postpartum.
- Effectiveness not affected by weight.
- Data links some of the non-contraceptive benefits associated with OCs with DMPA:
  - Decreased blood loss.
    - Less risk of anemia *(6)*.
    - Amenorrhea is an advantage to some users.

  - Less dysmenorrhea.
  - Decreased cyclic mood changes (for some users).
  - Decreased risk of endometrial cancer *(7)* and ovarian cancer.
  - Decreased risk of pelvic infection *(6)*.
  - Decreased risk of ectopic pregnancy.
- Compliance good when prescreening excludes women who are not prepared for bleeding changes.
- Depo-subQ is FDA-approved for management of pain associated with endometriosis.
  - Treatment every 3 months with depo-subQ is equivalent to leuprolide 11.25 mg (Lupron Depot) intramuscularly every 3 months in reducing endometriosis-associated pelvic pain, but with some fewer side effects.
    - Both treatment groups showed some bone mineral density (BMD) loss, but mean losses significantly less for women taking depo-subQ (0.3 versus 1.65%). BMD returned to pretreatment levels after discontinuing depo-subQ treatment for 12 months. Those who discontinued leuprolide continued to show BMD losses of 1.3% in the femur and 1.7% in the spine.
    - Depo-subQ users had significantly fewer vasomotor symptoms *(8)*.
- Decreased risk of sickle cell crisis.
- Decreased frequency of grand mal seizures in women with epilepsy *(9,10)*.

DISADVANTAGES OF LONG-ACTING PROGESTIN INJECTABLES

- Unpredictable, irregular, and frequent bleeding episodes.
- Amenorrhea common (disadvantage to some users who are reassured by the presence of menses).
  - 50% After 1 year of use.
  - 70% After 2 years of use *(11)*.
- Injection necessary every 3 months.
  - Office fees and co-pays may add significant cost.
- Return of fertility delayed; delay is minimally 3 extra months and is usually as long as 10 months *(3)*.
- Weight gain in some users linked to an increased appetite *(12)*.
  - 5–10 lb in first year of DMPA *(13)*.
  - In one comparative study, there was no difference in weight gain during the first year of DMPA, Norplant®, or OC use *(14)*.
- Provides no protection against STIs and HIV.
  - Concurrent condom use advised for women with risk of exposure to STIs.
- Local reaction or problems at injection site.
- Not possible to discontinue the method immediately if problems develop.

SIDE EFFECTS

The most common side effect is bleeding abnormalities, including irregular, heavy, or frequent bleeding or amenorrhea.

- Continuation rates are affected by bleeding problems and may be as low as 26–50% at 1 year *(11,15)*.
- Breast symptoms, tenderness, or galactorrhea.
- Headache is a commonly reported adverse effect (9%).
- Depression. Although the product labeling lists depression and mood changes as adverse effects of DMPA, several studies report that these occur in less than 5% of users.
- Emotional liability, nervousness, fatigue, depression, dizziness.
- Nausea.
- Allergic reaction.
- Change in cervix: erosion and secretions.
- Acne.
- Weight gain.
  - May be a problem in some users (5–10 lb/year), although studies report conflicting results *(13)*.
  - Some observational trials have reported no significant changes in weight gain in DMPA users over long periods of time *(16)*.
- Pain at injection site (5%), change in color of injection site.
- Increased sweating, muscle cramps, sexual problems, hot flushes.
- Labeling for DMPA and depo-subQ carries a black box warning regarding loss of BMD that is increased with long-term use.

Cardiovascular Disease Risk

All studies to date have shown that progestin-only methods of contraception do not increase the risk of the serious consequences attributed primarily to the estrogenic component of combination OC pills, including thrombophlebitis and pulmonary embolism (17,18).

- A World Health Organization study reports no change in hypertension, venous thromboembolism, or myocardial infarction after 2 years of use *(19)*.
- A slight deterioration of carbohydrate metabolism in long-term DMPA users is reported in some studies *(20,21)*.
- Cross-sectional studies generally report lower levels of high-density lipoprotein cholesterol, increases in low-density lipoprotein levels, and small or no changes in other parameters *(13)* in users. The long-term effect of these changes is unknown.

Risk of Bone Loss

In addition to blocking ovulation, DMPA also reduces ovarian estradiol production *(22,23)* that can lead to declines in BMD in users. There are at least 10 epidemiological studies and numerous prospective longitudinal documenting changes in BMD in DMPA users compared with controls *(24,25)*. Current DMPA users show some decrease of bone loss that is greater with longer duration of use *(26,27)*.

The bone loss appears to be reversible after stopping use *(28–30)* and use of low-dose estrogen supplementation (monthly estradiol cypionate injections) during use may prevent any BMD decline. In a 2-year double blind, randomized trial of 123 adolescents, the addition of low-dose estradiol supplementation to DMPA resulted in no decline in BMD *(31)*. A similar finding was also reported for adult users *(32)*. Smoking and low calcium intake may be contributory risk factors.

The loss in BMD during DMPA use may be similar to that seen in pregnant or lactating women *(33,34)*. This effect is transient and after weaning there is recovery of BMD to pre-pregnancy values *(35)*. There is no evidence that either prolonged lactation or use of DMPA in adolescents or adults results in an increased fracture risk.

Black Box Warning

Women who use medroxyprogesterone may lose significant bone mineral density. Bone loss is greater the longer the drug is used and may not be completely reversible. It is unknown if the use of medroxyprogesterone in adolescents or young adults will reduce bone mass and increase the risk for osteoporotic fracture in later life. Women should only use medroxyprogesterone as a long-term birth control method (longer than 2 years) if other birth control methods are inadequate.

Risk of Weight Gain

Weight gain of 5–10 lb/year has been reported in many studies. Many observational trials, however, have reported no significant changes in weight gain in DMPA users over long periods of time *(36)*. In one study, there was no difference in weight gain during the first year of use of either DMPA, Norplant, or OCs *(13)*.

However, DMPA has been linked to an increased appetite for some users *(12)* and a weight gain of 5–10 lb in first year of use of DMPA may occur *(13,37)*. Use of the lower-dose depo-subQ may result in a lower risk of side effects including weight gain. Research is ongoing.

Reproductive Effects

There is a delay in the return of ovulation in women discontinuing use of DMPA injections *(38)*. The minimal delay is 3 months and the average delay is 10 months.

Breast Cancer Risk

Two large case–control studies indicate the relative risk of diagnosis of breast cancer among all DMPA users is not significantly increased (relative risk [RR]: 1.2, confidence interval [CI]: 0.96–1.15; RR: 1.0, CI: 0.8–1.3, respectively)

(39,40). When data from these studies were pooled, the overall risk in long-term users (>5 years) was not increased (RR: 1.0, CI: 0.70–1.5) *(41)*.

However, in women who had started use within the past 5 years and were mainly younger than 35 years of age, there was a significantly increased risk of diagnosis of breast cancer (RR: 2.0, CI: 1.5–2.8). This finding is similar to that associated with use of OCs and women whose first-term pregnancy occurred at an early age. Thus DMPA, similar to other contraceptive steroids, does not change the overall incidence of diagnosis of breast cancer but may promote growth and detection of a pre-existing cancer *(42)*.

CONTRAINDICATIONS

MPA injections are safe for the majority of women of reproductive age, although there are certain contraindications:

- Known or suspected pregnancy.
- Before evaluation of genital bleeding.
- Acute or chronic hepatocellular disease with abnormal liver function.
- Liver tumors.
- Cancer of the breast (past or present).
- Hypersensitivity to any component of the product.

Relative Contraindications

- Stroke, ischemic heart disease, known vascular disease.
    - Multiple cardiovascular disease risk factors: age, smoking, diabetes, and hypertension.
- Uncontrolled hypertension.
- Current thrombophlebitis or thromboembolic disorders.
- Migraine headaches with localizing signs.

Benefits of iMPA use (with appropriate follow-up) generally outweigh the risks in the following conditions:

- Valvular heart disease.
- Controlled hypertension.
- Diabetes with no vascular disease.
- Hyperlipidemia.
- History of deep vein thrombosis/pulmonary embolism.
- Major surgery with prolonged immobilization.
- Migraine headaches without focal neurological symptoms.
- Depression or history of postpartum depression.
- Gall bladder disease, past OC- or pregnancy-related cholestasis.
- Use with rifampicin and certain anticonvulsants.
- Use with antiretroviral therapy.
- Adolescents under the age of 18.

- Cervical dysplasia or cancer.
- Endometrial cancer.

DRUG INTERACTIONS

> *Aminoglutethimide (Cytadren®) administered at the same time as medroxy-progesterone may decrease the effectiveness of iMPA.*

Some drugs can induce liver enzymes that may increase the conversion of steroids to more polar, less biologically active metabolites. For this reason, barbiturates, sulfonamides, griseofulvin, phenylbutazone, phenytoin, carbamazepine, cyclophosphamide, and rifampin *(43)* may affect the contraceptive efficacy. This should be taken into consideration when these drugs are used, although there is less of a concern when DMPA is used compared with the effect in OC users.

GOOD CANDIDATES FOR LONG-ACTING PROGESTIN INJECTABLES

- Women with iron deficiency anemia from heavy menstrual bleeding.
- Women who need short-term contraception, such as those getting a rubella vaccination, awaiting tubal sterilization, using Acutane, or immediately following Essure procedure or male partner vasectomy.
- Older women who can not use estrogen-containing contraceptives and who do not have known vascular disease.
- Breastfeeding women after 6 weeks postpartum.
- Women who find daily, weekly, monthly, or "at the time of intercourse" options difficult to use.
- Obesity (>30 body mass index).
    - iMPA is generally safe and effective for obese women, although further weight gain is a concern; assurance that use of iMPA should be accompanied by restriction of caloric intake and regular exercise.
- Heavy cigarette smoking (>15 cigarettes/day), regardless of age.
- Women with sickle cell disease.
- Women with epilepsy.
- Women with endometriosis-related pain or dysmenorrhea.

COUNSELING AND PATIENT SELECTION

Good candidates are women that are willing to:

- Accept changes in menstrual bleeding and a 5- to 10-month delay in return of fertility.
- Get adequate calcium intake.
- Limit their calorie intake.
- Get regular exercise.

Evaluation of a potential iMPA user includes the following. Bold items are conditions under which iMPA may be a particularly good choice because it may have a beneficial effect.

- Current gynecological issues.
  - **Menstrual cycle irregularities or anemia.**
  - **Endometriosis or fibroids.**
  - **Dysmenorrhea.**
  - **Problems with past use of OCs.**
  - **Cyclic problems or premenstrual syndrome.**
  - **History of pelvic inflammatory disease.**
  - **History of ectopic pregnancy.**
  - Exposure to STI or HIV (condom protection indicated).
  - Androgen excess, acne, hirsutism, or polycystic ovarian syndrome.
  - Recurrent ovarian cysts.
  - Current and future childbearing plans.
- Demographics.
  - Age, marital status, occupation.
- Family history.
- Concurrent problems, illnesses.
  - Smoking.
  - Medications.
  - Allergies.
  - Surgeries.
  - Medical problems.
    - Thromboembolic disease.
    - Cardiovascular disease.
    - Hypertension.
    - Diabetes.
    - Liver disease.
    - Sickle cell disease.
    - **Epilepsy.**
- Physical examination.
  - Vital signs and weight.
  - Breast and pelvic examination, cervical cytology.
- Laboratory assays as indicated.
  - Pregnancy test.
  - Cervical tests for STIs for women not in mutually monogamous relationships.
  - Screening for anemia, insulin resistance, or abnormal lipids as indicated.

INSTRUCTIONS TO USE

Instructions and training for home injections is provided by some health care providers; up to 1 year of coverage may be provided.

- The initial injection should be given within the first 5 days of menses.
  - 150 mg DMPA is given intramuscularly into the hip or arm once every 3 months (13 weeks).
  - 104 mg Depo-subQ is given by subcutaneous injection into the anterior thigh or abdomen once every 3 months (12–14 weeks). Depo-subQ is not formulated for intramuscular injection.
- Users should understand that their normal menstrual bleeding pattern will be altered following injection; abnormal, frequent, or infrequent bleeding/spotting may occur immediately.
  - The longer injections are used, the higher the frequency of amenorrhea; at 1 year, about 50% of users have amenorrhea.
- Users schedule a return visit in 3 months for the next injection.
  - If a dose of medroxyprogesterone contraceptive is missed or delayed past the recommended 3 month interval, another form of birth control should be used to ensure contraceptive protection.
  - A pregnancy test may be indicated before the next injection if the return visit is prolonged.

Timing of Initiation: Starting or Switching to iMPA

- Adolescents: after 3 regular menstrual cycles.
  - Because of the potential impact on bone density, use in adolescents under age 18 recommended only if benefits outweigh risks and there is no other acceptable method available.
- Switching from OCs: injection no later than day 5 of pill-free interval.
- Switching from intrauterine device: initiate immediately on day of removal.
- Switching from implant: initiate immediately on day of removal.
- Postabortion (spontaneous or induced): initiate immediately (if not started within 5 days, follow instructions for new starter and use back-up method in meantime).
- Postpartum non-breastfeeding: initiate as early as 5 days but generally 3–4 weeks postpartum.
- Fully breastfeeding: initiate 6 weeks or longer.
- Perimenopausal: begin by day 5 of menses. May give symptom relief and decrease amount of overall bleeding.

Switching From iMPA to Another Method

- Switching from iMPA to another method: begin new method on the Sunday before or on any day up to the day that the next injection is due.

Warning Signals

Patients should be instructed to contact their physician/health care provider if they have any of the following:

- Unusually heavy, prolonged bleeding, lightheadedness, fainting.
- Severe depression.

- Abdominal pain: rule out pregnancy, ectopic pregnancy, infection, or blood clot.
- Allergic reaction (difficulty breathing, tightness of throat, hives, or swelling of the lip, tongue, or face).
- Marked redness, pus, bleeding, or prolonged pain at injection site.

General Warning Signals

Although these are not commonly associated with iMPA use, they are important warning signals that should be reported immediately to a health care provider.

- Repeated, severe, or increased frequency of headaches.
  - High blood pressure.
  - Blurred vision.
  - Numbness in arm or leg.
- Chest pain, difficulty breathing.
- Yellowing of skin or eyes, nausea, abdominal pain (liver disease).

COUNSELING TIPS

- No rubbing of the injection site after administration.
- The abnormal bleeding patterns are not harmful.
- If the pattern of bleeding is excessive or worrisome, the user should contact the health care provider.
  - Medications are available for bothersome, prolonged bleeding problems (short-term OC pills, progestins, estrogens).
- iMPA offers no protection from STIs, although a decrease in upper tract pelvic inflammatory disease is reported in studies.
- Minor side effects of breast tenderness, nausea, mild depression, or headaches may decrease after several cycles.
- When discontinuing iMPA, it may take several months for regular menstrual cycles to return.
- The longer iMPA is used, the more common amenorrhea is.
- Limiting caloric intake and increasing exercise is important, especially for users complaining of weight gain. With continued weight gain after attempts to limit calorie intact and increase exercise have failed, switching to another contraceptive method may be advised.
- Smoking, low calcium intake, and lack of weight-bearing exercises may exacerbate bone loss in iMPA users and should be avoided. Calcium supplementation is an excellent choice, especially for those with a low calcium intake.
- Women selecting iMPA should be well-informed about the drug and know other options for birth control. (DMPA has received criticism in the past and it is important to insure that no iMPA user has been "pressured.")

OPTIONS AVAILABLE

Depo-Provera is available in 1-mL injection vials containing 150 mg MPA as a sterile, white, injectable suspension. It should be stored at room temperature

(15–30°C). Just before injection, the vial should be vigorously shaken so that a uniform suspension is administered.

- The recommended dose for contraceptive protection is 150 mg DMPA every 3 months (13 weeks) administered by deep intramuscular injection into the buttocks or upper arm.
  - It is recommended that this injection be given during the first 5 days after the onset of a normal menstrual period (or before the fourth to sixth week postpartum in a non-breastfeeding patient).
  - To increase assurance that the patient is not pregnant at the time of administration, a negative pregnancy test may be advised.
- The recommended dose of DMPA for endometriosis is 50 mg weekly or 100 mg every 2 weeks intramuscularly for at least 6 months. The resumption of ovulatory cycles is often significantly delayed following this regimen.

Depo-subQ is available in prefilled syringes each containing 0.65 mL (104 mg) of MPA sterile aqueous suspension for subcutaneous injection.

- Depo-subQ is given every 3 months (4 times a year) for contraceptive protection.
  - Same dose is given for treatment of pain associated with endometriosis.

REFERENCES

1. Ortiz A, Hirol M, Stanczyk FZ, et al. (1977) Serum medroxyprogesterone acetate (MPA) concentrations and ovarian function following intramuscular injection of depo-MPA. J Clin Endocrinol Metab 44:32–38.
2. Mishell DR Jr, Kharma KM, Thorneycroft IH, et al. (1972) Estrogenic activity in women receiving an injectable progestogen for contraception. Am J Obstet Gynecol 113:372–376.
3. Mishell DR Jr. (1996) Pharmacokinetics of depot medroxyprogesterone acetate contraception. J Reprod Med 41:381–390.
4. Croxatto HG. (2002) Mechanisms that explain the contraceptive action of progestin implants for women. Contraception 65:21–27.
5. World Health Organization Expanded Programme of Research, Development and Research Training in Human Reproduction Task Force on Long-Acting-Systemic Agents for the Regulation of Fertility. (1983) Multinational comparative clinical evaluation of two long-acting injectable contraceptive steroids: Norethisterone enanthate and medroxyprogesterone acetate final report. Contraception 18:1.
6. Cullins VE. (1996) Noncontraceptive benefits and therapeutic uses of depot medroxyprogesterone acetate. J Reprod Med 41:428–433.
7. World Health Organization Collaborative Study of Neoplasia and Steroid Contraceptives. (1991) Depot medroxyprogestonre acetate and the risk of endometrial cancer. Int J Cancer 49:186–190.
8. Sullivan MG. (2005) New treatment approved for endometriosis. OB Gyn News May 1.
9. Mattson RH, Cramer JA, Caldwell BVD, et al. (1984) Treatment of seizures with medroxyprogesterone acetate. Preliminary report. Neurology 34:1255–1258.
10. Mattson RH, Rebar RN. (1993) Contraceptive methods for women with neurologic disorders. Am J Obstet Gynecol 168:2027–2032.
11. Schwallie PC, Assenzo JR. (1973) Contraceptive use-efficacy study utilizing medroxyprogesterone acetate administered as a intramuscular injection once every 90 days. Fertil Steril 24:331–339.

12. World Health Organization (WHO). (1990) Injectable contraceptives: their role in family planning. Monograph. Geneva, Switzerland: WHO.
13. Westhoff C. (1996) Depot medroxyprogesterone acetate contraception. Metabolic parameters and mood changes. J Reprod Med 41:401–406.
14. Moore LL, Valuck R, McDougall C, et al. (1995) A comparative study of one-year weight gain among users of medroxyprogesterone acetate, levonorgestrel implants, and oral contraceptives. Contraception 52:25–29.
15. Polaneczky M, Guarnaccia M, Alon J, Wiley J. (1996) Early experience with the contraceptive use of depo-medroxypgrogesterone acetate in an inner-city population. Fam Plan Perspect 28:174–178.
16. Mainwaring R, Hales HA, Stevenson K, et al. (1995) Metabolic parameter, bleeding, and weight changes in U.S. women using progestin only contraceptives. Contraception 51:149–153.
17. McCann MF, Potter LS. (1994) Progestin-only contraception: a comprehensive review. Contraception Suppl 50:S1–S195.
18. Speroff L, Darney PD. (2001) A Clinical Guide for Contraception, 3rd ed. Philadelphia: Lippincott Williams & Wilkins.
19. Two-Year Multinational Comparative Trial. (1983) Multinational comparative clinical evaluation of two long-acting injectable contraceptive steroids: Norethisterone enanthate and medroxyprogesterone acetate final report. Contraception 28:1–20.
20. Lieu DFM, Ng CSA, Yong YM, et al. (1985) Long-term effects of Depo-Provera on carbohydrate and lipid metabolism. Contraception 31:51.
21. Virutamasen P, Wongsrichanalai C, Tangkeo P, et al. (1986) Metabolic defects of depot medroxyprogesterone acetate in long-term users: A cross-sectional study. Int J Gynaecol Obstet 24:291.
22. Westhoff C. (2003) Depot-medroxyprogesterone acetate injection (Depo-Provera): a highly effective contraceptive option with proven long-term safety. Contraception 68:75–87.
23. Kaunitz AM. (2001) Injectable long-acting contraceptives. Clin Obstet Gynecol 44:73–91.
24. Berenson AB, Breitkopf CR, Grady JJ, Rickert VI, Thomas A. (2004) Effects of hormonal contraception on bone mineral density after 24 months of use. Obstet Gynecol 103:899–906.
25. Berenson AB, Radecki CM, Grady JJ, Rickert VI, Thomas A. (2001) A prospective, controlled study of the effects of hormonal contraception on bone mineral density. Obstet Gynecol 98:576–582.
26. Banks E, Berrington A, Casabonne D. (2001) Overview of the relationship between use of progestogen-only contraceptives and bone mineral density. Br J Obstet Gynecol 108:1214–1221.
27. Clark MK, Sowers MR, Nichols S, Levy B. (2004) Bone mineral density changes over two years in first-time users of depot medroxyprogesterone acetate. Fert Steril 82:1580–1586.
28. Petitti DB, Piaggio G, Mehta S, et al. (2000) Steroid hormone contraception and bone mineral density: A cross-sectional study in an international population. Obstet Gynecol 95:736–744.
29. Orr-Walker BJ, Evans MC, Ames RW, et al. (1998) The effect of past use of the injectable contraceptive depot medroxyprogesterone acetate on bone mineral density in normal postmenopausal women. Clin Endocrinol 49:615–618.
30. Scoles D. LaCroix AZ, Ichikawa LE, Barlow WE, Ott SM. (2005) Change in bone mineral density among adolescent women using and discontinuing depot medroxyprogesterone acetate contraception. Arch Pediatr Adolesc Med 159:139–144.
31. Cromer BA, Lazebnik R, Rome E, et al. (2005) Double-blinded randomized controlled trial of estrogen supplementation in adolescent girls who receive depot medroxyprogesterone acetate for contraception. Am J Obstet Gynecol 192:42–47.
32. Cundy T, Ames R, Horne A, et al. (2003) A randomized controlled trial of estrogen replacement therapy in long-term users of depot medroxyprogesterone acetate. J Clin Endocrinol Metab 88:78–81.

33. Kalkwarf HJ, Specker BL. (1995) Bone mineral loss during lactation and recovery after weaning. Obstet Gynecol 86:26–32.
34. Holmberg-Marttila D, Sievanen H, Laippala P, Tuimala R. (2000) Factors underlying changes in bone mineral during postpartum amenorrhea and lactation. Osteoporos Int 11:570–576.
35. Polatti F, Capuzzo E, Viazzo F, Colleoni R, Klersy C. (1999) Bone mineral changes during and after lactation. Obstet Gynecol 94:52–56.
36. Mainwaring R, Hales HA, Stevenson K, et al. (1995) Metabolic parameter, bleeding, and weight changes in U.S. women using progestin only contraceptives. Contraception 51:149–153.
37. Moore LL, Valuck R, McDougall C, et al. (1995) A comparative study of one-year weight gain among users of medroxyprogesterone acetate, levonorgestrel implants, and oral contraceptives. Contraception 52:215–219.
38. Schwallie PC, Assenzo JR. (1974) The effect of depo-progesterone acetate on pituitary and ovarian function, and the return of fertility following its discontinuation: a review. Contraception 10:181–202.
39. World Health Organization Collaborative Study of Neoplasia and Steroid Contraceptives. (1991) Breast cancer and depot medroxyprogesterone acetate: a multinational study. Lancet 338:833–838.
40. Paul C, Skegg DCG, Spears GFS. (1989) Depot medroxyprogestereone (Depo-Provera) and risk of breast cancer. Br Med J 299:759–762.
41. Skegg DC, Noonan EA, Paul C, et al. (1995) Depot medroxyprogesterone acetate and breast cancer: a pooled analysis of the World Health Organization and New Zealand studies. JAMA 273:799–804.
42. Mishell DR. (2004) Contraception. In: Strauss J, Barbieri R, eds. Yen and Jaffe's Reproductive Endocrinologies. Philadelphia: Elsevier Saunders.
43. Back DJ, Breckenridge AM, Crawford, FE, et al. (1980) The effects of rifampicin on the pharmacokinetics of ethinyl estradiol in women. Contraception 21:135.
44. Henzl M. (1993) Evolution of steroids and their contraceptive and therapeutic use. In: Shoupe DS, Haseltine FP, eds. Contraception. New York: Springer-Verlag, pp. 1–16.

8 Contraceptive Implants

Introducing Implanon®

Philip D. Darney, MD, MSc

Contents

INTRODUCTION

Subdermal contraceptive implants offer women long-acting, controlled release of progestins. Over the past 20 years, they have been approved in more than 60 countries and used by more than 11 million women worldwide. Their high efficacy along with ease of use make them a good contraceptive option for women who require progestin-only methods because they should not use estrogen, teens who find adherence to a contraceptive regime difficult, as well as healthy adult women who desire long-term protection *(1)*. Norplant®, no longer marketed in the United States, garnered 1 million American users but was difficult to insert and remove *(2,3)*. Now, a highly effective and long-lasting single-rod etonogestrel subdermal implant (Implanon®) will make implant contraception available again in the United States.

BENEFITS OF IMPLANTABLE CONTRACEPTIVES

Implants offer a variety of benefits to women. They provide long-term, effective pregnancy prevention without the need for any action of the user. Implant contraception is cost-effective compared with short-acting methods or an unplanned pregnancy. The sustained administration of a low dose of progestin and maintenance

From: *Current Clinical Practice: The Handbook of Contraception: A Guide for Practical Management*
Edited by: D. Shoupe and S. L. Kjos © Humana Press, Totowa, NJ

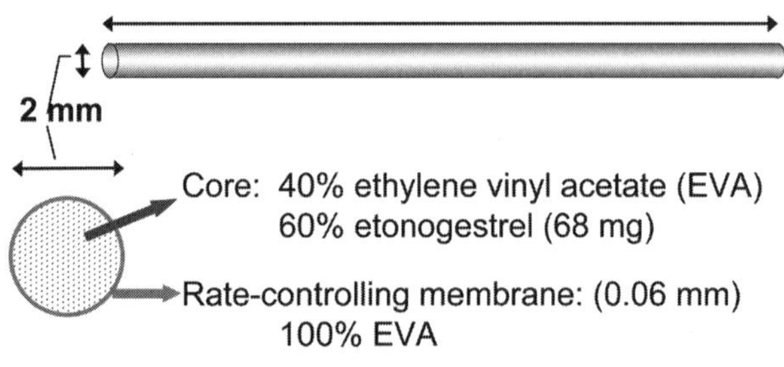

Fig. 1. Implanon. From Implanon package insert, Organon USA, Roseland, NJ, 2004.

of stable serum levels provide high efficacy, a long duration of action, a short fertility recovery time, and no cardiovascular effects.

Research and development of progestin-only subdermal implants began more than 35 years ago, but initial research with implants containing very low doses of progestins found that these implants were unsuccessful in preventing ectopic pregnancies. Development of Norplant, a six-capsule implantable system using the potent progestin levonorgestrel (LNG) followed. In 1991, it became the first US FDA-approved contraceptive implant. More than 1 million US women chose Norplant as their contraceptive. Norplant proved to be highly effective; over a 7-year duration of use, only about 1% of users became pregnant. Despite low rates of pregnancy and few serious side effects *(4–8)*, limited supplies of the silastic components and unwarranted negative media coverage led to Norplant's withdrawal from distribution in 2002, leaving no implant alternative for American women *(9)*.

The 15-year experience with Norplant instigated further development and improvements in implant design. A two-rod LNG system was approved in 1998, but never marketed in the United States. The US FDA is currently reviewing a contraceptive implant containing 68 mg of etonogestrel (ENG), the active metabolite of desogestrel, in a single rod made of ethylene vinyl acetate (EVA; Fig. 1). This one-implant contraceptive, called Implanon, is the most effective hormonal method of birth control ever developed and should soon become available in the United States. This implant is used by more than 2 million women in Europe and Asia. In Australia, one-fourth of all contracepting women are Implanon users.

ADVANTAGES OF PROGESTIN-ONLY CONTRACEPTION

Long-acting, progestin-only contraceptives, such as Implanon, Norplant, the Mirena® intrauterine contraceptive, and Depo-Provera, are highly effective and safer than oral contraceptive (OC) pills because they do not contain an estrogen

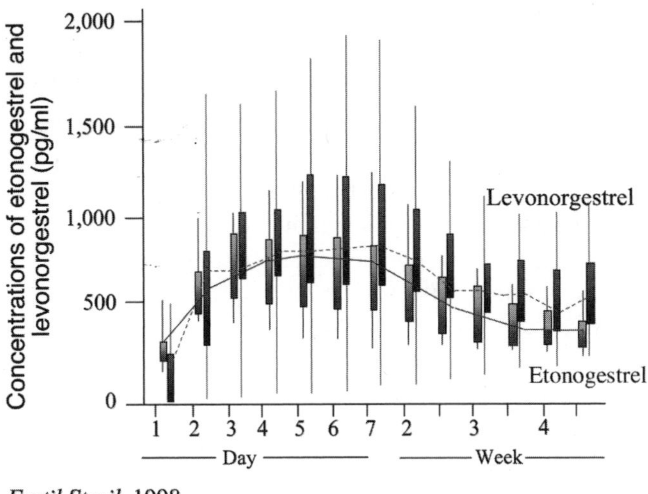

Fig. 2. Mean serum progestin concentrations in Norplant® and Implanon®.

that can provoke deep vein thrombosis. Progestin-only contraceptives offer women with contraindications to estrogen exposure and those who are breastfeeding an alternative to estrogen-containing methods, such as the combination OC pill, the contraceptive patch, and the vaginal ring.

LNG, the gonane progestin in Norplant, binds with high affinity to the progesterone, androgen, mineralocorticoid, and glucocorticoid receptors, but not to estrogen receptors. ENG (also known as 3-keto-desogestrel) has shown no estrogenic, anti-inflammatory, or mineralocorticoid activity, but has shown weak androgenic and anabolic activity, as well as strong antiestrogenic activity. Norplant, with six capsules, and the one-rod Implanon system result in nearly equivalent serum concentrations of LNG and ENG, respectively (Fig. 2). Unlike LNG, which is bound mainly to sex hormone-binding globulin, ENG is bound mainly to albumin, which is not affected by endogenous or exogenous estradiol concentrations. The overall safety of ENG has been demonstrated through studies of combined estrogen–progestin OCs and progestin-only OCs, both of which use desogestrel as a component.

MECHANISM OF ACTION

Progestin-containing implants have two primary mechanisms of action: inhibition of ovulation and restriction of sperm penetration through cervical mucus *(10)*. The LNG implants disrupt follicular growth and inhibit the ovulatory process through exerting negative feedback on the hypothalamic–pituitary axis, causing a variety of changes that range from anovulation to insufficient luteal function. A small number of women using LNG implants will have quiescent ovaries, but most will begin to ovulate as blood concentrations of LNG gradually fall after 2–3 years of implant use. The ENG implant suppresses ovulation by altering the hypothalamic–pituitary–ovarian axis and downregulating the luteinizing hormone surge, which is required to support the growth and maturation of ovarian follicles.

Even if follicles grow during use of progestin implants, oocytes are not fertilized. If the follicle ruptures, the abnormalities of the ovulatory process prevent release of a viable egg. Anti-estrogenic actions of the progestins affect the cervical mucus, making it viscous, scanty, and impenetrable by sperm. These ovarian and cervical mechanisms of action provide high contraceptive efficacy and occur before fertilization. No signs of embryonic development have been found among implant users, indicating that progestin implants have no abortifacient properties.

IMPLANON: THE SINGLE-ROD ENG IMPLANT

The high efficacy of Implanon, developed, manufactured, and marketed by Organon, results from the ability of a low dose of ENG to suppress ovulation, as well as the long duration of action of the implant. After subdermal insertion, users need do nothing more to have nearly complete protection from pregnancy for up to 3 years *(11)*. Implanon's one rod provides great improvements over the previously available six-capsule Norplant system in time and ease of insertion. In the US and European trials, which began 10 years ago, average insertion time of Implanon was 1 minute and removal time was 3 minutes—much faster than Norplant *(2,12)*.

Implanon's convenience is enhanced by other design features as well. The inserter is preloaded and disposable (*see* Fig. 3). Because only one rod is implanted, there is no chance of moving previously placed rods out of position during the insertion of subsequent ones. It is not necessary, as it was with Norplant, to create channels under the skin with local anesthetic, which made implants difficult to palpate after insertion. In addition, EVA, the plastic from which Implanon is made, is less likely then Norplant's Silastic to form a fibrous sheath that can prolong removals. These differences simplify the insertion and removal technique for Implanon. For patients, this simplicity means little discomfort at insertion or removal, an unobtrusive implant, and almost no scarring. For clinicians, it means simpler insertion and removal procedures of predictably short duration.

Implanon: Pharmacology

Implanon consists of one non-biodegradable rod of 40% EVA and 60% etonogestrel (40 × 2.0 mm) covered with a rate-controlling EVA membrane 0.06 mm thick. The rod contains 68 mg ENG, initially absorbed by the body at a rate of 60 μg per day and slowly declining to 30 μg per day after 2 years of use. The

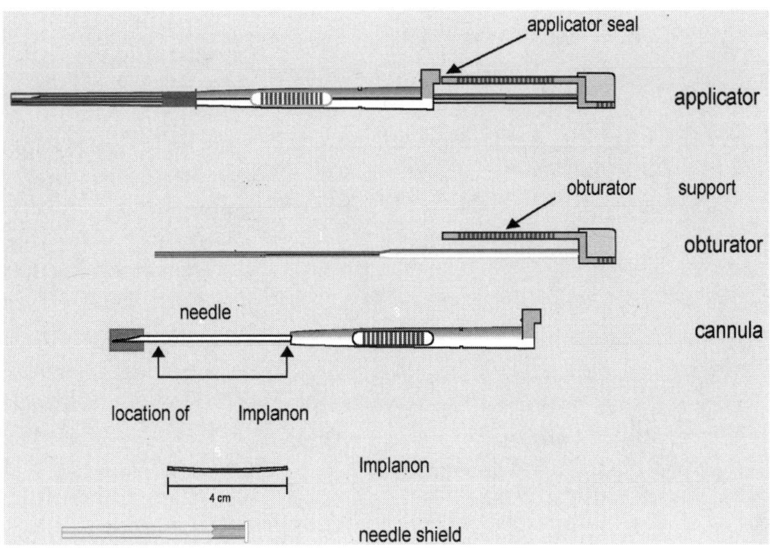

Fig. 3. Implanon insertion device.

high initial rate of absorption is probably because of a significant amount of ENG released from the uncovered ends of the implant. Peak serum concentrations (266 pg/mL) of ENG are achieved within 1 day after insertion, suppressing ovulation, which requires only 90 pg/mL or more *(10,11,13)*. Like other contraceptive steroids, serum levels of ENG are reduced in women taking liver enzyme-inducing drugs such as rifampicin, griseofulvin, phenytoin, and carbamazepine, but are not affected by antibiotics. Steady release of ENG into the circulation avoids first-pass effects on the liver. Bioavailability of ENG remains nearly 100% throughout 2 years of use. The elimination half-life of ENG is 25 hours compared with 42 hours for Norplant's LNG. After implant removal, serum ENG concentrations become undetectable within 1 week (*see* Fig. 4). Return of ovulation occurs in 94% of women within 3–6 weeks after method discontinuation *(8,11,13)*.

Implanon: Effectiveness

In clinical trials, the ENG implant demonstrated 100% contraceptive effectiveness with a Pearl Index of 0 per 100 woman-years (confidence interval: 0.00–0.08). The efficacy of the single-rod ENG implant was studied in clinical trials of 2043 women for a total of 74,000 months of use: 835 women completed 2–3 years and an additional 526 used the ENG implant for 3 years or longer. Neither intrauterine nor ectopic pregnancies were observed during these trials. Among the subjects were 365 women whose body weight was 154 lb (70 kg) or more, none of whom became pregnant, although serum concentrations were lower in heavier users (*see* Fig. 5) *(11)*.

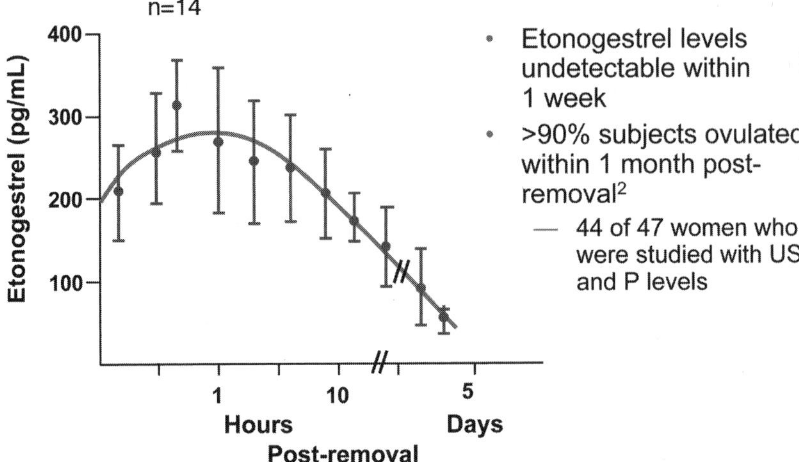

Fig. 4. Etonogestrel decline after Implanon® removal.

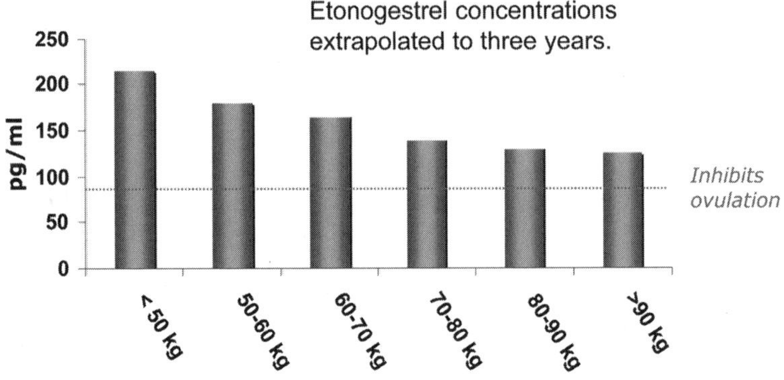

Fig. 5. Effect of weight on serum etonogestrel levels.

Implanon: Metabolic Effects

Published studies regarding the ENG implant indicate that metabolic effects are minimal and unlikely to be clinically significant. The ENG implant does not appear to have any clinically meaningful effect on lipid metabolism, carbohydrate metabolism, liver function, hemostatic factors, blood pressure, thyroid function, or adrenal function *(14–17)*.

Implanon: Safety

Overall, implants, including the ENG implant, are regarded as safe, with adverse event rates (including death, neoplastic disease, cardiovascular events, anemia, hypertension, bone density changes, diabetes, gall bladder disease, thrombocytopenia, and pelvic inflammatory disease) comparable with women not using implants *(18,19)*. The ENG implant reduced or eliminated menstrual pain in 88% of women previously experiencing dysmenorrhea; pain increased in only 2% of the ENG implant users *(20)*. In a study comparing 42 lactating mother–infant pairs using the ENG implant compared with 38 pairs using intrauterine devices, there were no significant differences between groups in milk volume, milk constituents, timing and amount of supplementary food, or infant growth rates *(21)*.

Low-dose progestin contraceptives have few contraindications. They may be less effective in obese women and in those using drugs that stimulate the liver's cytochrone metabolism of steroids (such as rifampin and phenytoin).

Implanon: Insertion and Removal

Although Implanon is designed to facilitate rapid and simple insertion and removal, clinicians should first be trained in the specific technique for Implanon *(22)*. Insertion of the ENG implant is less complex than insertion of the six-capsule LNG implant, with the average insertion time for the ENG implant ranging between 1 and 2 minutes. The disposable trocar comes preloaded. The tip of the needle has two cutting edges, with different slopes. The extreme tip has a greater angle and is sharp to allow penetration through the skin (*see* Fig. 6). The second, upper angle is smaller and unsharpened to reduce the risk of incorrectly placing the implant in the muscle. It is imperative that the implant be placed subdermally for efficacy and easy removal. Under aseptic conditions and with or without local anesthesia, the implant is inserted subdermally on the inner aspect of the nondominant arm, 6–8 cm above the elbow. After insertion, the implant may not be visible but must remain palpable.

Removal requires making a 2-mm incision at the distal tip of the implant and pushing the other end of the rod until it pops out *(23)* (*see* Fig. 7). Mean removal time is about 3 minutes (confidence interval: 2.6–5.4 minutes) *(24)*. Pain, swelling, redness, and hematoma have been reported following insertion and removal. Because return to ovulation is rapid following removal, women still desiring contraception should begin another method immediately or have a new rod inserted through the removal incision.

Implanon: Timing of Insertion and Removal

For women who either have not been using a contraceptive method or have been using a nonhormonal method, insertion should occur between days 1 and 5 of menses. For women presently using a combination OC, a progestin-only OC, or an intrauterine contraceptive device, the ENG implant can be inserted anytime, and the OCs continued until the pack is completed. For women changing from injectable contraception, insertion should occur on the day on which the next injection is scheduled. All women should be advised to use an additional barrier method of contraception for 7 days following insertion. If the ENG implant

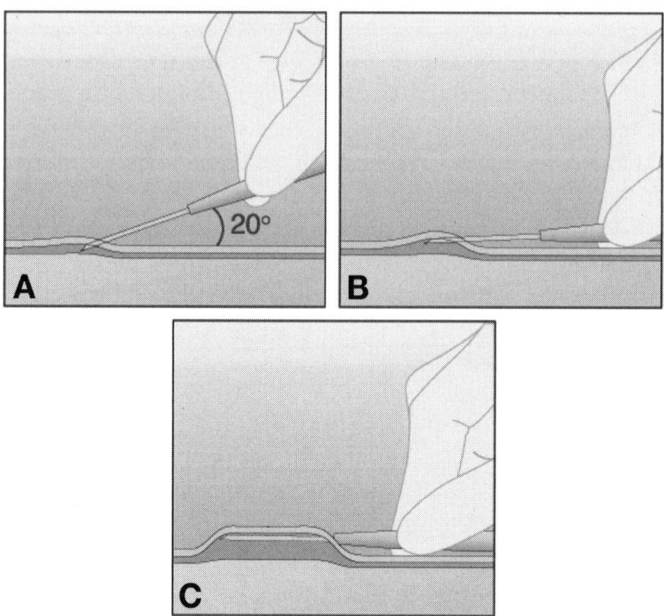

Fig. 6. Implanon insertion.

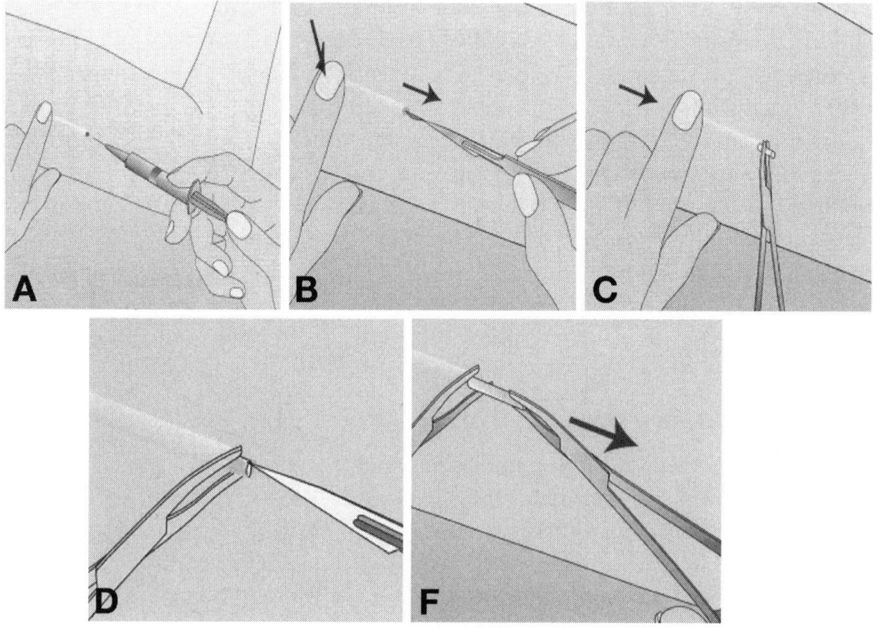

Fig. 7. Implanon removal.

is the contraceptive method selected following an abortion or delivery, it can be inserted immediately *(25)*; no additional contraceptive method is required. In all cases, pregnancy should be excluded before insertion, although there is no evidence that hormonal contraceptives cause birth defects.

The ENG implant can be removed at any time at the woman's discretion, but if left in place, remains effective for 3 years.

Implanon: Disadvantages

Although progestin-only contraceptives, such as Implanon, offer users a safe and effective method of preventing pregnancy, they have some drawbacks. Implants require a minor surgical procedure by trained clinicians for insertion and removal. Cost-effectiveness of the method depends on long-term use; early discontinuation negates this benefit *(26)*. Lack of protection against sexually transmitted infections (STIs) is a disadvantage of the ENG implants, as well as all nonbarrier contraceptive methods.

Side effects associated with the ENG Implanon implant include menstrual irregularities (infrequent bleeding [26.9%], amenorrhea [18.6%], prolonged bleeding [15.1%], frequent bleeding [7.4%]), weight gain [20.7%], acne [15.3%], breast pain [9.1%], and headache [8.5%]), but these symptoms rarely provoked discontinuation *(12,20,27)*. Women using any of the progestin-only methods will notice changes in bleeding patterns. A comparative study of bleeding patterns in single capsule ENG implant users and six-capsule LNG implant users found a statistically significant decrease in mean number of bleeding/spotting days for Implanon compared with Norplant (15.9–19.3 versus 19.4–21.6; $p = 0.0169$) *(28)*.

Because total uterine blood loss is reduced, users of progestin-only contraceptives (as well as OCs) are less likely to be anemic. However, the study also found that users of ENG implants had more variable bleeding patterns than users of the LNG implants *(28)*. Figure 8 shows the differences in bleeding between Norplant and Implanon, but it is impossible to predict which of these patterns a woman is likely to experience *(29)*. Despite side effects and dependence on clinicians to insert implants, most women using implantable contraception are satisfied with the method, citing its long duration of use, convenience, and high efficacy.

Implanon: Discontinuation Rates

Discontinuation rates for the ENG implant have varied by area of use, ranging from 30.2% in Europe and Canada to 0.9% in Southeast Asia *(20,24)*. Bleeding irregularities are cited as the most common reason for discontinuation of the ENG implant. A meta-analysis of 13 studies published between 1989 and 1992, found that among 1716 women using the ENG implant, 5.3% discontinued in months 1–6, 6.4% discontinued in months 7–12, 4.1% discontinued in months 13–18, and 2.8% discontinued in months 19–24. Overall, 82% of women continued to use the ENG implant for up to 24 months *(12)*.

Bleeding Pattern	Implanon	Norplant	Statistically Significant
Amenorrhea	+	–	Yes
Infrequent bleeding	+	–	Yes
Frequent bleeding	–	+	Yes
Prolonged bleeding	±	±	No

Fig. 8. Vaginal bleeding pattern: Implanon® versus Norplant® randomized, controlled trial.

Implanon: Counseling

Counseling women to expect bleeding irregularities reduces discontinuation owing to this problem. Prospective users should be provided with complete information about bleeding irregularities so they can make informed decisions regarding the side effects they are willing to accept to benefit from high contraceptive efficacy. Pre-insertion counseling and post-insertion follow-up are essential for continued use of implants. Satisfaction with the method increases with proper counseling and minimizes costly removals. Implant counseling should address the following *(30)*:

- Advantages and disadvantages of implants compared with other methods.
- Possible side effects, particularly altered bleeding patterns.
- Absence of inherent protection against STIs and measures to overcome this lack of protection.
- User-specific lifestyle and health issues.

Sexually active women are exposed to the risk of pregnancy as well as to the risk of STIs, such as HIV, hepatitis B, human papillomavirus, *Chlamydia trachomatis*, syphilis, and gonorrhea, whose sequelae may be life threatening. Implantable contraceptives neither increase the risk of nor offer protection against STIs *(31)*. Women counseled about contraception should also be informed about the risks of STIs. They should be advised that use of condoms concomitantly with an effective method of pregnancy prevention is the best means of protection against unintended pregnancy and STIs. It seems likely that Implanon, like OC pills and DMPA, reduces the risk of pelvic inflammatory disease (PID).

Clinical experience with the ENG implant has reinforced that method effectiveness and satisfaction are closely associated with patient education and provider training. The ENG implant was introduced to Australia in May 2001. During the first 18 months of use, an unexpectedly high number of adverse incidents were reported and 100 unintended pregnancies occurred *(32)*. Almost universally, these events were traced to improper insertion by untrained clinicians, and poor patient selection, timing, and counseling. Policies that adequately document the process, procedure, and patient consent were initiated by the Royal Australian College of General Practitioners and have corrected the problems.

SUMMARY

Progestin-only contraceptive implants provide safe, convenient, and highly effective long-term contraception with high continuation rates. The six-capsule LNG implant and the single-rod ENG implant have been used successfully by millions of women worldwide. The introduction of Implanon to US women and their clinicians will provide an additional contraceptive that offers effectiveness independent of user adherence to a routine action, long duration of effectiveness, absence of estrogen, ease of use, reversibility, and overall safety. Implanon will contribute to clinicians' ability to offer a wider choice of contraceptive options, so that each woman can select a method that best fits her circumstances, preferences, and lifestyle.

REFERENCES

1. Darney PD, Atkinson E, Tanner S, MacPherson S, Hellerstein S, Alvarado A. (1990) Acceptance and perceptions of Norplant among users in San Francisco, USA. Stud Fam Plann 21:152–160.
2. Bromham DR, Davey A, Gaffikin L, Ajello CA. (1995) Materials, methods and results of the Norplant training program. Adv Contracept 11:255–262.
3. Dunson TR, Amatya RN, Krueger SL. (1995) Complications and risk factors associated with the removal of Norplant implants. Obstet Gynecol 85:543–548.
4. Fu H, Darroch JE, Haas T, Ranjit N. (1999) Contraceptive failure rates: new estimates from the 1995 National Survey of Family Growth. Fam Plann Perspect 31:56–63.
5. Meirik O, Farley TM, Sivin I, for the International Collaborative Post-Marketing Surveillance of Norplant. (2001) Safety and efficacy of levonorgestrel implant, intrauterine device, and sterilization. Obstet Gynecol 97:539–547.
6. Diaz S, Herreros C, Juez G, et al. (1985) Fertility regulation in nursing women: influence of Norplant levonorgestrel implants upon lactation and infant growth. Contraception 32:53–74.
7. Sivin I, Mishell DR Jr, Diaz S, et al. (2000) Prolonged effectiveness of Norplant® capsule implants: a 7-year study. Contraception 61:187–194.
8. Diaz S, Pavez M, Cardenas H, Croxatto HB. (1987) Recovery of fertility and outcome of planned pregnancies after the removal of Norplant subdermal implants or copper-T IUDs. Contraception 35:569–579.
9. Kuiper H, Miller S, Martinez E, Loeb L, Darney PD. (1997) The double paradox: urban adolescent females and the decline of contraceptive implants. Fam Plann Perspect 29:167–172.
10. Brache V, Faundes A, Johansson E, Alvarez F. (1985) Anovulation, inadequate luteal phase, and poor sperm penetration in cervical mucus during prolonged use of Norplant implants. Contraception 31:261–273.
11. Croxatto HB, Mäkäräinen L. (1998) The pharmacodynamics and efficacy of Implanon. Contraception 58:91S–97S.
12. Croxatto HB, Urbancsek J, Massai R, Coelingh Bennink H, van Beek A. (1999) A multicentre efficacy and safety study of the single contraceptive implant Implanon. Implanon Study Group. Hum Reprod 14:976–981.
13. Makarainen L, van Beek A, Tuomiyaara L, Asplund B, Bennink HC. (1998) Ovarian function during the use of a single contraceptive implant (Implanon) compared with Norplant. Fertil Steril 69:714–721.

14. Mascarenhas L, van Beek A, Bennink H, Newton J. (1998) Twenty-four month comparison of apolipoproteins A-1, A-II and B in contraceptive implant users (Norplant and Implanon) in Birmingham, United Kingdom. Contraception 58:215–219.
15. Biswas A, Viegas OA, Bennink HJ, Korver T, Ratnam SS. (2000) Effect of Implanon use on selected parameters of thyroid and adrenal function. Contraception 62:247–251.
16. Biswas A, Viegas OA, Coeling Bennink JH, Korver T, Ratnam SS. (2001) Implanon contraceptive implants: effects on carbohydrate metabolism. Contraception 63:137–141.
17. Biswas A, Viegas OA, Roy AC. (2003) Effect of Implanon and Norplant subdermal contraceptive implants on serum lipids—a randomized comparative study. Contraception 68:189–193.
18. Meckstroth K, Darney PD. (2000) Implantable contraception. Obstet Gynecol Clin North Am 27:781–815.
19. Meirik O, d'Arcangues C, for the WHO Consultation on Implantable Contraceptives for Women. (2003) Implantable contraceptives for women. Hum Reprod Update 9:49–59.
20. Affandi B, Korver T, Geurts TB, Coelingh Bennink JH. (1999) A pilot efficacy study with a single-rod contraceptive implant (Implanon) in 200 Indonesian women treated for< or = 4 years. Contraception 59:167–174.
21. Reinprayoon D, Taneepanichskul S, Bunyavejchevin S, et al. (2000) Effects of the etonogestrel-releasing contraceptive implant (Implanon) on parameters of breastfeeding compared to those of an intrauterine device. Contraception 62:239–246.
22. Mascarenhas L. (2000) Insertion and removal of Implanon: practical considerations. Eur J Contracept Reprod Health Care 5:29–34.
23. Zieman M, Klaisle C, Walker D, Bahisteri E, Darney P. (1997) Fingers versus instruments for removing levonorgestrel contraceptive implants (Norplant). J Gynecol Tech 3:213–217.
24. Smith A, Reuter S. (2002) An assessment of the use of Implanon in three community services. J Fam Plann Reprod Health Care 28:193–196.
25. Shaaban MM, Salem HT, Abdullah KA. (1985) Influence of levonorgestrel contraceptive implants, Norplant, initiated early postpartum, upon lactation and infant growth. Contraception 32:623–635.
26. Trussell J, Leveque JA, Koenig JD, et al. (1995) The economic value of contraception: a comparison of 15 methods. Am J Public Health 85:494–503.
27. Alvarez-Sanchez F, Brache V, Thevenin F, Cochon L, Faundes A. (1996) Hormonal treatment for bleeding irregularities in Norplant implant users. Am J Obstet Gynecol 174:919–922.
28. Zheng SR, Zheng HM, Qian SZ, Sang GW, Kaper RF. (1999) A randomized multicenter study comparing the efficacy and bleeding pattern of a single-rod (Implanon®) and a six-capsule (Norplant®) hormonal contraceptive implant. Contraception 60:1–8.
29. Darney PD, Taylor RN, Klaisle C, Bottles K, Zaloudek C. (1996) Serum concentrations of estradiol, progesterone, and levonorgestrel are not determinants of endometrial histology or abnormal bleeding in long-term Norplant implant users. Contraception 53:97–100.
30. Sivin I, Mishell Jr DR, Darney P, Wan L, Christ M. (1998) Levonorgestrel capsule implants in the United States: a 5-year study. Obstet Gynecol 92:337–344.
31. Darney PD, Callegari LS, Swift A, Atkinson ES, Robert AM. (1999) Condom practices of urban teens using Norplant contraceptive implants, oral contraceptives, and condoms for contraception. Am J Obstet Gynecol 180:929–937.
32. Harrison-Woolrych M, Hill R. (2005) Unintended pregnancies with the etonogestrel implant (Implanon): a case series from postmarketing experience in Australia. Contraception 71:306–308.

9

Intrauterine Devices

Comparison of the Copper T Intrauterine Device With the Levonorgestrel Intrauterine System

Angela Y. Chen, MD, MPH
and Susie Baldwin, MD, MPH

Contents

INTRODUCTION

Intrauterine devices offer safe, effective, long-term contraception and should be considered for all women who seek a reliable, reversible contraception that is effective before coitus (1).

From: *Current Clinical Practice: The Handbook of Contraception: A Guide for Practical Management*
Edited by: D. Shoupe and S. L. Kjos © Humana Press, Totowa, NJ

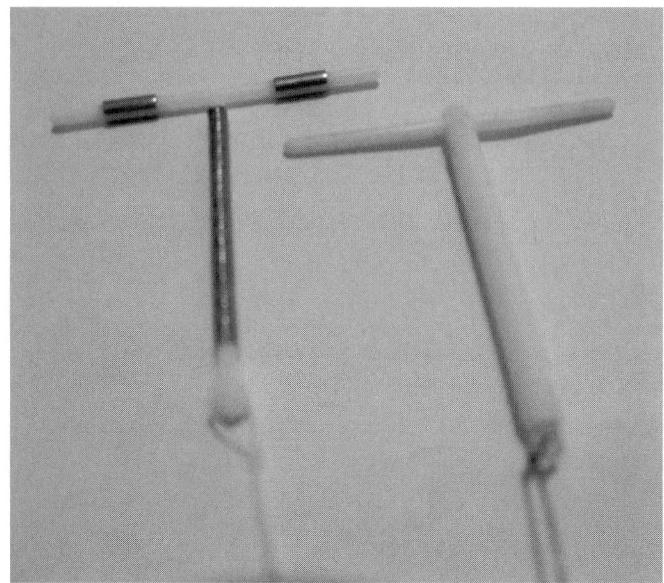

Fig. 1. A side-to-side comparison of the TCu380A IUD with the LNG-IUD.

Women in the United States currently may choose between two forms of intrauterine contraception (IUC): the 380 mm^2 copper T intrauterine device (IUD) (TCu380A, marketed as ParaGard®) and the levonorgestrel intrauterine system (LNG-IUS, sold as Mirena®) (Fig. 1). Both devices offer excellent, reversible, long-term contraception, but each manifests a unique profile of benefits and side effects. Generally speaking, women using the copper IUD maintain their menstrual cycles, but are more likely to experience menorrhagia. With the LNG-IUS, endometrial suppression results in an alteration of bleeding patterns and 20% of users become amenorrheic within 1 year of use and the majority of users become amenorrheic by 5 years *(2,3)*.

The LNG-IUS releases 20 μg LNG every 24 hours during 5 years of use. After 5 years, the device releases 14 μg LNG per day *(4)*, which is sufficient for it to remain efficacious for 2 additional years *(5)*. The TCu380A is approved for 10 years of use, but provides effective contraception for as long as 12 years *(6)*.

HISTORICAL PERSPECTIVE

At the peak of IUD popularity in the 1960s and 1970s, approximately 11% of women using a contraceptive method were using one of the many available IUDs *(7)*. But after the Dalkon shield was linked to septic abortion and serious pelvic infections, many US manufacturers withdrew their product from the market, and by 1988, only one IUD remained available. Despite continued studies demonstrating the safety and effectiveness of current IUDs, many US providers and potential users remain concerned about the risk of infection. In the world today, IUDs continue to be the most popular reversible method of contraception and currently the choice of more than 90 million women *(1)*.

MECHANISM OF ACTION

Experimental evidence suggests that IUC affects events before fertilization *(2)* and implantation *(8)*. The primary mechanism of action for the copper TCu380A and the LNG-IUS is preventing sperm from fertilizing ova *(9)*. While using a copper IUD, the copper ions reduce sperm motility and viability, so sperm rarely reach the fallopian tubes *(10)*. The TCu380A also causes increases in white blood cells, enzymes, and prostaglandsin in the uterine fluids that also impairs sperm function as well as implantation. Inhibition of implantation is a secondary mechanism of action for the copper T. Additionally, the copper IUD inhibits development of ova *(10)*. The LNG-IUS inhibits fertilization by thickening cervical mucus and causing changes in uterotubal fluid that impair sperm migration *(2)*. Inhibition of implantation by alteration of the endometrium is the secondary mechanism of action for the LNG-IUS. All of the antifertility actions of IUDs occur before implantation.

EFFICACY OF IUC

IUC has an extremely high efficacy rate compared with other methods of contraception. IUC should be thought of as reversible sterilization because the methods are as effective as, or more effective than, female sterilization. In the first year of use, the copper IUD has failure rate of 0.6% in perfect use and 0.8% in typical use. The cumulative failure rate over the 10-year use of the IUD is 2.1–2.8%. The failure rate for the LNG-IUS in the first year of use is 0.1% for perfect and typical use. The cumulative failure rate over 5 years of use is 0.7%, and 1.1% over 7 years of use. Unlike most of the other forms of reversible contraception, IUC does not rely on patient participation for correct usage, thus the failure rates of typical and perfect use are similar.

During the last 20–30 years, a number of researchers have conducted head-to-head trials of copper versus LNG intrauterine contraceptives. In the 1980s, the Population Council conducted a 7-year, randomized trial comparing the TCu380A with the LNG-IUS, and found that the devices had similar rates of failure (1–1.4 pregnancies per 100 woman-years). Expulsion of the contraceptive occurred less frequently with the copper IUD than with the LNG-IUS (8.4 versus 11.7 per 100 users), while rates of pelvic inflammatory disease (PID) among users were similar (3.6/100 women). More users of the LNG-IUS terminated use because of amenorrhea, but TCu380A users were more likely to terminate the method because of pain and "other menstrual events" *(4)*.

A 5-year, Swedish trial of 2758 women compared a 200 mm^2 copper IUD with the LNG-IUS, and found a significantly higher failure rate among the copper IUD users (5.9 versus 0.5 per 100 women).* Expulsion occurred with equal frequency between the two groups, as did reports of pain. Significantly more women with the copper IUD had the device removed because of heavy and prolonged menstrual flow, whereas significantly more women with the LNG-IUS terminated the method because of amenorrhea. Discontinuation because of hormonal side effects was also more common among LNG-IUS users *(11)*.

Another randomized comparative trial conducted in several European countries inserted intrauterine contraceptives in women immediately after surgical abortion procedures and followed them for 5 years. The pregnancy rate was significantly higher among users of the 200 mm^2 copper IUD than among users of the LNG-IUS (9.5 versus 0.8 per 100 women). In both of the pregnancies that occurred in LNG-IUS users, the contraceptive had been unknowingly expelled. Expulsion rates did not significantly vary between the two methods, but the overall rate of expulsion was significantly higher than expected. There were no significant differences in method termination rates because of bleeding problems, pain, or amenorrhea, but significantly more users of the LNG-IUS discontinued use of the method because of hormonal complaints *(12)*.

BARRIERS TO IUC

Unlike the rest of the world, IUC, IUD, or intrauterine contraceptive device (IUCD) is underused in the United States. IUC is so effective that it can be considered reversible sterilization. Although changing with the growth of evidence-based practice, there are still persistent misconceptions that unduly restrict greater use of this very effective contraceptive.

A 2002 survey of members of the American College of Obstetricians and Gynecologists showed positive regard for IUC. Ninety-five percent agreed that the method is safe and 98% agreed that it is effective *(13)*. A lower rate of IUC insertion was correlated with the degree to which the respondent believed that IUC caused PID *(13)*. There was a statistically significant correlation between fear of litigation and lower number of IUC insertions *(13)*. This study suggests that belief that IUC causes PID is a contributor to the underuse of IUC in the United States *(13)*. Although American practitioners are unlikely to promote use of the IUC to their patients, statistics show that a greater proportion of female Obstetrician (Ob)/Gynecologist (Gyn) physicians use IUC as compared with the general population *(14,15)*.

---

*Importantly, IUDs now available in the United States have significantly more copper than the older models, and a dose–response relationship exists between the amount of copper and contraceptive activity.

The persistence of misperceptions continues in both professional and lay press. According to a review of obstetrics and gynecology textbooks in the United States and United Kingdom, IUD disadvantages are often inflated and the advantages minimized *(16)*. Both provider- and consumer-oriented websites inaccurately reported that the risk of ectopic pregnancy and PID increase with IUD use *(17)*.

SIDE EFFECTS AND CONCERNS

PID, Infertility, and IUC

One comparative study examined the presence of *Actinomyces*-like organisms in the pap smears of IUC users, and found significantly higher rates in the women with a copper IUD compared with those with the LNG-IUS *(18)*. This result was concerning, because many physicians regarded the presence of *Actinomyces*-like organisms as a harbinger of severe pelvic infection in users of IUC. However, current evidence does not support this notion. In the absence of clinical signs of pelvic infection, *Actinomyces* are regarded as normal inhabitants of the female genital tract and are their presence on a pap smear does is not a harbinger of pelvic infection *(5)*.

In fact, when bias is controlled and confounders removed, current studies indicate that the IUC is not correlated with PID *(19)*. Earlier studies selected inappropriate control groups for comparison with the IUD user leading to incorrect conclusions. PID incidence in IUC users is not different from non-IUC users. There is a small risk of infection within the first 20 days of insertion, suggesting that pre-existing infection or contaminations is responsible for infection, not the IUC *(20)*. In a well-done case–control study of nulliparous IUC users, tubal infertility was positively correlated with the presence of *Chlamydia* antibodies, not the IUC *(21)*.

If the diagnosis of genital tract infection is suspected, antibiotics should be promptly administered per Center for Disease Control and Prevention guidelines to the woman and her partner. The woman may retain her IUC if she desires. A randomized control trial showed no added benefit to IUD removal during treatment for acute salpingitis *(22)*. Multiple trials have demonstrated that prophylactic antibiotics have little to no benefit at the time of insertion *(23)*.

Return to Fertility and IUC

Previous studies impugned IUC with falsely elevated rates of PID and hence the fear of infertility was raised. Following removal of the copper IUD and the LNG-IUS, fertility returns at comparable rates. Among 110 women who discontinued use of these methods to become pregnant, more than 90% in both groups conceived within 1 year *(24)*.

Ectopic Pregnancy and IUC

The IUC is so effective at preventing pregnancy that the incidence of both intrauterine and ectopic pregnancies are reduced *(25,26)*. But should pregnancy be suspected, attention should be made to investigate for ectopic as well as intrauterine pregnancy. The rate of ectopic pregnancy with a copper-bearing IUD is 0.09 per 100 women at 1 year and 0.89 per 100 women cumulatively over 10 years *(27)*. Ectopic pregnancy rate among LNG-IUS users is 0.045 per 100 women at 1 year and 0.22 per 100 women at 5 years *(28)*. The rate of ectopic pregnancy with IUC is still lower than the rate in women not using any contraceptive method (0.325–0.525 per 100 woman-years) *(29,30)*.

Nulliparity and IUC

Although insertion may be more difficult, nulliparity does not preclude from usage of a highly effective contraceptive. A World Health Organization medical criteria guideline states that the benefits still generally outweigh the risk for the nullipara who wishes to have IUC *(31)*. Current product labeling for IUC in the United States recommend use for women who are parous *(32,33)*. However, studies showed no increase in risk and actually showed a decrease in the expulsion rate among nulliparas *(34)*. In properly selected nulliparous women, an IUC may be a better option than other lesser effective forms of contraception.

HIV and IUC

The World Health Organization has classified the use of either a TCu380A or LNG-IUS for HIV-positive women or those with AIDS as a category 3; that is, that the risks generally outweigh the benefits *(35)*. Several studies have looked at viral shedding in HIV-positive users of IUC and have found no increased risk *(36,37)*. This would suggest that IUC use is safe for the patient as well as her partner. As with any patient with sexually transmittable illness, regardless of contraceptive method chosen, a barrier method, such as condom, should be promoted in conjunction to reduce transmission.

IUD AS EMERGENCY CONTRACEPTION

Emergency insertion of the copper IUD within 7 days of unprotected sex has been demonstrated to be safe and effective as postcoital contraception (*see* Chapter 12). The purported mechanism of action is most likely interference with implantation. One study documented the failure rate to be less than 0.1% *(38)*. A recent study of more than 1000 women, including 170 nulliparous women, reported a 0.2% pregnancy rate and an 86% continutation rate in parous women and an 80% rate in nulliparous women *(39)*. The LNG-IUS has not been studied for use as an emergency contraceptive and it is not recommended.

THERAPEUTIC USES OF THE LNG-IUS

Menorrhagia and Bleeding Disorders

Although there is strong evidence that supports use of the LNG-IUS for indications other than contraception, such use of the LNG-IUS is considered "off-label" because the device is approved in the United States only for contraception. Off-label prescribing is legal and ethical when these alternate indications for drugs or devices are grounded in scientific evidence. In Europe, the LNG-IUS is explicitly approved for the treatment of menorrhagia.

Numerous studies of the LNG-IUS have documented an increase in blood hemoglobin and serum ferritin levels among users, resulting from the inhibitory effects of the LNG-IUS on the endometrium and the resulting decrease in menstrual blood loss *(3,11,40–43)*. This characteristic of the LNG-IUS confers its therapeutic properties, applicable to the treatment of many common gynecological disorders including menorraghia *(44–46)*.

Menorrhagia, defined as menstruation of excessive flow and duration, is an extremely common gynecological complaint, and the most common cause of iron deficiency anemia. Studies have demonstrated a reduction in blood loss of up to 94% after 3 months of use, and reductions of 80–96% after 12 months *(42,45,47,48)*.

Results from a Chinese study of 34 women with menorrhagia, ages 27–43, reported and increase in mean hemoglobin from 12.2 g/dL pre-insertion to 13.6 g/dL after 36 months, and increase of ferritin levels from 21.9 ng/mL to 92.8 ng/mL after 3 years *(49)*. Although irregular spotting is common during the first few months after insertion, most patients with menorrhagia find prolonged spotting and light bleeding preferable to cyclical, heavy monthly bleeding.

The therapeutic properties of the LNG-IUS on the endometrium make it an excellent form of contraception in women with bleeding disorders, who commonly suffer from menorrhagia. A small British study of women with von Willebrand's disease and other inherited disorders demonstrated that the LNG-IUS was well-tolerated in this population, effectively reduced menstrual bleeding, and brought about significant improvements in hemoglobin levels *(50)*.

The use of a LNG-IUS is often as effective in treating menorragia as various surgical treatments and may avoid the necessity of such procedures. In Scandinavia, a randomized, comparative trial of the LNG-IUS with transcervical endometrial resection in 60 women found similar reductions in blood loss and number of bleeding and spotting days with the two treatments. Improvements in hemoglobin and serum ferritin concentrations were also comparable, but women treated with the LNG-IUS reported less menstrual pain in the first 90 days after treatment than did women in the resection group *(42)*.

A randomized comparative trial of the LNG-IUS compared with hysterectomy in 236 Finnish women, ages 35–49, found similar improvements in hemoglobin and serum ferritin concentrations in both treatment groups, as well as similar improvements in health-related quality of life and levels of depression and anxiety. Significant improvement in general health status occurred only in the hysterectomy group, whereas costs were significantly lower in the LNG-IUS group after both 1 and 5 years of follow-up *(44,51)*.

The LNG-IUS reduces menorrhagia associated with adenomyosis, as demonstrated in an Italian study of 25 women. Although one adenomyosis patient expelled the IUD 2 months after insertion and another requested removal of the device after 4 months because of irregular bleeding, the remaining 23 women experienced resolution of menorrhagia. Hemoglobin, serum iron, and ferritin levels improved significantly, and uterine volume decreased slightly but significantly *(52)*. Case reports have also demonstrated that the LNG-IUS reduces leiomyoma size and menorrhagia in women with uterine fibroids *(44,53)*.

A Cochrane evidence-based review concluded that the LNG-IUS is more effective for the treatment of heavy menstrual bleeding than oral progesterone taken over 21 days of the cycle. Women using the LNG-IUS have more side effects than those receiving oral therapy, but nonetheless are more satisfied with treatment and willing to continue it. Compared with transcervical endometrial resection, the LNG-IUS results in smaller reductions in menstrual blood loss but equivalent improvements in quality of life *(54)*.

Endometriosis and Pelvic Pain

A few studies have demonstrated the efficacy of the LNG-IUS as a treatment for endometriosis. A clinical trial in Brazil randomized 82 women with chronic pelvic pain resulting from endometriosis to treatment with either LNG-IUS or the gonadotropin-releasing hormone (GnRH) analog, Lupron Depot®. Chronic pelvic pain decreased equivalently in both groups and quality of life improved similarly in both groups. Women in the GnRH analog group became amenorrheic in shorter time period and reported less bleeding overall than did women with the LNG-IUS *(55)*. One advantage of LNG-IUS over GnRH analog, however, is that it does not induce a hypoestrogenic state, sparing patients uncomfortable vasomotor symptoms and risks to their bone health.

Other observational studies have demonstrated that the LNG-IUS reduces chronic pelvic pain and dyspareunia in women with endometriosis and can improve the staging of endometriosis with accompanying symptom reduction *(56–58)*. Studies of the LNG-IUS in endometriosis patients have also demonstrated a decrease in extension of recto-vaginal septum lesions as evaluated by ultrasonography, and a decrease in the severity of lesions identified at laparoscopy *(58)*. It has been postulated that the therapeutic effects of the LNG-IUS in endometriosis are mediated through estrogen and progesterone receptors on endometriotic implants, which are downregulated in the presence of LNG. No correlation has been noted between symptom improvement in endometriosis and the level of LNG in the serum or peritoneal fluid *(59)*.

Progestin Therapy to Prevent or Treat Endometrial Hyperplasia

The LNG-IUS has been studied in the treatment of endometrial hyperplasia as a means of delivering potent progestin directly to the uterus. Belgian researchers treated 12 women with biopsy-confirmed endometrial hyperplasia with a frameless LNG device that secreted 14 μg LNG per day. The patients were monitored with transvaginal ultrasound and repeat endometrial biopsies during 3–4 years of follow-up. After an initial period of spotting, bleeding stopped in all women, and measurements of the endometrium in all but one woman decreased to less than 5 mm thickness. All patients were considered cured by use of the device *(60)*.

The LNG-IUS also can serve as an alternative to hysterectomy in women in whom surgery is contraindicated. One case report describes successful treatment of an endometrial cancer, staged as at least IB, with a combination of the LNG-IUS and oral progestin therapy. The patient in this case was a woman whose multiple comorbidities made her a poor surgical candidate, and whose enormous body habitus (body mass index of 58) precluded her from fitting into a linear accelerator to receive radiation therapy. The tumor, a well-differentiated endometrioid adenocarcinoma arising within atypical complex hyperplasia, responded completely to hormonal treatment. After 13 months of follow-up, the patient had no evidence of hyperplasia or carcinoma of the endometrium and her bleeding completely resolved *(61)*.

Finally, the LNG-IUS is also increasingly used as hormone therapy in menopausal women, to balance the proliferative effects of estrogen on the endometrium. A number of trials have demonstrated that various LNG-releasing IUDs are effective and well-tolerated in menopausal women receiving concomitant oral or transdermal therapy with conjugated equine estrogen or estradiol *(62–64)*. Similarly, the LNG-IUS has been demonstrated to successfully protect the endometria of breast cancer patients against the proliferative effects of tamoxifen *(44,65)*.

GOOD CANDIDATES FOR IUC USE

- Multiparous women at low risk for sexually transmitted infections (STIs) who want long-term reversible contraception.
  - Nulliparous women at low risk for STIs are candidates, although insertion may be more difficult.
- Women with medical conditions that are poor candidates for other methods.
  - Women over 35 years of age with risk factors for cardiovascular disease, such as smoking, long-standing obesity, diabetes *(66)*, or thromoboembolism.

- Immediately after a first-trimester spontaneous or induced abortion.
- Women on medications that affect liver enzymes (rifampicin, griseofulvin, phyenytoion, cargamazepine, barbiturates, primidone).

Good Candidates for TCu380A

- Postpartum women, breastfeeding or not, after 4 weeks.
- Women with liver disease, hepatitis.
- Women with breast cancer.
- Women with hypertension, hyperlipidemia.
- Women with current or history of ischemic heart disease, stroke.
- Women with multiple risk factors for cardiovascular disease.
    - Women with uncomplicated valvular heart disease.
- Women with current deep vein thrombosis/pulmonary embolism.
- Women who have had major surgery.
- Women with migraines with or without focal neurological symptoms.
- Women with gall bladder disease or history of pregnancy-related cholestasis.

GOOD CANDIDATES FOR LNG-IUS

- Women with menorrhagia, dysmenorrhea, or endometriosis.
- Women with bleeding disorders or on anticoagulation therapy *(67)*.
    - Women with thalassemia, sickle cell disease, or iron-deficiency anemia.
- Breastfeeding women after 4–6 weeks postpartum.

CONTRAINDICATIONS TO IUC USE

- Women with current or recent history (within the last 3 months) of PID.
    - Women with past PID with subsequent pregnancy and no known current risk factors for STIs may use either IUD.
        - Women with past PID without a subsequent pregnancy and currently at low risk of STIs may be considered for IUD.
- Women with current STI.
    - Women with purulent cervicitis.
- Women with pelvic tuberculosis.
- Women who are currently pregnant (other than when used as emergency contraception as discussed in "IUD as Emergency Contraception").
- Women with recent post-septic abortion or puerperal sepsis.
- Women with uterine abnormalities or fibroids distorting the endometrial cavity.
- Women with undiagnosed genital bleeding.
- Women with allergy to any component of the IUD.
    - Women with Wilson's disease (for copper-containing IUD).

COUNSELING GUIDELINES

Women should be counseled regarding the risks and benefits of IUC and other contraceptive methods. Women should understand that the risk of infection is slightly increased during the first month following insertion. Use of IUC is very safe in both multiparous and nulliparous women who do not have risky sexual behavior. Amenorrhea is common in women with a LNG-IUS and heavy menses is common in women with a TCu380Ag. Women who miss a period while using the TCu380A should get a pregnancy test. Women should understand the warning signs of pelvic infection.

INSERTION INSTRUCTIONS

Because the devices vary in size, shape, and inserter mechanism, it is important to read the product instructions before insertion.

- Pretreatment with ibuprofen or nonsteroidal anti-inflammatory drugs is often beneficial in reducing pain.
  - Current data do not support routine pre-insertion screening for STIs in women at low risk; the presence of STIs is an important predictor of subsequent upper genital tract infection and is a contraindication to insertion.
- First, a bimanual pelvic exam is done to determine the size, shape, and position of the uterus and to exclude pelvic infection.
- A sterile speculum is inserted and an antiseptic, such as iodine, may be applied to the cervix.
  - Use of a paracervial block (not to exceed 2 mg/lb or 300 mg of lidocaine) or pretreatment with 2% intracervical lignocaine gel *(68)* or other cervical dilators may increase the ease of insertion and decrease the associated pain.
- Open the sterile package and put on (sterile, when appropriate) gloves.
- Load the IUC device into the inserter with sterile preparation.
  - For the TCu380A, no more than 5 minutes before insertion, bend the arms of the IUD and slide the inserter tube over the bent arms (using either sterile gloves or complete within the sterile package on a flat surface), place inserter rod into the inserter tube, and advance until it is contact with the IUD.
  - For the LNG-IUS, release the threads so that they hang loosely, and slide the inserter into the top of the inserter tube, against the bottom of the IUS. Make sure the arms of the IUS lie evenly on either side of the inserter tube, pull on both threads evenly, and pull the IUS into the insertion tube. Make sure the knobs (located at the ends of the arms) evenly cover the open end of the inserter and fix the threads in the cleft at the end of the inserter.
- Apply the tenaculum to obtain stabilization of the cervix and draw traction to straighten the axis of the uterus. Paracervical block with local anesthesia is optional.

- Sound the uterus to determine the appropriate depth of insertion of the device. Uterine depth of at least 6–9 cm is desirable because lengths less than that may be associated with an increased risk of expulsion.
  - For the TCu380A, set the flange to the appropriate depth desired for insertion and the direction that the arms should open and check that the axis of the horizontal arms of the IUD and the long axis of the flange are the same.
  - For the LNG-IUS, set the flange on the inserter to the depth measured by the sound.
- Gently insert the device and deploy within the uterus according to manufacturer's instruction. Be careful not to exceed the depth of the sound.
  - For the Cu380A, advance the IUD until the flange is at the cervix. Withdraw the insertion tube about 0.5 in. while holding the insertion rod in place (this will release the arms of the IUD above the tube). Move the insertion tube gently upward until resistance at the fundus is noted (this places the IUD as high as possible in the fundus) and withdraw the inserter rod and the insertion tube.
  - For the LNG-IUS, holding onto the top of the handle, advance the insertion tube into the uterus until the flange is at a distance of about 1.5–2 cm from the external cervical os (this allows space for the arms to open), hold the inserter steady, and pull the insertion tube back until the top of the IUD is released (top of the slider reaches the horizontal line on the handle). Gently push the inserter into the uterine cavity until the flange reaches the cervix (this pushes the IUD to the correct fundal portion of the uterus). Hold the inserter in place and pull the slider down (the threads will be released automatically). Remove the slider and inserter.
- Trim the visible strings to about 2–3 cm long (1 in.; documenting the length of strings is optional).
- Instruct the woman on how to check her own strings, checking after next menses and then periodically after a menses.
  - Routine use of prophylactic antibiotics for insertions confers little benefit but it may be appropriate in certain patients, especially if the insertion was particularly difficult. (The American Heart Association does not recommend subacute bacterial endocarditis antibiotic prophylaxis for either IUD insertion or removal *[69]*.)

COUNSELING TIPS

- Further routine visits are not mandatory, although a 1-month check-up to make sure the IUD is in place may be appropriate, especially in women who have concerns or who may not be able to check themselves.
- If a woman is unable to feel her strings, she should return to the clinic and use back-up protection in the meantime.
- Counseling on changes in menstrual flow: either heavy menstrual flow, intermittent bleeding, or spotting may occur with the TCu380A. Less flow and possible amenorrhea may occur with the LNG-IUS.

- Use on anti-inflammatory or hormonal medications to control bleeding or pain may help promote continued use.
- As with all forms of contraception, it is advised that users who engage in risky sexual activity also use a condom.
- Women using a TCu380A should get a pregnancy test if they miss a period.
- The Food and Drug Administration recommends that the IUD be removed if a user becomes pregnant, if it can be removed without an invasive procedure.
- The IUD should be removed in postmenopausal women. Waiting for 1 year of amenorrhea (to ensure menopausal status) before removing the device may be appropriate.

MANAGING PROBLEMS

- Excessive bleeding. Treat with non-steroidal anti-inflammatory medications; rule out other disorders, such as polyp, pregnancy, or endometritis; consider small catheter pipelle endometrial biopsy.
- Partial expulsion (presence of a hard plastic in the cervix or vagina, lengthening of the string, pain, and cramping). Rule out pregnancy, remove misplaced device; immediate re-insertion is an option.
- Cramping and pain. Treat with oral non-steroidal anti-inflammatory medications.
- Perforation. Copper IUD outside the uterus should be removed immediately.
- Missing strings. Probe cervix with brush to locate strings or confirm the presence of an IUD inside the endometrial cavity with ultrasound. If IUD is in place, no further action is necessary.
  - To remove an IUD within the uterine cavity but with no visible strings, gentle exploration with an alligator forceps or endometrial biopsy instrument (a paracervical block may be useful). Overnight cervical dilators (400 μg misoprostol vaginally or orally, or 400–600 μg cyctotec vaginally) may be helpful.
  - Rarely, hysteroscopy is necessary for removal.
- Pregnancy. Confirm that the pregnancy is intrauterine and not ectopic. Remove the IUD if it is easy to do so, regardless of her desire to keep or terminate the pregnancy.
- Pelvic infections. Removal of IUD may be indicated, although it may not improve treatment response *(22)*. Use two antibiotics for best spectrum coverage and refer male partner for potential treatment.
- *Actinomyces*-like organisms on pap smear. Notify user about finding. If she is asymptomatic, no further action is necessary. If she has evidence of infection, the device should be removed and a course of antibiotics should be started (penicillin is a good option).

REMOVAL

Slow steady traction on the IUC strings will allow for easy removal. Application of the tenaculum to straighten the axis of the uterus is rarely required. If the strings are not visible, gentle probing with a hook or endocervical brush inside the cervical canal can often find the wayward strings. Ultrasound can be used to confirm intrauterine position and also guide the use of the IUD hook or alligator forceps for removal of the device. Liberal use of paracervical local anesthesia or medical dilators (misoprostol, cytotec) for patient comfort may be helpful if cervical dilation or uterine exploration is required for IUD removal.

CURRENTLY AVAILABLE IUCS

- The TCu380A IUD, marketed as ParaGard®, is a T-shaped polyethylene rod, wrapped with copper around the arms and stem. It is approved for 10 years of continuous use (Fig. 1).
- The LNG-IUS, sold as Mirena®, is a T-shaped polydimethylsiloxane rod containing 52 mg LNG. The LNG-IUS is approved for 5 years of use (Fig. 1).

REFERENCES

1. ACOG Practice Bulletin. (2005) Clinical Management Guidelines for Obstetrician-Gynecologists, No. 59.
2. Hidalgo M, Bahamondes L, Perrotti M, Diaz J, Dantas-Monteiro C, Petta C. (2002) Bleeding patterns and clinical performance of the levonorgestrel releasing intrauterine system (Mirena) up to two years. Contraception 65:129–132.
3. Hatcher RA, Zieman M, Cwiak C, Darney PD, Creinin MD, Stosur HR. (2004) A Pocket Guide to Managing Contraception. Tiger, GA: Bridging the Gap Foundation.
4. Sivin I, Stern J, Coutinho E, et al. (1991) Prolonged intrauterine contraception: a seven-year randomized study of the levonorgestrel 20 mcg/day (LNg 20) and the Copper T380 Ag IUDs. Contraception 44:473–480.
5. Ronnerdag M, Odland V. (1999) Health effects of long-term use of the levonorgestrel-releasing system. Acta Obstet Gynecol Scand 78:716–721.
6. Hatcher RA, Trussell J, Stewart F, et al. (2004) Contraceptive Technology, 18th ed. New York: Ardent Media.
7. Piccinnino LJ, Mosher WD. (1998) Trends in contraceptive use in the United States. Fam Plann Perspect 30:4–10, 46.
8. Alvarez F, Brache V, Fernandez E, et al. (1988) New insights on the mode of action of intrauterine contraceptive devices in women. Fertil Steril 49:768–773.
9. Rivera R, Yacobson I, Grimes D. (1999) The mechanism of action of hormonal contraceptives and intrauterine contraceptive devices. Am J Obstet Gynecol 181:1263–1269.
10. Ortiz ME, Corxatto H. (1987) Mode of action of IUDs. Contraception 36:37–53.
11. Andersson K, Odlind V, Rybo G. (1994) Levonorgestrel-releasing and copper-releasing (Nova T) IUDs during 5 years of use: a randomized comparative trial. Contraception 49:56–72.
12. Pakarinen P, Toivonen J, Luukkainen T. (2003) Randomized comparison of levonorgestrel and copper releasing intrauterine systems immediately after abortion, with 5 years' follow-up. Contraception 68:31–34.
13. Stanwood NL, Garrett JM, Conrad TR. (2002) Obstetrician-gynecologists and the intrauterine device: a survey of attitudes and practice. Obstet Gynecol 99:275–280.
14. Population Reference Bureau. (2002) Family Planning Worldwide 2002 Data Sheet.
15. The Gallup Organization. (2003) A survey of female ob-gyns on health issues and concerns. Conducted for The American College of Obstetricians and Gynecologists, Princeton, NJ. ACOG Today. 2004;48:1,6–7.

16. Espey E, Obgurn T. (2002) Perpetuating negative attitudes about the intrauterine device: textbooks lag behind the evidence. Contraception 65:389–395.
17. Weiss E, Moore K. (2004) An assessment of the quality of information available on the internet about the IUD and the potential impact on contraceptive choices. Contraception 68:359–364.
18. Merki-Feld G, Lebeda E, Hogg B, Keller PJ. (2000) The incidence of Actinomyces-like organisms in Papanicolaou-stained smears of copper and levonorgestrel releasing intrauterine devices. Contraception 61:365–368.
19. Buchan H, Villard-Mackintosh L, Vessey M, Yeates D, McPherson K. (1990) Epidemiology of pelvic inflammatory disease in parous women with special reference to intrauterine device use. Br J Obstet Gynaecol 97:780–788.
20. Farley TM, Rosenberg MJ, Rowe PJ, et al. (1992) Intrauterine devices and pelvic inflammatory disease: an international perspective. Lancet 339:785–788.
21. Hubacher D, Lara-Ricalde R, Taylor DJ, Guerra-Infante F, Guzman-Rodriguez R. (2001) Use of copper intrauterine devices and the risk of tubal infertility among nulligravid women. N Engl J Med 345:561–567.
22. Soderberg G, Lindgren S. (1981) Influence of an intrauterine device on the course of an acute salpingitis. Contraception 24:137–143.
23. Grimes DA, Schulz KF. (1999) Prophylactic Antibiotics for intrauterine device insertion: a metaanalysis of the randomized controlled trials. Contraception 60:57–63.
24. Chi I. (1993) The Tcu-380A, MLCu375, and Nova T IUDS and the IUD daily releasing 20μg levonorgestrel—4 pillars of IUD contraception for the nineties and beyond? Contraception 47:325–347.
25. Ory HW. (1981) Ectopic pregnancy and intrauterine contraceptive devices: new perspectives. The Women's Health Study. Obstet Gynecol 57:137–144.
26. Penny G, Brechin S, deSouza A, et al. (2004) The copper intrauterine device as long-term contraception. J Fam Plann Reprod Health Care 30:29–41, quiz 42. Erratum in: J Fam Plann Reprod Health Care 2004;30:134.
27. Ganacharya S, Bhattoa HP, Batar I. (2003) Ectopic pregnancy among non-medicated and copper-containing intrauterine device users: a 10-year follow-up. Eur J Obstet Gynecol Repod Biol 111:78–82.
28. Backman T. Rauramo I, Huhtala S, Koskenvuo M. (2004) Pregnancy during the use of levonorgestrel intrauterine system. Am J Obstet Gynecol 190:50–54.
29. Franks AL, Beral V, Cates W Jr, Hogue CJ. (1990) Contraception and ectopic pregnancy risk. Am J Obstet Gynecol 163:1120–1123.
30. Sivin I. (1991) Dose- and age-dependent ectopic pregnancy risks with intrauterine contraception. Obstet Gynecol 78;291–298.
31. World Health Organization (WHO). (2004) Improving Access to Quality Care in Family Planning:Medical Eligibility Criteria of Contraceptive Use, 3rd ed. Geneva, Switzerland: WHO.
32. Mirena (package insert). (2000) Montville, NJ: Berlex Laboratories.
33. Paragard T380 Intrauterine Copper Contraceptive (package insert). (2003) North Todawanda, NY: FEI Products.
34. Duenas JL, Albert A, Carrasco F. (1996) Intrauterine contraception in nulligravid vs parous women. Contraception 53:23–24.
35. World Health Organization. (2004) Medical Eligibility Criteria for IUDS, 3rd ed. Available from: http://www.who.int/reproductive-health/publications/mec/iuds.html. Accessed: March 11, 2006.
36. European Study Group on Heterosexual Transmission of HIV. (1992) Comparison of female to male and male to female transmission of HIV in 563 stable couples. BMJ 304:809–813.
37. Sinei SK, Morrison CS, Sekkadde-Kigondu, Allen M, Kokonya D. (1998) Complications of use of intrauterine devices among HIV-1 infected women. Lancet 351:1238–1241.

38. Trusell J, Ellerston C. (1995) Efficacy of emergency contraception. Fert Control Rev 4:8–11.
39. Zhou L, Xiao B. (2001) Emergency contraception with Multiload CU-375 SL IUD: a multicenter clinical trial. Contraception 64:107–112.
40. Luukkainen T, Allonen H, Haukamaa M, et al. (1987) Effective contraception with the levonorgestrel-releasing intrauterine device: 12 month report of a European multi-center study. Contraception 36:169–179.
41. Chi IC. (1991) An evaluation of the levonorgestrel-releasing IUD: its advantages and disadvantages when compared to the copper-releasing IUDs. Contraception 44:573–588.
42. Rauramo I, Elo I, Istre O. (2004) Long-term treatment of menorrhagia with levonorgestrel intrauterine system versus endometrial resection. Obstet Gynecol 104:1314–1321.
43. Hurskainen R, Teperi J, Rissanen P, et al. (2004) Clinical outcomes and costs with the levonorgestrel-releasing intrauterine system or hysterectomy for treatment of menorrhagia. JAMA 291:1456–1463.
44. Hubacher D, Grimes D. (2002) Noncontraceptive health benefits of intrauterine devices: a systematic review. Obstet Gynecol Surv 57:120–128.
45. Stewart A, Cummings C, Gold L, Jordan R, Phillips W. (2001) The effectiveness of the levonorgestrel-releasing intrauterine system in menorrhagia: a review. BJOG 108:74–86.
46. Hurskainen R, Paavonen J. (2004) Levonorgestrel-releasing intrauterine system in the treatment of heavy menstrual bleeding. Curr Opin Obstet Gynecol 16:487–490.
47. Banu NS, Manyonda IT. (2005) Alternative medical and surgical options to hysterectomy. Best Prac Res Clin Obstet Gynecol 19:431–449.
48. Soysal S, Soysal ME. (2005) The efficacy of levonorgestrel-releasing intrauterine devices in selected cases of myoma-related menorrhagia: a prospective controlled trial. Gynecol Obstet Invest 59:29–35.
49. Xiao B, Wu S, Chong J, Zeng T, Han L, Luukkainen T. (2003) Therapeutic effects of the levonorgestrel-releasing intrauterine system in the treatment of idiopathic menorrhagia. Fertil Steril 79:963–969.
50. Kingman CEC, Kadir RA, Lee CA, Economides DL. (2004) The use of levonorgestrel-releasing intrauterine system for treatment of menorrhagia in women with inherited bleeding disorders. BJOG 111:1425–1428.
51. Hurskainen R, Teperi J, Rissanen P, et al. (2001) Quality of life and cost-effectiveness of levonorgestrel-releasing intrauterine system versus hysterectomy for treatment of menorrhagia. Lancet 357:273–277.
52. Federle L, Bianchi S, Raffaelli R, Portuese A, Dorta M. (1997) Treatment of adenomyosis-associated menorrhagia with a levonorgestrel-releasing intrauterine device. Fertil Steril 68:426–429.
53. Grigorieva V. (2003) Use of a levonorgestrel-releasing intrauterine system to treat bleeding related to uterine leiomyomas. Fertil Steril 79:1194–1198.
54. Lethaby AE, Cooke I, Rees M. (1999) Progesterone/progestogen releasing intrauterine systems for heavy menstrual bleeding. Cochrane Database Syst Rev 2:CD002126.
55. Petta CA, Ferriani RA, Abrao MS, et al. (2005) Randomized clinical trial of a levonorgestrel-releasing intrauterine system and a depot GnRH analogue for the treatment of chronic pelvic pain in women with endometriosis. Hum Reprod 20:1993–1998.
56. Vercellini P, Aimi G, Paonazza S, DeGiorgi O, Pesole A, Crosignani PG. (1999) A levonorgestrel-releasing intrauterine system for the treatment of dysmenorrhea associated with endometriosis: a pilot study. Fertil Steril 72:505–508.
57. Lockhat FB, Emembolu JO, Konje JC. (2004) The evaluation of the effectiveness of intrauterine-administered progestogen (levonorgestrel) in the symptomatic treatment of endometriosis and in the staging of the disease. Hum Reprod 19:179–184.

58. Federle L, Bianchi S, Zanconato G, Portuese A, Raffaelli R. (2001) Use of a levonorgestrel-releasing intrauterine device in the treatment of rectovaginal endometriosis. Fertil Steril 75:485–488.
59. Lockhat FB, Emembolu JE, Konje JC. (2005) Serum and peritoneal fluid levels of levonorgestrel in women with endometriosis who were treated with an intrauterine contraceptive device containing levonorgestrel. Fertil Steril 83:398–404.
60. Wildemeersch D, Dhont M. (2003) Treatment of nonatypical and atypical endometrial hyperplasia with a levonorgestrel-releasing intrauterine system. Am J Obstet Gynecol 188:1297–1298.
61. Giannopoulos T, Butler-Manuel S, Tailor A. (2004) Levonorgestrel-releasing intrauterine system (LNG-IUS) as a therapy for endometrial carcinoma. Gynecol Oncol 95:762–764.
62. Varila E, Wahlstrom T, Rauramo I. (2001) A 5-year follow-up study on the use of a levonorgestrel intrauterine system in women receiving hormone replacement therapy. Fertil Steril 76:969–973.
63. Raudaskoski T, Tapanainen J, Tomas E, et al. (2002) Intrauterine 10 microgram and 20 microgram levonorgestrel systems in postmenopausal women receiving oral oestrogen replacement therapy: clinical, endometrial and metabolic response. BJOG 109:136–144.
64. Wildermeersch D, Schacht E, Wildemeersch P, Calleweart K, Pylyser K, De Wever N. (2004) Endometrial safety with a low-dose intrauterine levonorgestrel-releasing system after 3 years of estrogen substitution therapy. Maturitas 48:65–70.
65. Gardner FJ, Konje JC, Abrams KR, et al. (2000) Endometrial protection from tamoxifen-stimulated changes by a levonorgestrel-releasing intrauterine system: a randomised controlled trial. Lancet 356:1711–1717.
66. Kimmerle R, Weiss R, Berger M, Jurz KH. (1993) Effectiveness, safety and acceptability of a copper intrauterine device [Cu safe 300] in type 1 diabetic women. Diabetes Care 16;1227–1230.
67. Siegel JE, Kouides PA. (2002) Menorrhagia from a haematologist's point of view. Part II: Management. Haemophilia 8:339–347.
68. Oloto EJ, Bromham DR, Murty JA. (1997) Pain and discomfort perception at IUD insertion-effect of short-duration, low-volume, intracervical application of two per cent lignocaine gel—a preliminary study. Br J Fam Plann 22:177–180.
69. Dajani AS, Taubert KA, Wilson W, et al. (1997) Prevention of bacterial endocarditis. Recommendations by the American Heart Association. JAMA 277:1794–1801.

10 Barrier Contraceptives

Male Condoms, Vaginal Spermicides, and Cervical Barrier Methods

Donna Shoupe, MD

CONTENTS

MALE CONDOMS

> *Latex condoms, when used consistently and correctly, are highly effective in preventing the sexual transmission of HIV, the virus that causes AIDS (1).*

Introduction

Male condoms are a popular contraceptive method. Additionally, they also play an integral role in US public health programs designed to prevent the spread of HIV and other sexually transmitted infections (STIs). Since the 1986 report from the US Surgeon General advocating the use of condoms to help prevent the spread of AIDS, awareness of the benefits of condom use has continued to increase. The percentage of reproductive-age women choosing condoms for contraceptive protection increased from 13% in 1988 to around 20% today. Use among sexually active adolescents is dependent on a variety of factors, including race and ethnicity, but averages around 45% *(2,3)*.

Although correct and consistent use of the male latex condom reduces the risk of HIV and STI transmission in at-risk persons, no method is 100% effective. The best way to avoid transmission of STIs is to abstain from sexual intercourse or to be in a long-term, mutually monogamous relationship with a partner who is known to be uninfected.

From: *Current Clinical Practice: The Handbook of Contraception: A Guide for Practical Management*
Edited by: D. Shoupe and S. L. Kjos © Humana Press, Totowa, NJ

Effectiveness

Contraceptive Efficacy

- The male condom prevents pregnancy by acting as a physical barrier to sperm movement and is most effective if used from "beginning to end" on every sexual contact.

If used correctly on each act of sexual intercourse, only about 2–3% of couples will experience unintended pregnancy during the first year of use. However, typical first-year failure rates are about 15% because many couples fail to use condoms with each act. Both US consumer surveys *(4)* and tightly controlled trials *(5)* document that couples using condoms for their sole method of contraception report using condoms correctly and consistently in less than 50% of cycles.

Protection From STIs and HIV

- In vitro studies show that latex condoms are impermeable to a large number of bacterial and viral STIs, including HIV *(6)*.
- Genital areas not covered by the condom, improper or inconsistent use of the condom, or damage to a condom are factors that may allow viral or bacterial transmission.

Several clinical studies of heterosexual couples who consistently used latex condoms to prevent transmission of HIV from an infected individual to their non-infected partner, reported around a 90% success rate *(7,8)*. A meta-analysis of 25 studies report efficacy rates for condoms preventing the transmission of HIV ranging from 87 to 96% *(9)*. The success rate of the condom's ability to protect from transmission of other STIs have been more variable, but studies generally confirm reductions in gonorrhea, genital herpes, chlamydia, syphilis, and trichomoniasis *(10–15)*.

Advantages of Male Condoms

- Effective at preventing pregnancy when used correctly and consistently.
- Compared with other barrier methods, the male condom is considered to be the most effective for prevention of the transmission of STIs and HIV.
- One of the most cost-effective contraceptive options now available, especially in view of the fact that condoms also offer protection against STI and HIV transmission *(16)*. Prices vary from as low 25¢ per condom to more than $1 in cost. Some publicly funded organizations offer condoms at very low or no cost to certain users.
    - Latex condoms are generally the cheapest type.
- Relatively easy to get, easy to use, highly portable, and can be bought in a variety of stores without a prescription.
- Do not have systemic side effects.
- Offer better hygiene because the semen is collected and discarded with the condom following use.

Table 1
Oil-Based Products That May Degrade Latex Condoms, Latex Diaphragms, or Cervical Caps

Vaseline petroleum jelly
Hand lotions
Cold cream
Baby oil
Peanut oil
Suntan oil
Corn or sunflower oil
Massage oil
Whipping cream
Vaginal yeast medications: Femstat®, Monistat®, Vagisil®
Estrogen cream

- By blocking the movement of gonorrhea and other STIs, female partners of users have a lowered risk of developing pelvic inflammatory disease and tubal-factor infertility *(17)*.
- Provide some limited protection from spread of human papillomavirus (HPV) *(18)* and their use is associated with a lowered rate of cervical dysplasia and cancer *(19)*.
  - Although condoms do not appear to provide as much protection from HPV as from other STIs, the Centers for Disease Control and Prevention recommends condom use as a way to reduce the risk of HPV and herpes infections *(20)*.
- During use, some men are able to sustain erection longer.
- Come in many sizes, colors, flavors, and styles.
  - Available with and without ribbing, studs, and lubrication or spermicide.

Disadvantages of Male Condoms

- During vaginal or anal intercourse, condom breakage is reported to occur about 2% of the time.
- Although rates vary, condom slippage off of the penis occurs in about 2% of vaginal intercourse.
  - Improper placement or incorrect withdrawal technique may increase this risk.
  - Partial slippage during intercourse may allow skin-to-skin transmission and increased risk of STI transmission.
- Efficacy is compromised with re-use of a condom, inconsistent use, improper use, concomitant use of latex condom with oil-based lubricants or vaginal medications (Vaseline® [petroleum jelly], suntan oil, whipped cream, Crisco®, baby oil, hand lotions, vaginal yeast medications, or massage oil; Table 1) *(21)*.
  - Polyurethane condoms are not affected by oil-based products.
  - Condoms tear easily with fingernails, a ring, teeth, or anything sharp.

- Polyurethane condoms may be necessary in persons with latex allergies.
- The man must pull out soon after ejaculation.
  - If the man loses his erection, the condom can fall off and protection is lost.
- Animal membrane condoms are not as effective at protecting against infection as latex or polyurethane condoms.

User Complaints

- Unless the partner puts it on as a part of foreplay, the condom interrupts sex.
  - "It spoils the spontaneity" or alters the "mood."
  - May imply a lack of trust.
- Fear that one may face rejection if he or she insists on condom use.
- Less sensation and pleasure.
- Difficult to use if the male partner is unable to maintain an erection.
- Embarrassment when purchasing condoms over the counter.

Patient Counseling

> *Unless a sexually active person is in a mutually monogamous relationship, they are at risk for the transmission of STIs and HIV/AIDS.*

Condom use is strongly recommended for sexually active women and men who are not in mutually monogamous relationships. Dual use of a condom plus another contraceptive method, such as oral contraceptives, is the "gold standard" and is a good option for sexually active adolescents, young singles, or others at risk for STIs and unintended pregnancy.

Many of the problems experienced by condom users are usually resolved as users become more experienced. The different brands and types of condoms offer a variety of options and advantages. The counselor should encourage users to try different brands should problems develop.

- STIs impact millions of people in the United States each year, especially young people.
- Half of all people with HIV were infected before they were 25 years old.
- STIs can be painful, cause infertility, and lead to serious health problems, including death.
- STIs may be silent and unknown to the infected individual.
- Using condoms properly every time:
  - Reduces the risk of STI and HIV/AIDS transmission.
  - Reduces the risk of pregnancy.
  - May protect the future fertility of the female.
- Condoms are designed to give pleasure, protection, and freedom from worry.
- There are many different styles of condoms, and they are easy to find in stores and easy to use.
- Using a water-based lubricant (such as Very Private® Intimate Moisture, Astroglide®, or MyPleasure® Personal Lubricant Gel) may decrease the risk of condom breakage.

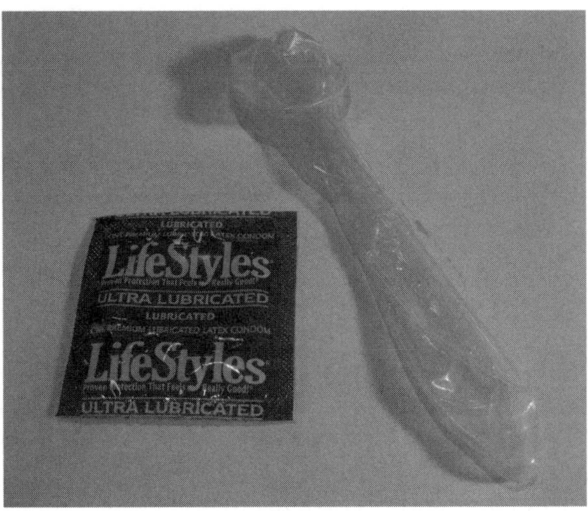

Fig. 1. Ultra-lubricated male condom with a reservoir-tip and container pouch.

Patient Counseling Techniques

Be ready to explain the benefits of condom use to your partner.

A potential user should be ready to respond to any partner objections with the following statements about condom use:

- It is a smart thing to do.
- It is a responsible act that demonstrates maturity.
- It shows respect for a partner.
- It is evidence that the users care about the safety of others.
- It will improve the "mood" because both partners will feel more secure.

Instructions Regarding Proper Use of Condoms

- Select an appropriate size and style of condom at a pharmacy. Note the expiration date and have condoms readily available.
- Before intercourse, discuss condom use with partner. Be ready to explain that condom use is smart, responsible, and will improve the "mood."
- A new condom is used "beginning to end" for every act of intercourse.
- As soon as the penis is erect, open the package and compress the tip of the condom to remove any excess air. Check the condom to make sure it is not dried out or torn. Use another condom if damage is detected or if the condom appears old.
- Place the open end of the condom, ring side up, on to the head of the penis.
- Roll the condom down the shaft of the penis until the condom is completely unrolled. The condom should cover the entire shaft of the penis and fit smoothly. There should be a small space left or a reservoir tip at the tip for collection of semen (Fig. 1).

- Right after ejaculation, hold the top rim of the condom firmly against the still-erect penis and make sure it remains in place as the penis is withdrawn.
- The condom is removed after the penis is withdrawn.
  - The condom is checked for holes or damage.
  - If condom damage is noted or if slippage occurred during intercourse, consider emergency contraception (within 72 hours) and STI follow-up/treatment.
- Condom is disposed in a trash container.

Options

There are more than 100 different condoms on the US market today. A user can chose a condom with or without lubricants or spermicides, reservoir tip, and ribbing. They come in a variety of thicknesses, colors, sizes, shapes, and scents (including mint). The majority of condoms are made of latex (rubber-based), but they are also available in polyurethane (synthetic) or natural membrane (intestinal caecum of lambs). A unisex condom has also been introduced. The unisex condom is a modified condom that has a hoop at the base. It is made of a very thin, hypoallergenic plastic, and is designed to be used with a lubricant. It may be used by either women or men and is thinner than most latex condoms.

Newer model condoms made of polyurethane may be more comfortable, less constricting than latex condoms, and are not affected by oil-based lubricants. Polyurethane condoms offer similar protection against STIs and small viruses as latex condoms. The polyurethane condom is a good option for the 1% of the US population with a latex allergy *(22)*. Some users prefer the soft, "natural" feel of the natural membrane condoms but these condoms contain small pores, and thus do not protect against HIV and STI transmission. The latex condoms tend to have the lowest cost.

With so many options available, dissatisfied users should be encouraged to shop around and try different types. Many of the problems encountered by condom users may be solved as they become more experienced and find the right condom.

Condoms are considered a medical device and regulated by the US Food and Drug Administration (FDA). Condoms must meet minimum thickness and width standards, and are periodically subjected to laboratory testing for leakage, strength, and packaging standards.

VAGINAL SPERMICIDES

Introduction

Vaginal spermicides are relatively inexpensive and available over the counter. Like other barrier methods, the contraceptive effectiveness of vaginal spermicides is highly dependent on the user's ability to use the method consistently and properly. Spermicides are placed immediately before each sexual contact and effectiveness lasts only 1 hour. When used alone, vaginal spermicides may provide limited protection against the transmission of STIs and do not protect against HIV infection. They are most effective when used with other barrier methods, such as the male condom, diaphragm, or cervical caps.

Effectiveness

Vaginal spermicides, when used alone, have highly variable typical use failure rates that range from 5 to 50%. It is difficult to compare different spemicides because their effectiveness is highly dependent on the user's ability to use the method consistently and properly. Correct placement of the spermicide against the cervix and adequate time for dispersion are critical factors that may not always be fulfilled. Generally, failure rate for spermicides is around 20–30% for typical use and 6–18% for perfect use. Use of a spermicide with other barrier methods significantly increases effectiveness and is strongly recommended.

- Use of a spermicide with a condom is associated with a 1-year failure rate as low as 0.1%.

Advantages of Vaginal Spermicides

- Are low cost and available over the counter.
- Can be used by wide range of users and rarely have systemic effects.
- Are easy to transport and can be readily available.
- Can be a unilateral decision not requiring partner approval.
- May provide additional lubrication during intercourse.
- Can be used with a variety of other barrier methods.
- Are useful a variety of situations including:
  - Temporary use while waiting to use another method.
  - During breastfeeding.
  - After missing two or more pills in a cycle.
  - Suspicion that an intrauterine device has been expelled.
  - Infrequent sexual activity.
  - Mid-cycle to augment other methods.
- May provide some limited protection against gonorrhea and chlamydia.

Disadvantages of Vaginal Spermicides

- Lasts only 1 hour after insertion.
- Typical failure rates range from 20 to 30% (but are substantially reduced if vaginal spermicides used with other methods).
- Although nonoxynol-9 is lethal to many organisms, including trichomoniasis, chlamydia, syphilis, genital herpes, and HIV, clinical trials have reported mixed results regarding STI protection from use of vaginal spermicides *(23–26)*.
  - If used more than twice per day, spermicides may damage the vaginal mucosa and increased rates of HIV transmission are reported in some studies *(27)*.

- Some users complain about the messiness, taste, necessity of having to touch the genitals, wait time necessary for the suppositories to dissolve, or excessive lubrication.
- Spermicide use can result in local vaginal and vulvar irritation, especially with frequent use. If an allergy or sensitivity is suspected, another contraceptive method should be considered.
- Use of spermicides is associated with higher rates of:
  - Urinary tract infections *(28)*.
  - Vaginosis.
  - Yeast vaginitis when used with a diaphragm.
- Although there is concern, several studies report no causal association between fetal defects and use of spermicides *(29,30)*.
- Women with vaginal or uterine prolapse, or those with a vaginal deformity, such as a septum, are poor candidates because they may not be able to correctly place the spermicide.

Patient Counseling

> *One applicator or suppository is necessary for each act of intercourse and is effective for only 1 hour.*

Vaginal spermicides are a good choice for women who are highly motivated to use the method properly and consistently on each sexual act. Use of vaginal spermicides with other barrier methods significantly improves contraceptive effectiveness. Women with risky sexual behaviors who are especially prone to STI exposure should use the vaginal spermicide plus a condom.

- User should read the product instructions.
- The spermicide must cover and coat the cervix to ensure contraceptive effectiveness.
  - High placement in vagina near the cervix necessary.
  - If a suppository, tablet, or film is used, it is necessary to wait at least 15 minutes to ensure adequate dispersion of the spermicide.
  - Spermicide must be left in place for at least 6 hours after intercourse.
- No douching for at least 6–8 hours.
- Keep adequate supplies available.
- Women with a vaginal abnormality that may interfere with proper placement of the spermicide should check with a health care provider.
- If irritation occurs, changing to another product may be advisable.
- In case the spermicide is used incorrectly, emergency contraception should be considered.

Proper Use of Vaginal Spermicides

- Foam. The aerosol can must be shaken at least 20 times. The applicator is placed on top of the aerosol container and pressed down. This causes the applicator to fill with foam. The applicator is then inserted high into the vagina. At elevations higher than 3500 ft, it is necessary to use two applicators. Contraceptive protection begins immediately and remains effective for 1 hour.

- Gel or cream. Open the tube. Place the open end of the applicator over the opening and squeeze the spermicide into the applicator. The applicator is then inserted high into the vagina near the cervix. The applicator is held still and the plunger is pushed to release the product. Contraceptive protection begins immediately and lasts up to 1 hour.
- Vaginal contraceptive film. Hands must be clean and dry before touching the film. A small thin sheet is removed from the wrapper, folded in half, and inserted as high as possible onto the back wall of the vagina. The film should rest on or near the cervix. Contraceptive protection begins 15 minutes after insertion and remains effective for about 1 hour.
- Suppository or tablet. The wrapper is removed and the suppository or tablet is inserted high into the vagina near the cervix. Contraceptive protection begins 10–15 minutes after insertion and remains effective for about 1 hour.

Options

Spermicidal preparations have two components: the base (gel, foam, cream, film, suppository, or tablet) and the spermicidal chemical that kills sperm.

Nonoxynol-9, a surfactant that disrupts the cell membrane of the sperm, is the active agent in most spermicidal products marketed in the United States. A few spermicides contain octoxynol. Other surfactants, available in other parts of the world include menfegol and benzalkonium chloride. Many new spermicidal products are under testing and evaluation.

Vaginal spermicides come in a variety of options including foam, film, suppository, tablets, coated latex condoms, creams, gels, and jellies (some of the available brands include Ortho-Gynol®, Ortho-Cream®, Gynol II®, Preceptin®, Kormex II®, Conceptrol®).

CERVICAL BARRIER METHODS: COMPARISON OF THE DIAPHRAGM, FEMALE CONDOM, CERVICAL CAP AND SHIELD, AND VAGINAL SPONGE

Introduction

Cervical barrier methods are effective when they are used consistently and properly. They are popular with many women because they provide convenience, safety, and sexual spontaneity. Depending on the method, there are limited degrees of protection from STI and HIV transmission, although there is a growing body or research suggesting that covering the cervix may potentially play an important role. The contraceptive sponge was the largest-selling over-the-counter female contraceptive in the United States until it was abruptly taken off the market in 1995. Becuase of a high demand for its return, it was re-introduced in 2005.

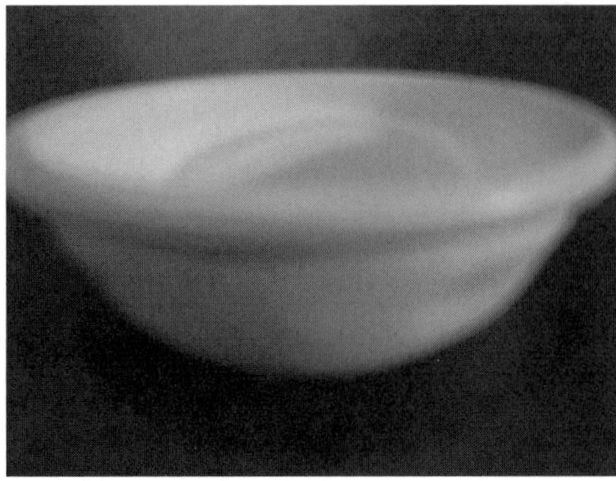

Fig. 2. Side view of a diaphragm.

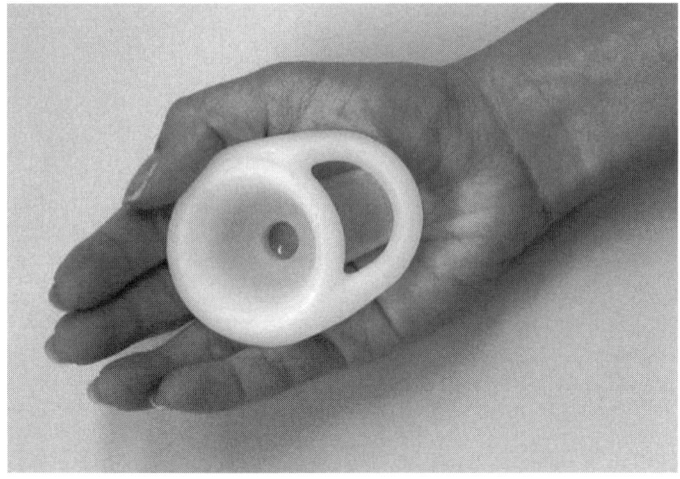

Fig. 3. Lea's Shield. (Reproduced with permission from Yama, Inc.)

The sponge and female condom are available over the counter. The female condom shares many of the same advantages and disadvantages as the male condom. The diaphragm is used with a spermicide, must be fitted by a health care provider, and is available by prescription only (Fig. 2).

In March 2002, the US FDA approved a new female barrier contraceptive, Lea's Shield® by prescription only (Fig. 3). The shield has been available over the counter since 1993 in Germany, Austria, Switzerland, and Canada. The second-generation FemCap™, currently available in Germany, France, the United Kingdom, Austria, Switzerland, and the Netherlands, was approved for marketing by the US FDA in March 2003 (Fig. 4). Lea's Shield is "one size fits all" and

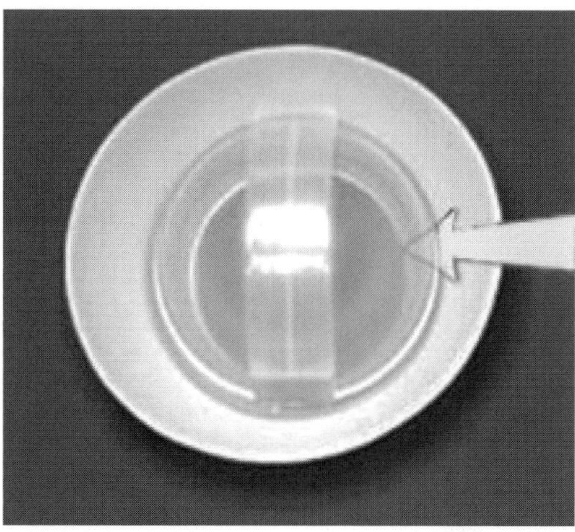

Fig. 4. Second-generation FemCap with removal strap. (Reproduced with permission from FemCap, Inc. and Alfred Shihata, MD.)

the size selection of the second-generation FemCap is determined by obstetrical history. Both Lea's Shield and FemCap are used with a spermicide and are available by prescription only.

Mechanism of Action

The cervical barrier methods prevent pregnancy by acting as a physical, and in some cases, chemical barrier to sperm movement.

The internal sheath of the female condom prevents sperm from entering the cervix and protects the vagina and cervix from STI exposure. The external ring also physically protects a large part of the perineum from STI exposure. The cervical cap, shield, contraceptive sponge, and diaphragm physically occlude the cervical os and hold a spermicide against it for added protection.

Lea's Shield is not held in place by the cervix, but rather by the vaginal wall, therefore cervical size does not play a role. Once inserted, the air trapped between the cervix and the shield escapes through the one-way valve, creating a tight fit between the vaginal wall and the shield (Fig. 5). The bowl of Lea's Shield is large enough to accommodate any normal-sized cervix. The second-generation FemCap is also held in place by the muscular walls of the vagina so it does not need to fit snugly around the cervix or hinge behind the pubic bone. The portion of the cap facing away from the cervix is shaped like an inverted funnel that directs sperm into the groove where the spermicide is stored.

The diaphragm is anchored in place between the pubic bone and the posterior fornix. This distance varies from woman to woman, and thus the diaphragm must be fitted and correctly sized. A spermicide is placed inside the dome before insertion.

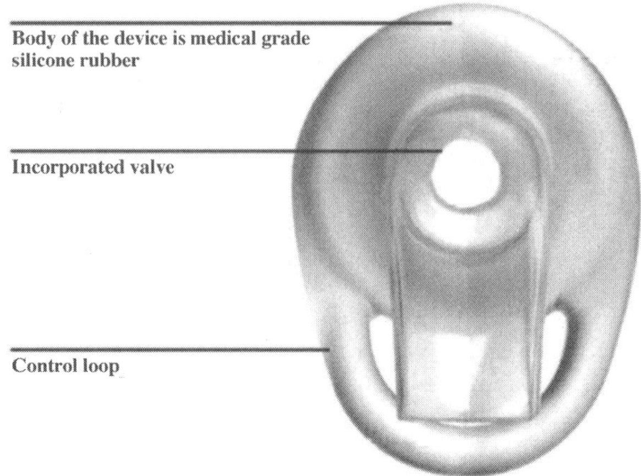

Fig. 5. Lea's Shield. (Reproduced with permission from Yama, Inc.)

The sponge is made from polyurethane foam that absorbs semen before the sperm have a chance to enter the cervix. It also contains a spermicide.

Effectiveness of Cervical Barrier Methods

As with all barrier methods, cervical barrier methods are most effective if used from "beginning to end" on every sexual contact. It is estimated that at least half of the pregnancies occurring in women who claim they were using a cervical barrier contraceptive are the result of improper or inconsistent use of the method. Both perfect use and typical use failure rates for cervical barriers are also affected by other factors including intercourse frequency and user fecundity. Some of the older cervical caps had much higher failure rates in parous compared with nulliparous women *(32)*. However, newer-generation products are designed to grossly cover the cervix and upper vagina (rather than fit tightly around the cervix) and newer reports show very little differences in failure rates between parous and nulliparous women.

Because of the large number of variables that can affect failure rates of barrier methods, large differences in failure rates are reported in the literature. To reflect some of this variability, the effectiveness rates noted below are given as ranges.

Effectiveness of the Diaphragm

Data from several studies *(33–35)* demonstrates a modest increase in effectiveness when comparing diaphragm use with and without a spermicide.

- For perfect use of the diaphragm, 2–8% of users will have an accidental pregnancy during the first year.
- In "normal" populations in which use is not always consistent or proper, the typical use failure rate is between 6 and 28% diaphragm users *(36,37)*.

Effectiveness of the Female Condom

- If used correctly on each act of sexual intercourse (perfect use), about 5% of female condom users will experience an unintended pregnancy during the first year of use.
- In "normal" populations in which use is not always consistent or proper, the typical use failure rates are 12–22% for female condom.

Effectiveness of the Cervical Cap and Shield

- For perfect use, cap failure rates (primarily based on older and no-longer-available models) are 8–15% in nulliparous users and 20–30% in parous women *(38)*.
  - Failure rate for Lea's Shield is around 9–14%; 6-month failure rate of 6.4 per 100 women with a spermicide and 12.2 per 100 women when used without.
    - FemCap (first-generation, now obsolete) was 86.5% successful in preventing pregnancy in the 6-month clinical trials. The increased dimensions of the brim are designed to increase the stability and effectiveness of the second-generation FemCap.
      - Based on the small studies to date of the second-generation FemCap, the typical failure rate is estimated to be 7.6%. For perfect use, it is estimated that the failure rate is 2–4%. Perfect use includes using FemCap correctly every time, applying spermicides with each act of intercourse, and using emergency contraception as back-up if the cap is used incorrectly *(39)*.

Effectiveness of the Vaginal Sponge

In older studies, when the vaginal sponge was used correctly, about 9–14% of nulliparous and 9–27% of parous women became pregnant. Typical failure rates in nulliparous sponge users range from 9 to 21% and from 10 to 40% in parous users.

- Some newer studies of the Today® Sponge report lower failure rates in all women, regardless of their previous child-bearing history (91% effective in nulliparous women and 89.9% effective for parous women *[40–42]*).

Advantages of Cervical Barrier Methods

The cervical barrier methods have many advantages and are particularly good for motivated women who need intermittent protection. There are no systemic side effects and they can be backed up with emergency contraception to improve efficacy rates. Generally, these methods do not require more than limited partner involvement and are relatively easy and inexpensive to buy. Depending on the method, there are variable degrees of protection from STIs.

Advantages of the Diaphragm

- Allows better sexual spontaneity and more sexual sensation than male condom use *(43)*.
- Easy to use, reversible, affordable.

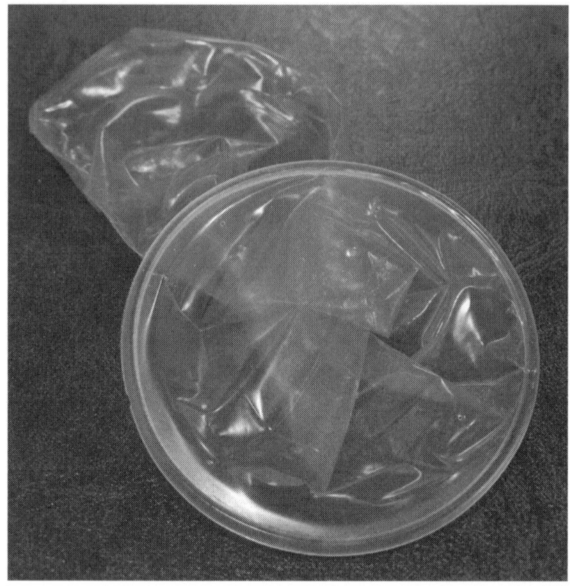

Fig. 6. Female condom showing outer ring with inner sheath and inner ring.

- Female-controlled contraception.
- The diaphragm is a barrier that may offer limited protection of the cervix from STIs *(44,45)*.
  - Observation trials have had variable results regarding protection from chlamydia, gonorrhea, and trichomoniasis *(46)*.
  - Several observation trials have reported that the diaphragm users have a lower risk of cervical dysplasia and cancer *(47–49)*.

Advantages of the Female Condom

- The polyurethane material making up the sheath of the female condom is impenetrable to HIV virus and to other STIs *(50)*. The inner and outer ring of the female condom prevents contact between the penis and the vagina and perineum (Fig. 6).
  - The female condom may offer as much protection (51) as the male condom, although more studies are needed.
  - Failure of protection occurs if the condom is torn or if the penis is not placed correctly inside the condom.
- The female condom can be placed in the vagina up to 8 hours before intercourse.
- The polyurethane material in the female condom is stronger than a male condom and less likely to tear or break.
  - It can be stored for long periods of time.
  - It does not deteriorate when exposed to an oil-based lubricant.

Advantages of the Second-Generation FemCap and Lea's Shield

- The current labeling gives cervical caps the longest duration of use of all the cervical barrier methods, that is, up to 48 hours of protection.
- No effects on sexual desire or pleasure.
- Can be inserted up to 42 hours before sexual intimacy.
- Safe and highly acceptable to many women and men.
- Easy to learn and simple to use (patient instructional brochure and video tape provided).
- Minimum training time for a health care provider.
- Fitting not necessary and usable by most women.
  - FemCap comes in three sizes and obstetrical history determines the size.
  - Lea's Shield is a one-size-fits-all product.
- Inexpensive and reusable for 1 year.
- No effect on fertility, instantly reversible when pregnancy is desired.
- No effects with breastfeeding or breast milk.
- Woman can have full control (no male involvement necessary).
- Portable with discrete cover.
- May offer similar protection from STIs as the diaphragm, although further studies needed. Protecting the cervix (covering the cervix plus use of an appropriate microcide) may be an important factor in preventing disease transmission *(52)*.
  - FemCap provides a microbicide reservoir on the vaginal side that provides immediate contact of any STI/HIV virus with the microbicide *(53)*.
- Made of durable, latex-free material that is easy to clean.
- Although acceptability ratings have varied, in some studies 87% of women said that they would recommend Lea's Shield and 55% of male partners said they liked the device. Of women who express an opinion regarding the diaphragm, 84% reported they preferred Lea's Shield *(54)*.

Advantages of the Sponge

- Contraceptive protection lasts for up to 24 hours no matter how many sexual contacts occur.
- One size fits all.
- Easy to use, inexpensive, portable.
- Over-the-counter availability.
- May provide limited protection from some STIs (gonorrhea, chlamydia) *(55)*.

Disadvantages

The most common disadvantages to cervical barrier methods are related to local irritation or physical discomfort. When used with a spermicide, the nonoxyl-9 can be very irritating, especially if used frequently. Increases in vaginal discharge, urinary tract infections, bacterial vaginosis, and candidiasis are problems related to use. A certain amount of preplanning and interruption of sexual activity may be necessary. Importantly, cervical barrier methods are not as effective as many other methods of contraception including oral contraceptive pills, intrauterine devices, implants, and injectables.

Disadvantages of the Diaphragm

- The diaphragm must be fitted by a trained health care worker.
  - Refitting may be necessary following childbirth, significant weight gain (usually >10–15 lb), vaginal or pelvic surgery, or if the current size is associated with bothersome vaginal irritation.
  - Women with poor vaginal tone, cystocele, rectocele, or uterine prolapse may not be able to use a diaphragm.
- Wearing a diaphragm for more than 24 hours may increase the risk for toxic shock syndrome (2.4 cases per 100,000 women using diaphragms *[56]*).
- Urinary tract infection more common in users *(57,58)*.
- Although not common, rectal, bladder, or uterine discomfort may occur.
  - Dyspareunia is rarely reported.
- Vaginal abrasion or laceration may occur, but is not common.
- Latex allergies are rare but are more common in health care workers who may have repeated exposure to latex gloves over many years.
  - Those with hypersensitivity to latex may use wide-seal rim diaphragm.
- Side effects of spermicides include irritation to either partner especially with frequent use, allergy to nonoxyl-9, and concerns over potential teratogenic effects if a fetus is incidentally exposed, although studies report no relationship *(59)*.

Disadvantages of the Female Condom

- The female condom may be physically uncomfortable to either the female user or male partner.
  - Occasionally, it may irritate the vagina or penis.
- Some couples complain that it decreases sensation.
- Some may find the appearance of the female condom unappealing or awkward, especially at first.
- A certain amount of "buy-in" from the male partner may be necessary.

Disadvantages of Cervical Cap and Shield

- Needs a prescription.
- Newer caps fit most nulliparous and parous women, although those with significant uterine or vaginal prolapse may not be good candidates.
- A few weeks needed to learn how to use the device properly; a back-up method is recommended during this time.
- Women may need to squat down to insert.
- The cap and shield provides up to 48 hours of contraceptive protection after placement, but this length of use may be associated with odor and discharge.
  - Longer use may increase the risk of toxic shock syndrome.

- Women may forget and leave the cap in longer than 48 hours because they are unable to feel its presence. Women may find that monitoring insertion and removal with a calendar may avoid this problem.
- Vaginal dryness, vaginal abrasion or laceration, dysparunia, penile irritation, bladder pain, or cramps may occur.
- Side effects of spermicides as listed in "Disadvantages of the Diaphragm" section.
- Planning necessary before sexual intimacy; must be placed before sexual arousal to avoid interruption of spontaneity and misplacement of the cap.
- Rarely, the male partner may have a sense of awareness and may object to its use.

Disadvantages of Vaginal Sponges

- Sponge must be placed just before intercourse and may interrupt sexual intimacy.
  - The sponge must be moistened with water before insertion.
- Sponge removal may be problem, especially in new users.
- The sponge must be left in place for at least 6 hours after intercourse.
- Foul odor or vaginal discharge common if the sponge left in place for more than 24 hours.
- Conflicting data suggests the sponge may be less effective in parous women (new studies report the sponge has similar effectiveness in parous and nulliparous).
- Side effects of spermicides as listed in "Disadvantages of the Diaphragm" section.

Good Candidates for Cervical Barrier Methods

- Motivated women who need intermittent protection.
- Women who cannot or prefer not to take hormonal contraceptives.
  - Women over 35 who smoke or have known cardiovascular disease or clotting problems or those with significant risk factors for cardiovascular disease.
- Women who need a back-up method, such as when pills are missed, during first month of pill use, or while using drugs that interfere with pill effectiveness.

Candidates for the Diaphragm, Cervical Cap, and Shield: Additional Considerations

Women with an allergy to latex are candidates for the cervical barriers made with silicone including the wide-seal rim diaphragm, cervical cap, and shield. Women with a history of frequent urinary tract infections or those that develop frequent urinary tract infections when using a diaphragm may find the cervical cap or shield a good option.

The diaphragm, cap, and shield are generally not recommended for women with the following:

- Significant vaginal abnormalities that interfere with placement.
  - Severe uterine prolapse, vaginal septum.
- During first 4–6 weeks after childbirth because of lochia or during heavy bleeding.
- Allergy or sensitivity to spermicides.
- History of toxic shock syndrome.

- Unstable, unpredictable, spontaneous sexual habits.
- Women uncomfortable with genital manipulation or inserting and removing foreign devices from their vaginas.

Additionally, the cervical cap is not recommended for women with:

- Current cervicitis or vaginal infection.
- Current pelvic, tubal, or ovarian infection.
- Polyurethane allergy.
- Abnormal/unresolved pap smear.

Candidates for the Female Condom: Additional Considerations

- Women with significant uterine or vaginal prolapse may be limited to the female or male condom.
- Women at risk for STIs or HIV transmission are good candidates for condom use (not as much data to support protection with female condoms as there is for the male condom).

Candidates for the Vaginal Sponge: Additional Considerations

Any woman who is comfortable using tampons or other vaginal contraceptives is a candidate for the sponge. Women should not use the sponge if:

- Either a woman or her partner have a sensitivity to:
  - Sulfa drugs. A very small number may be allergic to the metabisulfite preservative in the sponge.
  - Spermicide (Nonoxynol-9).
  - Polyurethane.
- She has a significant vaginal abnormality.
- She cannot risk any chance of pregnancy whatsoever.
- She has a risk of exposure to STIs or HIV (sponge may be used with a condom).
- She has had toxic shock syndrome.
- Within 4–8 weeks of a vaginal delivery.
- During menstruation.
- During a current vaginal infection.

Patient Counseling

The most common problems related to cervical barrier methods are local irritation, foul odor, or discharge. These usually abate within a few days after removing the method. When trying to select the best cervical barrier for a motivated user, consider the timing and style of protection she needs. Vaginal spermicides give 1 hour of protection, the diaphragm provides 6 hours of protection, the sponge provides 24 hours, and the cervical cap provides 48 hours of protection after insertion. The female condom is the method of choice in women with risk of STI exposure but may be more cumbersome and requires some partner cooperation. The diaphragm, cap, and shield must be cleaned and stored,

Table 2
Danger Signs of Toxic Shock Syndrome

Especially concerning if a barrier method has been in place for a prolonged period of time (longer than 24–30 hours).
High fever
Sore throat
Rash
Diarrhea or vomiting
Dizziness, fainting
Weakness, muscle aches

are used with a spermicide, and require a prescription. The diaphragm must be fitted by a health care provider. The female condom and sponge are readily available over the counter. Those who often use oil-based lubricants or medications are not good candidates for a latex diaphragm (Table 1).

A serious, although rare, side effect of cervical barriers is toxic shock syndrome. The danger signs are listed in Table 2. A comparison of barrier methods is giving in Table 3.

Diaphragm: Instructions for Use

Instructions on how to use a diaphragm are included with the diaphragm. Some women find squatting the easiest position, whereas others find lying down or standing with one foot on a chair the best position.

Inserting a Diaphragm Without An Inserter: An Arcing-Spring (All-Flex) or Coil-Spring Diaphragm (Fig. 7)

- After a contraceptive cream or jelly is placed in the center of the cup (some recommend that it be placed on both sides of the diaphragm) the diaphragm is folded together so that the cream or jelly is held inside. Some women find placing some on the rim makes insertion easier. The folded diaphragm is gently inserted into the vagina with the edges facing forward/upward. The diaphragm is then pushed as high as comfortably possible so that the lower rim rests behind the public bone and the higher rim slides up behind the cervix into the fornix. With proper placement, the dome of the diaphragm should completely cover the cervix, placing the spermicide directly against the cervix.
    - The patient should be taught how to locate the cervix behind the dome of the diaphragm to insure proper placement. The cervix feels like a "nose" that should be covered completely by the diaphragm.
- If placed properly, the diaphragm provides 6 hours of protection. It must be kept in place for 6 hours after intercourse but no longer than 24 hours. For repeated acts of intercourse within the first 6 hours, the diaphragm should not be removed, but additional spermicide should be placed vaginally.

Table 3
Barrier Methods Time Comparisons

Method	*May insert before intercourse*	*Protection after insertion lasts for*	*After last intercourse, leave in place for at least*	*Remove within*
Diaphragm	30 minutes to less than 6 hours prior	6 hours (Additional spermicide added for each additional intercourse.)	6 hours	24 hours
FemCap™ (second generation)	Should be inserted 15 minutes (up to 42 hours) before the start of sexual activity	48 hours (Check the position of FemCap and insert additional spermicide without removing the cap before each repeated intercourse within the next 48 hours.)	6 hours	48 hours
Lea's Shield®	Should be inserted before the start of sexual activity	48 hours (Additional spermicide needed if intercourse occurs after 8 hours.)	8 hours	24 hours
Sponge	Up to 90 minutes prior	24 hours	6 hours	24 hours
Female condom	0–8 hours prior	While in place	Immediate removal after intercourse	
Male condom	After erection	While in place	Removal while penis still erect	
Vaginal spermicides	5–60 minutes depending on type	1 hour	6 hours	

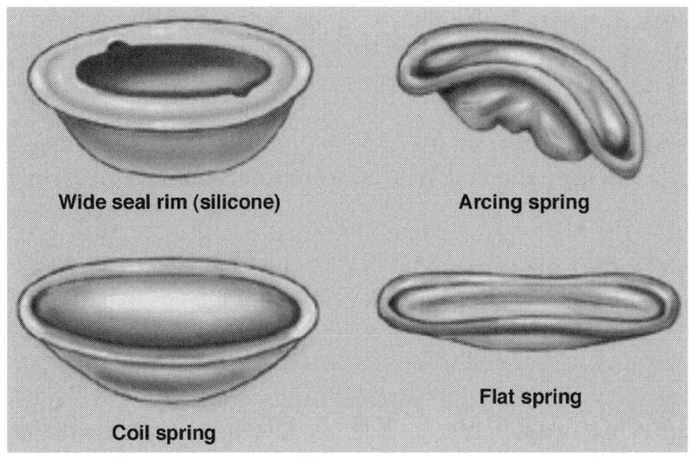

Fig. 7. Types of diaphragm rims. (Reproduced with permission from Marie Dauenheimer, MA, CMI.)

- To remove the diaphragm, the front rim is either grasped using two fingers or hooked using one finger. For removal it is sometimes necessary to pull the diaphragm away from the underlying vaginal tissue because a slight suction may hold the diaphragm in place.
  - The diaphragm should be cleaned with mild soap and air-dried.
  - Check the diaphragm for holes or tears by visual inspection and by holding it up to the light.

Inserting a Diaphragm With An Inserter: Flat- or Coil-Spring Diaphragm (Fig. 7)

- This diaphragm comes with a special plastic applicator that has a series of small notches, corresponding to the size in centimeters of a diaphragm. The diaphragm rim, with the dome facing upward, is hooked into the large notch at the end of the applicator. The other end of the rim is hooked into the notch corresponding to the size of the diaphragm. By doing this, the diaphragm is stretched into a flat oval with the dome puckered into folds. The spermicide is placed into these folds and a small amount placed around the rim. With the spermicide facing upward, the applicator is placed into the vagina and angled toward the small of the back. It is slid into the small space between the cervix and the rear wall. When pushed as far as it will go, the applicator is twisted to release the diaphragm and then removed. With one finger, the front edge is pushed up behind the pubic bone. Finally, a check is made to make sure that the diaphragm covers the cervix.

Instructions for Use: Female Condom

- The female condom is available as an over-the-counter product and is marketed for one-time use.
- The female condom can be inserted up to 8 hours before intercourse.

- It should not be used with a male condom because the two condoms may stick to each other and cause discomfort or displacement.

Instructions for insertion:

- For insertion, the inner, smaller ring is squeezed and inserted into the vagina. The outer rim is placed evenly over the introitus.

INSTRUCTIONS FOR USE: CERVICAL CAPS

To ensure correct placement, the FDA has strongly advised women to insert the FemCap before sexual arousal. FDA also recommends that a back-up method be used during the learning phase and that emergency contraception be used as a back-up method, if needed, in case the woman has not used the FemCap or has used it incorrectly. There is an instructional video supplied with the FemCap.

After removing a cap, wash the device with a mild soap, air-dry, and store it in its original container in a cool, dry place. Before using the device again, inspect it for weak spots or pinholes by holding it up to a light or by filling it with water.

All prescription barrier devices eventually wear out. Diaphragms and cervical caps often need to be replaced after 1–2 years of use, and a cervical shield may last 6 months to 2 years. A new fitting for a diaphragm may be necessary after a pregnancy, significant weight gain or loss, or abdominal or pelvic surgery. A change in FemCap size may be necessary after a pregnancy, including miscarriage, induced abortion, or delivery.

Insertion/Removal of FemCap

The FemCap has an asymmetrical rim designed so that the larger rim fits into the top of the vagina. Spermicide is placed on the inner and outer surfaces. It may be necessary to tip the rim of the cap to release the suction for removal.

- Knowing the position of the cervix is very important because the cervix is the target, and knowing where it is helps to determine how deep to place the FemCap. To check the position of the cervix, it may be easiest to squat down and bear down and insert a finger deep into the vagina. The cervix feels like the tip of a nose.
- Apply a very small amount of spermicide (about 1/4 tsp.) in the bowl of the FemCap and spread a thin layer over the outer brim (but not over the area where the cap is being held). Turn the cap over and apply the bulk of spermicide (about 1/2 tsp.) in the groove between the brim and the dome. (This is the area that faces outward from the cervix and collects most of the sperm when placed correctly (Fig. 8).
- The squeezed, flattened cap is inserted into the vagina with the bowl facing upward and the long brim entering first.
- FemCap is pushed downward toward the rectum and slid as high into the vagina as possible.
- After placement, a finger should be used to make sure the cap is pushed all the way in and covers the cervix completely. Make sure that it is not partway between the vaginal opening and the cervix.

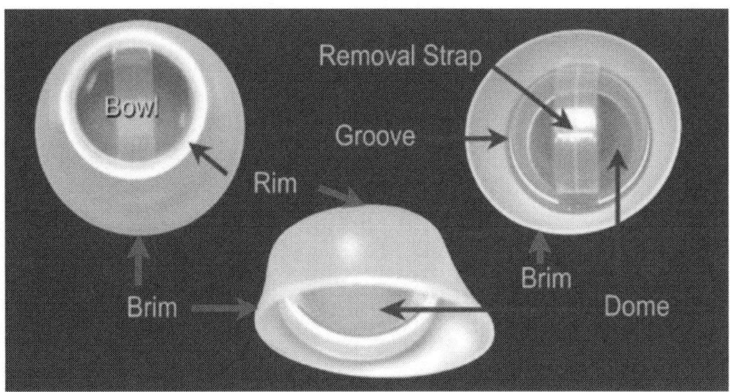

Fig. 8. The bowl of the second-generation FemCap is placed over the cervix. It is designed to cover the cervix completely. The brim forms a seal against the vaginal wall and funnels the ejaculate fluid into the groove. (Reproduced with permission from FemCap, Inc. and Alfred Shihata, MD.)

 - ◦ If the FemCap is placed correctly, women are rarely aware of its presence during either daily activities or during intercourse. Men also are usually unaware of it presence and it should not interfere with sexual pleasure.
- Wait at least 6 hours after the last act of intercourse before removing the cap. To remove the cap, it is best to squat and bear down. This will bring the cap closer to the vaginal opening.
  - ◦ Rotate the FemCap in any direction, or push the tip of a finger against the dome to dimple it. These maneuvers help to break the suction and allow a finger to fit between the dome and the removal strap. Hook the removal strap with the tip of a finger and gently pull it down and out of the vagina.
  - ◦ Wash the FemCap with soap and rinse it with tap water. Pat dry and allow the cap to air-dry.
  - ◦ Store the cap in its plastic storage container.

Insertion of Lea's Shield

Lea's Shield is much like a diaphragm, although it is designed to fit around the cervix. It has a central one-way valve that allows for cervical mucus to pass. It is one size fits all so that fitting in not required. It is not necessary to form suction with the cervix when using Lea's Shield.

Insertion of Lea's Shield is almost as easy as insertion of a tampon. Studies showed that the average woman can learn how to insert and remove the Lea's Shield just by reading the Lea's Shield user manual. Lea's Shield consists of a cap-shaped appendage and a "control loop" that together form an elliptical device. The shield is placed behind the pubic bone, as far as it can comfortably go. The loop aids in insertion and removal of the shield and stabilizes the device. When in place, the lower tip of the cap is positioned under the cervix (with the cervix resting in the interior of the cap) while the control loop extends toward the posterior aspect of the pubic symphysis.

- Spermicide should be applied to the rim and the bowl (one-third full) of the device before insertion.
- Squeeze the device.
- Insert it and push it in as far as it can go. It "settles in place" and automatically completely covers the cervix.
- Additional spermicide is only required if sex occurs more than 8 hours after insertion. If more spermicide is required, it should be placed in the vagina without removing Lea's Shield.
- For removal, grasp the loop with one finger and remove the device.
- Lea's Shield should be washed thoroughly with mild liquid soap for approximately 2 minutes, dried, and then stored in its silk pouch (*see* user manual).
- It is recommended that Lea's Shield be replaced if it shows any signs of wear or deterioration.

Insertion of Prentif™ Cavity Rim (Currently Unavailable Because of Manufacturing Difficulties)

Before use, a spermicide is placed in the cervical cap, filling it to about one-third full. The cap is placed against the cervix with the lower rim fit snugly placed under the cervix. As the cap is placed, it is unfolded. As the dome expands, suction is produced that holds the cap in place. It may be necessary to tip the rim of the cap to release the suction for removal.

Instructions for Use: Vaginal Sponge

- Remove the sponge from its pouch. Moisten it with about 2 tbsp. tap water and gently squeeze to activate the spermicide.
- Fold the foamy sponge in half with the dimple side facing upward. Holding the sponge between two fingers, insert it deep into the vagina, up to and against the cervix. The dimple should face the cervix and the loop should face away from the cervix. Palpate around the sponge to make sure it completely covers the cervix.
- After intercourse, wait at least 6 hours before removal.
  - For removal, place a finger into the vagina and reach upward to find the loop.
  - Bear down and push the sponge toward the vaginal opening. Hook the finger around the loop or grasp the sponge between fingers.
  - Withdraw the sponge from the vagina. If the vaginal muscles are tight and removal is difficult, relax, wait a few minutes, and try again.

Selecting Available Options, Fitting, and Counseling

Selecting the Correct Diaphragm

There are four major types of diaphragms as determined by the rim flexibility, degree of arch, spring strength, and width (Fig. 7). The arching-spring diaphragm is the easiest type to insert because it has a firm rim that forms an arch when folded. The arching spring is a good choice for women with decreased vaginal tone or pelvic relaxation. Latex diaphragms are available in all rim styles and silicone diaphragms are available as wide-seal rims in either the arching or coil spring type. Diaphragms fitting rings come in sizes 60–90, although actual diaphragms are available from size 50–105 mm in diameter. The all-flex diaphragm is very popular and allows a moderate, even, and usually comfortable spring strength. The most common size diaphragm is 75 mm.

Diaphragm manufacturers supply a set of fitting diaphragms or fitting rings that come with a variety of rim spring strengths. It is generally best for the patient to practice insertion and removal with the fitting diaphragm and be given a prescription for the same size and same rim style.

- Coil-spring diaphragm (coiled wire).
  - Soft, flat, flexible rim with intermediate spring strength.
  - Intended for women with average vaginal tone (average strength of the vaginal muscles) and no genital abnormalities. Good for those who feel the arching-spring diaphragm to be too firm.
  - Folds flat when folded for insertion and can be inserted with an introducer.
  - Products: Koromex®, sizes 50–95, latex; Ortho®, sizes 50–100, latex; Ramses® Flexible Cushioned, sizes 50–95, gum rubber.
- Arching-spring diaphragm (combination metal spring).
  - Very firm, sturdy rim with firm spring strength.
  - Can be used by all women; also intended for women with weak vaginal tone, moderate descent of bladder or rectum (cystocele or rectocele), or with their uterus bent far forward or backward, average pubic notch.
  - Very popular because it offers the easiest insertion because it bends everywhere and forms an arch when folded.
  - May be less comfortable than the other two styles after insertion.
  - Products: Koroflex®, sizes 60–95, latex; Allflex®, sizes 55–95, latex; Ramses Bendex, sizes 65–95, gum rubber.
- Wide-seal rim.
  - Has a flexible, 1.5-cm wide flange attached to the inner edge of the rim. The flange holds the spermicide inside the diaphragm and forms a tight seal between the vaginal wall and the diaphragm, providing increased suction action, which minimizes risk of diaphragm dislodging during intercourse.
    - Available with either an arcing or coil spring (Omniflex).
  - Distributed directly to clinic or directly from the manufacturer.
  - Products available:
    - Milex® Wide-Seal Arching, sizes 60–95, latex; Milex Omniflex Coil Spring, sizes 60–95, latex.
    - Milex Wide-Seal Silicone Arching and Omniflex.

    - Silicone associated with longer shelf life, does not absorb odors or secretions, can be autoclaved, hypoallergenic.
- Flat-spring diaphragm (flat metal band).
    - Thin, flat, delicate rim with gentle spring strength (similar to coil spring but thinner).
    - Intended for women with very firm vaginal tone, nulliparous, a shallow pubic arch, or those with a shallow notch behind the public bone.
    - May not be stocked in all pharmacies.
    - Folds flat for insertion and can be inserted with a diaphragm introducer.
    - Products: Ortho-White® Diaphragm, sizes 55–95, latex.

Women who are not satisfied with a particular style diaphragm may find that another style is significantly more acceptable. In a study in college students, overall satisfaction throughout 1 year of use was significantly better with the coil-spring diaphragm compared with the arching-spring diaphragm. The study results demonstrate that certain diaphragm styles may improve women's use of and satisfaction with the diaphragm *(60)*.

Diaphragm Fitting and Counseling

Proper fitting and patient education along with user motivation are the keys to success (61). (See Table 3.)

An extended visit may be needed for proper fitting and counseling. Diaphragm-fitting rings can be obtained from the manufacturer. Examinaton gloves and vaginal lubricating gel are used during the fitting. Optimally, the patient should do at least one insertion and removal while still in the clinic in case she experiences problems. Practicing again at home before use is advisable.

- A middle and index finger (or measuring instrument) are used to measure the distance from the bottom of the pubic bone to the posterior fornix of the vagina. Before the fingers are removed, the thumb (or an instrument) is used to mark the spot where the public arch touches the top of the index finger. This measurement is then used to select a diaphragm size (75 mm is a common size).
- The selected size is lubricated, folded in half, and then placed in the vagina with the two rims touching and facing upwards. Holding the vulva open with one hand, the health care provider uses the other hand to insert the folded diaphragm into the vagina and to direct it into the posterior fornix. The correct placement of the diaphragm is then confirmed by palpating the cervix through the dome of the fitting diaphragm. The anterior rim is then checked to see that it fits snugly and directly behind the public bone.
    - The size that best fits is the one that completely covers the cervix and extends into the posterior vaginal fornix while fitting securely/gently behind the public symphysis. Generally, the proper fit is the largest diaphragm that is comfortable for the client.

      - Checking that the proper size has been selected by checking the fit of one size larger or one size smaller may be helpful.
        - A too-small diaphragm will not fit up snugly behind the pubic bone and it will fall out when the patient sits on the toilet, ambulates, or does a Valsalva's manueuver.
        - A too-large diaphragm will rest improperly in front of the public bone and be uncomfortable; it may interfere with urination.
- The diaphragm is removed by "hooking" the anterior rim with a finger and pulling the diaphragm down and out of the vagina.
- After the correct size is determined, the patient should be taught:
  - How to place about 1 tsp. of the spermicide into the dome of a diaphragm (for added efficacy, jelly can be applied around the rim).
  - How to insert the folded diaphragm.
  - How to feel for the cervix through the dome.
  - How to remove the diaphragm.
  - Instructions: the diaphragm must remain in place for at least 6 hours after intercourse but not for more than 24 hours.
    - For additional acts of intercourse, the diaphragm remains in place and additional spermicide jelly is inserted.
    - The diaphragm is washed and checked periodically for holes, but many last several years.

One Available Option: Female Condom

Reality®, the only female condom on the US market today, was approved by the FDA in 1993. The female condom consists of two flexible polyurethane rings and a loose-fitting polyurethane sheath. One ring is at the base of the sheath and is used for insertion and for holding the top of the sheath in place at the top of the vagina. The other ring forms the external opening and holds the outer portion of the sheath over the perineum. The inner lining of the sheath is coated with a lubricant and an additional lubricant can be use on the exterior for easier insertion. The female condom contains no spermicide.

Selecting the Proper Cervical Cap or Shield

- Lea's Shield was approved by the FDA in 2002. Lea's Shield can be ordered from YAMA, Inc. (Millburn, NJ; http://www.birthcontrol.com/leabody.html). It is a one-size-fits-all oval cap containing a central valve that allows passage of cervical mucus or discharge. It has an attached loop that helps with removal. It is used with a spermicide and is similar in use to a diaphragm. It is made of medical-grade silicone rubber.
- The second-generation FemCap comes in three sizes as determined by the inner diameter of the rim (FemCap Inc., Del Mar, CA, www.femcap.com). The fit of the FemCap is determined by the obstetrical history of the potential user. Women who have never been pregnant will use the 22-mm FemCap; women who have

been pregnant but never delivered vaginally (miscarried or had caesarian section) will use the 26-mm FemCap; and women who have vaginally delivered a full-term baby will use the 30-mm FemCap. If in doubt, the medium size is recommended.

  - The FemCap is made with silicone rubber and has an asymmetrical rim that flares outward. The cap fits over and completely covers the cervix and the rim fits into the vaginal fornices, the larger brim fitting into the back of the vagina. The FemCap has a brim, a dome, a groove between the dome and the brim, and a removal strap.
  - The retail price is around $50 for a single FemCap and it should last 2 years. The FemCap kit contains an FDA-approved instructional videotape. It is recommended that a back-up method be used during the first few weeks of use.
- The Prentif Cavity Rim cervical cap is a deep cap made of rubber that has a solid round rim. It is designed to fit firmly around the cervix. A small groove, located along the inner rim is designed to improve the seal between the cap and the cervix. A spermicide is placed to partially fill the cap before insertion. The Prentif Cavity-Rim cervical cap was previously available in sizes 22, 25, 28, and 31 mm. Because of manufacturing difficulties and low sales, this cervical cap is no longer available in the United States.

One Available Option: Vaginal Sponge

Today sponge has been recently reintroduced into the US over-the-counter market (Allendale Pharmaceuticals). The availability of the sponge may be currently limited. The sponge is a one-size-fits-all, small, round polyurethane sponge containing nonoxynol-9 spermicide. The concavity on one side is designed to fit over the cervix. On the other side is a loop that helps with removal of the sponge after use.

In Europe, there is a tablet called Pharmatex that uses the spermicide benzalkonium chloride. Another sponge, called Protectaid® is manufactured in Canada. It is designed to cause less vaginal irritation by incorporating three different spermicides in low concentrations.

REFERENCES

1. Centers for Disease Control and Prevention, National Center for HIV, STD, and TB Prevention. (2003) Fact Sheet for Public Health Personnel: Male Latex Condoms and Sexually Transmitted Diseases. www.cdc.gov/hiv/pubs/facts/condoms.htm. Accessed March 11, 2006.
2. Centers for Disease Control and Prevention. (1998) Trends in sexual risk behaviors among high school students—United States, 1991–1997. MMWR Morb Mortal Wkly Rep 47:749–752.
3. American Academy of Pediatrics Committee on Adolescence. (2001) Condom use by adolescents. Pediatrics 107:1463–1469.
4. Mosher WD, Pratt WF. (1993) AIDS-related behavior among women 15–44 years of age: United States, 1988 and 1990. Adv Data 22:1–15.
5. Walsh TL, Frezieres FG, Peacock K, Nelson AL, Clark VA, Bernstein L. (2003) Evaluation of the efficacy of a nonlatex condom: results from a randomized, controlled clinical trial. Perspect Sex Reprod Health 35:79–86.

6. Carey RF, Herman WA, Retta SM, Rinaldi JE, Herman BA, Athey TW. (1992) Effectiveness of latex condoms as a barrier to human immunodeficiency virus-sized particles under conditions of simulated use. Sex Transm Dis 19:230–234.
7. Davis KR, Weller SC. (1999) The effectiveness of condoms in reducing heterosexual transmission of HIV. Fam Plann Perspect 31:272–279.
8. Pinkerton SD, Abramson PR. (1997) Effectiveness of condoms in preventing HIV transmission. Soc Sci Med 44:1303–1312.
9. Cates W Jr, Holmes KK. (1996) Re: condom efficacy against gonorrhea and nongonococcal urethritis. Am J Epidemiol 143:843–844.
10. Zenilman JM, Weisman CS, Rompalo Am, et al. (1995) Condom use to prevent incident STIs: the validity of self-reported condom use. Sex Transm Dis 22:15–21.
11. Wald A, Langenberg AG, Link K, et al. (2001) Effect of condoms on reducing the transmission of herpes simplex virus type 2 from men to women. JAMA 285:3100–3106.
12. Warner L, Newman DR, Austin HA, et al. (2004) Condom effectiveness for reducing transmission of gonorrhea and chlamydia: the importance of assessing partner infection status. Am J Epidemimiol 159:242–251.
13. Cates W, Stone KM. (1992) Family planning, sexually transmitted diseases and contraceptive choice: a literature update—part I. Fam Plann Perspect 24:75–84.
14. Cramer DW, Goldman MB, Schiff I, et al. (1987) The relationship of tubal infertility to barrier method and oral contraceptive use. JAMA 257:2446–2450.
15. Lytle CED, Routson LB, Seaborn GB, Dixon LG, Bushar HF, Cyr WH. (1997) An in vitro evaluation of condoms aas barriers to sa small virus. Sex Transm Dis 24:161–164.
16. Wang PD, Lin RS. (1996) Risk factors for cervical intraepithelial neoplasia in Taiwan. Gynecol Oncol 62:10–18.
17. Centers for Disease Control and Prevention. (1998) 1998 Guidelines for the treatment of sexually transmitted diseases. MMWR 47:1–116.
18. Voeller BV, Coulson A, Bernstein GS, Nakamura R. (1989) Mineral oil lubricants cause rapid deterioration of latex condoms. Contraception 39:95–101.
19. Fisher AA. (1987) Condom dermatitis in either partner. Cutis 39:284–285.
20. Roddy RE, Zekeng I, Ryan KA, Ubald T, Tweedy KG. (2002) The effect of nonoxynol-9 gel on urogential gonorrohea and Chlamydia infection. JAMA 287:1117–1122.
21. Louv WC, Austin H, Alexander WJ, Stagno S, Cheeks J. (1988) A clinical trial of nonoxynol-9 for preventing gonococcal and chlamydial infections. J Infect Dis 158:518–523.
22. Barbone F, Austin H, Louv WC, Alexander WJ. (1990) A follow-up study of methods of contraception, sexual activity and rates of trichomoniasis, candidiasis, and bacterial vaginosis. Am J Obstet Gynecol 163:510–514.
23. Van Damme L, Ramjee G, Alary M, et al. (2002) Effectiveness of COL-1492, a nonoxynol-9 vaginal gel, on HIV-1 transmission in female sex workers: a randomized controlled trial. Lancet 360:971–977.
24. Van Damme L, Ramjee G, Alary M, et al. (2001) Effectivenss of COL-1492, a nonoxynol-9 vaginal gel, on HIV-1 transmission in female sex workers: a randomized controlled trial. Sex Transm Dis 28:394–400.
25. Hooton TM, Scholes D, Hughes JP, et al. (1996) A prospective study of risk factors for symptomatic urinary tract infection in young women. N Engl J Med 335:468–474.
26. Simpson JL, Phillips OP. (1990) Spermicides, hormonal contraception and congenital malformations. Adv Contracept 6:141–167.
27. Einarson TR, Koren G, Mattice D, Schechter-Tsafriri O. (1990) Maternal spermicide use nad adverse reproductive outcome: a meta-analysis. Am J Obstet Gynecol 162:655–660.
28. Harrison T, Backes K. (2004) A potential new role for cervical barrier methods. Southern Africa HIV/AIDS Information Dissemination service, 10:1–3.

29. Trussell J, Sturgen K, Stricker J, Dominik R. (1994) Comparative contraceptiive efficacy of the female condom and other barrier methods. Fam Plann Perspect 26:66–72.
30. Cook I, Nanda K, Grimes DA. (2003) Diaphragm versus diaphragm with spermicides for contraception. Cochrane Datbase Syst Rev 1:CD002031.
31. Smith C, Farr G, Feldblum PJ, Spence A. (1995) Effectiveness of the non-spermicidal fit-free diaphragm. Contraception 51:289–291.
32. Bounds W, Guillebaud J, Dominik R, Dalberth BT. (1995) The diaphragm with and without spermicide. A randomizecd, comparative efficacy trial. J Reprod Med 40:764–774.
33. Lane ME, Arceo R, Sobrero AJ. (1976) Successful use of the diaphragm and jelly by a young population: report of a clinical study. Fam Plann Perspect 8:81–86.
34. Shihata A. (2004) New FDA-approved woman-controlled, latex-free barrier contraceptive device "FemCap." In: Daya S, Gunby J, Pierson R, eds. Research Papers in Fertility and Reproductive Medicine, 1271. Toronto: Elsevier, pp. 303–306.
35. McClure DA, Edelman DA. (1985) Worldwide method effectiveness of the Today® vaginal contraceptive sponge. Adv Contracept 1:305–311.
36. North BB, Vorhauer BW. (1985) Use of the Today® contraceptive sponge in the United States. Int J Fertil 30:81–84.
37. Edelman DA, North BB. (1987) Updated pregnancy rates for Today® contraceptive sponge. Am J Obstet Gynecol 157:1164–1165.
38. Rieder J, Coupey SM. (1999) The use of nonhormonal methods of contraception in adolescents. Pediatr Clin North Am 46:671–694.
39. Kelaghan J, Rubin GL, Ory HW, Layde PM. (1982) Barrier-method contraceptives and pelvic inflammatory disease. JAMA 248;184–187.
40. Rosenberg MJ, Davidson AJ, Chen HJ, Judson FN, Douglas JM. (1992) Barrier contraceptives and sexually transmitted diseases in women: a comparison of female-dependent methos and condoms. Am J Public Health 82:669–674.
41. d'Oro LC, Parazzini F, Naldi I, La Vecchia C. (1994) Barrier methods of contraception, spermicides, and sexually transmitted diseases: a review. Genitourin Med 70:410–417.
42. Peters RK, Thomas D, Hagan DG, Mack TM, Henderson BE. (1986) Risk factors for invasive cervical cancer among Latinas and non-Latinas in Los Angeles county. J Natil Cancer Inst 77:1063–1077.
43. Parazzini F, Negri E, La Vecchia C, Fedele L. (1989) Barrier methods of contraception and the risk of cervical neoplasia. Contraception 40:519–530.
44. Hildesheim A, Brinton LA, Malin K, et al. (1990) Barrier and spermicidal contraceptive methods and risk of invasive cervical cancer. Epidemiology 1:266–272.
45. Drew WL, Blair M, Miner RC, Conant M. (1990) Evaluation of the virus permeability of a new condom for women. Sex Transm Dis 17:110–112.
46. Soper DE, Shoupe D, Shangold GA, Shangold MM, Gutmann, Mercer L. (1993) Prevention of vaginal trichomononiasis by compliant use of the female condom. Sex Transm Dis 20:137–139.
47. Moench TR, Chipato T, Padian NS. (2001) Preventing disease by protecting the cervix: the unexplored promise of internal cervical barrier devices. AIDS 15:1–8.
48. Mauck C, Glover LH, Miller E, et al. (1996) Lea's Shield®: a study of the safety and efficacy of a new vaginal barrier contraceptive used with and without spermicide. Contraception 53:329–335.
49. Moench TR, Chipato T, Padian NS. (2001) Preventing disease by protecting the cervix; the unexplored promise of internal vaginal barrier devices. AIDS 15:1595–1602.
50. Schwartz B, Gaventa S, Broome CV, et al. (1989) Nonmenstrual toxic shock syndrome associated with barrier contraceptives: report of a case-control study. Rev Infect Dis 11:S43–S48.

51. Fihn SD, Latham Rh, Roberts P, Running K, Stamm WE. (1985) Association between diaphragm use and urinary tract infection. JAMA 254:2540–2245.
52. Foxman B. (1990) Recurring urinary tract infection: incidence and risk factors. Am J Public Health 80:331–333.
53. Food and Drug Administration (FDA). (1986) Data does not support association between spermicides, birth defects. FDA Bulletin, pp. 11–21.
54. Loucks A. (1989) A comparison of satisfaction with types of diaphragms among women in a college population. J Obstet Gynecol Neonatal Nurs 18:194–200.
55. Allen RE. (2004) Diaphragm fitting. Am Fam Physician 69:97–100, 103, 105–106.

11 Behavioral Methods of Contraception

Jennefer A. Russo, MD *and Anita L. Nelson,* MD

CONTENTS

INTRODUCTION

A surprising number of couples rely on behavioral methods of contraception, at least intermittently. Abstinence promotion usually targets adolescents, but abstinence is used by women of all ages. Natural family planning (NFP) and fertility awareness methods (FAMs) are critically important for many couples for whom this is the only religiously, culturally, or socially acceptable method. *Coitus interruptus* has a typical failure rate comparable with the more effective female barrier methods. This chapter provides information about the techniques found to enhance the success of each of these methods.

CANDIDATES FOR NFP OR FAMS

Only women with regular cycles are appropriate candidates for NFP techniques. This typically excludes women with polycystic ovary syndrome and women who have menstrual disruptions because of breastfeeding, as well as postpartum and perimenopausal women and those currently or recently using medications and herbs that affect their menstrual cycling. Success requires that both members of the couple agree to abstain or use protection during the data collection periods and during the at-risk days. In clinical trials, the greatest source of failures has been that couples decide to have intercourse despite clear indications of ovulation *(1)*. Given such realities, NFP users should be extensively counseled about emergency contraception and offered kits by advance prescription.

From: *Current Clinical Practice: The Handbook of Contraception: A Guide for Practical Management*
Edited by: D. Shoupe and S. L. Kjos © Humana Press, Totowa, NJ

EFFICACY AND CONTINUATION RATES

Typical use failure rates are reported to be 25%. The typical use failure rates vary little among the currently available NFP and FAM, mostly because of routine violation *(2)*. However, failure rates associated with consistent and correct method use do vary, depending on whether pre-ovulation intercourse is permitted or excluded. The calendar method has a 9% failure rate with correct and consistent use, compared with 3% for ovulation detection, 2% for symptothermal method, and 1% for post-ovulation method *(3)*.

Continuation rates with NFP methods in well-supported programs after 1 year range between 52 and 74% *(3)*. Advantages of NFP are wide-ranging: no exogenous devices or drugs are routinely used, most couples learn a great deal about their own reproductive physiology, and NFP may be the only method accepted by various religions and cultural groups. The same techniques for identifying at-risk days can be used by couples seeking pregnancy to conceive. There are no direct medical side effects from use of the method, although the psychosocial implications of avoiding intercourse for significant periods of time should be taken into account by couples considering use of these methods.

TRAINING

With the exception of the standard days method with CycleBeads™, couples need extensive formal training to effectively practice periodic abstinence or fertility awareness. Because it is quite time-consuming to provide couples with all of the needed information in a busy office practice, it may be helpful to have available community resources to provide more detailed education. The organizations listed in Table 1 can provide advice, charts, and teaching plans.

OPTIONS: BEHAVIORAL METHODS OF CONTRACEPTION

Abstinence

Worldwide, it has been estimated that 200 million reproductive-aged women use abstinence as their method of birth control, where abstinence is defined as the avoidance of penile-insertive vaginal intercourse. For some women, this is a permanent choice, but for others it may be a temporary one. This latter situation accounts for the variable success rate of abstinence. If practiced, abstinence should be 100% effective, but when declared as a method at one point of time (such as an annual visit) but not practiced consistently until the next visit, "abstinence" carries with it a measurable risk of pregnancy.

Much effort has been invested in developing programs to encourage abstinence among adolescent men and women. The benefits are obvious: abstinence provides the only truly effective way to prevent pregnancy and sexually transmitted infections (STIs). It can help promote self-esteem and maintain a young

Table 1
Natural Family Planning Resources for Advice, Charts, Teaching Plans, and Referrals

Billings Ovulation Method Association, NFP Office
316-N 7th Avenue
St. Cloud, MN 56303
Phone no.: (888) 867-6371

Calgary Billings Centre of Natural Family Planning
Room 1
1247 Bel-Aire Dr SW
Calgary, AB T2V 2C1
Phone no.: (403) 252-3929
Website: www.billings-centre.ab.ca

California Association of Natural Family Planning
1010 11th Street
Suite 200
Sacramento, CA 95814
Phone no.: (877) 332-2637
Website: www.canfp.org

The Couple to Couple League International
PO Box 111184
Cincinnati, OH 45211-1184
Phone no.: (513) 471-2000
Website: www.ccli.org

Institute for Reproductive Health
Georgetown University Medical Center
3 PHC, Room 300r
3800 Reservoir Road NW
Washington, DC 20007
Phone no.: (202) 687-1392
Website: www.dml.georgetown.edu/depts/irh

National Center for Women's Health
Pope Paul VI Institute
6901 Mercy Road
Omaha, NE 68106-2604
Phone no.: (402) 390-6600
Website: www.popepaulvi.com

Family of the Americas Foundation, Inc.
PO Box 1170
Dunkirk, MD 20754-1170
Phone no.: (800) 443-3395
Website: www.familyplanning.net

(continued)

Table 1 *(Continued)*
Natural Family Planning Resources for Advice, Charts, Teaching Plans, and Referrals

Natural Family Planning Center of Washington DC
8514 Bradmoor Drive
Bethesda, MD 20817-3810
Phone no.: (301) 897-9323

Northwest Family Services
4805 NE Glisan Street
Portland, OR 97213
Phone no.: (503) 230-6377
Website: www.nwfs.org

Twin Cities NFP Center
HealthEast, St. Joseph's Hospital
69 W Exchange Street
St. Paul, MN 55102
Phone no.: (651) 232-3088
Website: www.tcnfp.org

woman's options for self-growth and financial self-sufficiency. In the United States, however, only about half of all adolescents choose this method. In a 2004 review of data from the 2002 National Survey of Family Growth, Abma et al. found that 47% of female adolescents and 46% of male adolescents reported that they had engaged in sexual intercourse at least once in their lives. For the age group of 15–17, there was a decrease in sexual behavior from 1995 to 2002, with 30% of girls and 31% of boys reporting sexual activity in 2002 versus 38% of girls and 43% of boys in 1995 *(4)*.

Risk factors for early and/or unprotected intercourse among adolescents have been identified. Low income, poor school performance, siblings with teen pregnancies, early puberty, and other risk-taking behaviors have all been demonstrated to be associated with an adolescent's risk for unintended pregnancy. However, teen sexual activity and adolescent pregnancy are not restricted to these high-risk groups; adolescent pregnancy is an epidemic that cuts across all socioeconomic and ethnic groups. Even parent–family connectedness and perceived school connectedness were not found to protect against pregnancy *(5)*.

Abstinence-promoting programs must be broad-based. They must also recognize that, for many adolescents, the risk of an unintended pregnancy is minor compared with other risks that they face on a daily basis. For example, in 2004, the Center for Disease Control and Prevention estimated that 33% of adolescents had been in a physical fight in the last 12 months and 17% had carried a weapon in the last 30 days *(6)*.

Experience with a wide variety of abstinence-promoting programs has provided important insights. Programs based on a "just say no" approach or that threatened young women with STIs or unintended pregnancies if they engage in sexual activity ("scare them straight" approach) have been shown to have no effect on either sexual behavior or contraceptive use. Analysis of the "Postponing Sexual Involvement" curriculum used in 31 California counties showed no effect on sexual behavior of 7340 students participating in the program. Such programs do not delay the onset of sexual activity, but they do result in higher pregnancy rates than controls *(7,8)*.

A didactic program that only discussed human sexuality and encouraged young people to seek family planning services if they needed them did not change sexual behavior *(9)*. This is consistent with other research showing that knowledge-based approaches are not effective in reducing adolescent negative health behaviors *(10,11)*. Programs that strongly encourage abstinence but also provide information about available methods for birth control and STD protection have been shown to increase contraceptive utilization by 70–80% *(12,13)*. Providing teen women with concrete examples of how to decline sexual advances is also important; translating abstinence principles into action in different situations is not a skill most adolescents have mastered. The realities of adolescent life involve the rejection of adult authority, relatively low self-esteem, and foreshortened time frames. In addition to the limited future alternatives many teens anticipate for themselves and the short-term gains many teens achieve with pregnancy, teens' motivations for seeking pregnancy are complex and must be addressed when developing pregnancy-prevention programs.

In a similar vein, some adolescent women may not be in a position to select abstinence; the 2002 National Survey of Family Growth revealed that 10% of women reported that their first sex was nonvoluntary *(4,5)*. Victims of sexual abuse may need provider assistance not only in preventing pregnancy, but also in dealing with their hazardous environment.

One model outreach family planning center from Atlanta, GA implemented a "social inoculation" program, which exposed young teens to samples of peer pressure and other negative influences, enabling them to examine those forces and develop skills to resist their lure. Older teens were used to instruct younger teens. Overall, a statistically significant lower percentage of young people who were enrolled in the program initiated sexual activity after eighth grade compared with controls *(9)*. Another study in South Carolina demonstrated importance of a multidisciplinary, community-based program that involved medical personnel but also community groups to create other immediate activity options and long-term career options for the teens *(14)*.

Physicians have a role to play in promoting abstinence among young people. High school students were asked whether their physician had discussed sexuality issues with them, including the question, "Has your physician discussed with you how to say no when you don't want to have sex?" Only half of the students had discussed sex or abstinence with their physician, and many more reported that they would like to have this discussion with their physician *(15)*. An office-based intervention to reduce risky sexual activity among adolescents has been shown to reduce STD rates *(16)*. Even when physicians may not be able to conduct these interventions in their offices, they can provide pivotal leadership to help establish effective adolescent programs in their communities.

NFP Methods

Couples practicing periodic abstinence (NFP methods) avoid coitus during the days of a woman's cycle when she is fertile. Couples practicing FAMs use contraceptive methods (usually barriers) during the identified at-risk days. In 2000, it was estimated that 2.6% of women were using periodic abstinence as contraception, or 27 million women worldwide *(17)*.

Calendar or Rhythm Method

Several techniques have been developed to identify fertile days. For the "calendar" or "rhythm" method, it is assumed that sperm last 1–3 days and an egg is vulnerable to fertilization up to 24 hours after ovulation. The fertile window includes, at least, the 5 days before ovulation and the day after. To use this method using traditional approaches, it is necessary to obtain information about the woman's spontaneous menstrual cycling for at least 6 months. The first day of abstinence is calculated by subtracting 18 from the number of days in the woman's shortest cycle. The latest day of her fertile period is calculated by subtracting 11 from the number of days in her longest cycle. Tables such as Table 2 can be consulted to confirm the calculations. For example, a woman whose 6-month data showed that her cycle length varied between 26 and 30 days would be required to abstain from coitus between days 8 and 19 each month; the couple may engage in intercourse on cycle days 1–7 and from day 20 to menses.

The need to document cycle lengths was recently highlighted in a prospective study of low-literacy Mayan women who were self-declared to be "regularly cycling." Quite surprisingly, only 46% of these women were found to have regular cycles (26–32 days), even for 3 consecutive months *(18)*. Clearly, approaches such as blanket days 9–19 of abstinence will result in higher than expected failure rates when such dramatic inherent variation in cycle length exists. The traditional calculation requires an average of 13 days of abstinence a month for the general population and provides 67.8% coverage of peak risk days *(19)*. Even when women have regular cycles, they may ovulate earlier or later than expected using these calculations. In one study of 221 health women attempting to conceive, 10% of women with regular cycles were in their fertile window on any given day between days 6 and 21 *(20)*.

Standard Days Method Using CycleBeads

The standard days method was developed by Georgetown investigators particularly for women desiring to start a simple method immediately and for those

Table 2
Calculation of Fertile Period

Shortest cycle (days)	*First fertile (unsafe) day*	*Longest cycle (days)*	*Last fertile (unsafe) day*
21	3	21	10
22	4	22	11
23	5	23	12
24	6	24	13
25	7	25	14
26	8	26	15
27	9	27	16
28	10	28	17
29	11	29	18
30	12	30	19
31	13	31	20
32	14	32	21
33	15	33	22
34	16	34	23
35	17	35	24

Day 1 = First day of menstrual bleeding.
(Adapted from ref. *2*.)

living in areas of low literacy *(21)*. It is designed for women who have cycle lengths lasting 26–32 days. Women are given CycleBeads (Figs. 1 and 2), a device designed to assist women in monitoring their cycles and determining their fertile days. The first bead is red, which represents the first day of menses. The next six beads are brown, representing non-fertile days. Fertile days are represented by the following twelve white beads, which are followed by another thirteen brown "infertile" beads. The patient advances a moveable ring one bead a day to determine her fertility. The at-risk white beads even glow in the dark. There are two black beads at days 27 and 32. If the woman's menses starts before she reaches the first bead, then she learns that her cycle length is too short to rely on the CycleBeads. Similarly, if she reaches the 32nd (black) bead without having started her menses, her cycle is too long to use the standard days method. A back-up calendar is provided to allow for the woman to record that she has moved the elastic band every day as directed. CycleBeads are available via the Internet. One study of women using this technique in the Philippines, Peru, and Bolivia found a first-year pregnancy rate of 4.8% with correct use, meaning no intercourse days 8–19 of the cycle. Of the participants in this study, 28% had two cycles out of the 26- to 32-day range and were excluded from the results. The probability of pregnancy was 12% with typical use *(21)*.

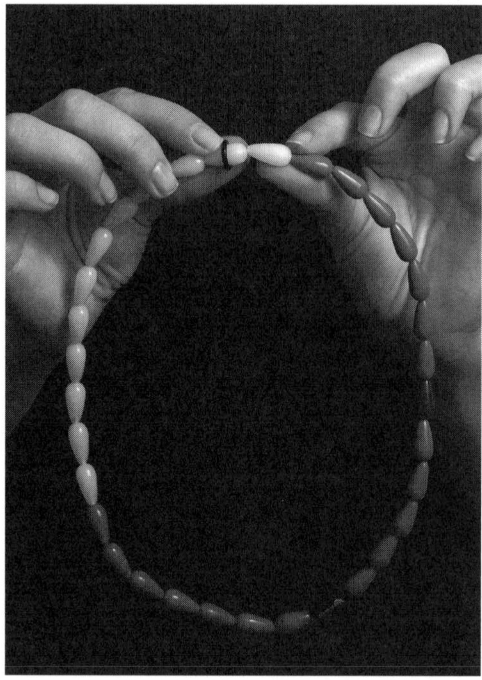

Fig. 1. CycleBeads™. (Courtesy of Cycle Technologies; www.cyclebeads.com.)

Basal Body Temperature Method

Other techniques are available to predict ovulation. Basal body temperature (BBT) measurements are used to detect ovulation and, more importantly, to indicate when the risk of pregnancy has passed for a given cycle. Patients are instructed to measure their temperatures at the same time each day before arising. Ovulation is identified by an average temperature increase of about 0.4–0.8°F (usually following a slight dip in BBT). Studies have shown that ovulation occurs within 48 hours of either side of the temperature shift *(22)*. Inaccuracies in measurements may be introduced if the woman gets out of bed at night, has an infection, or varies the time of day the temperatures are taken. Intercourse is prohibited for at least 3 days following the temperature rise. However, this does not protect against exposure to semen when intercourse immediately precedes the BBT rise. In practice, only 80% of women have interpretable BBT patterns. Therefore, the best use of BBT is as a post-ovulatory method or in combination with some other technique that can better predict ovulation.

Billings Technique

The Billings technique of ovulation detection relies on changes in cervical/vaginal secretions that reflect the hormonal swings of the menstrual cycle. Each

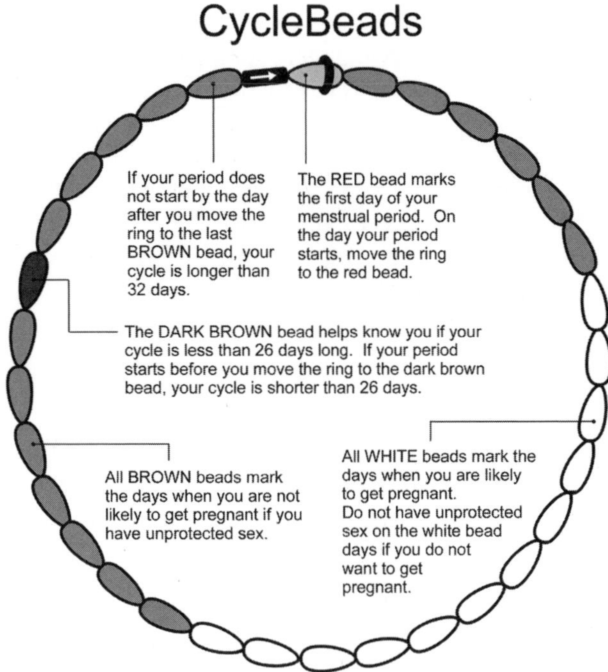

Fig. 2. CycleBeads™ (Courtesy of Cycle Technologies; www.cyclebeads.com.)

day, the woman touches a piece of paper or her finger against her vaginal introitus before urination to test the quantity and character of those secretions. During the days following menses, cervical mucus is scant and the introital testing will be negative. As the follicular phase advances, the secretions increase slightly, but they are still viscous. The pre-ovulatory estrogen surge dramatically increases the amount of these secretions and makes them more clear and elastic (creating the maximal finger-to-thumb Spinnbarkeit sign) *(23)*. After ovulation, the mucus again thickens under the influence of progesterone, and coitus may be permitted only after 3 days of dry secretions.

A woman wanting to use the Billings method must first learn about her cycles. Data are best gathered during a period of 6–9 months of abstinence. After a woman learns how to interpret her mucus patterns, the couple should forego coitus at least every other day to permit a woman to assess her fertility without having her measurements confused by seminal fluid or vaginal secretions resulting from the woman's own sexual arousal. Other external factors can also confound these measurements. A woman's introital moisture may be changed by vaginal infections or vaginal therapies. Douching may result in misreading, either directly—by eliminating important evidence—or indirectly, by disrupting her vaginal defense system and inducing vaginal infections.

Two-Day Method

A simpler technique using cervical secretions, called the two-day method, has recently been proposed. A woman relies on the presence or absence of cervical secretions to determine whether or not she is fertile each day, asking herself, "Did I note secretions today?" and "Did I note secretions yesterday?" She considers herself fertile if she notices cervical secretions of any type on that day or the day before, avoiding intercourse on these days. The first-year pregnancy rate in one study using this method was 3.5% with correct use of the method and 13.7% with typical use, with 96.4% of participants saying that they had no difficulty in detecting secretions after the third cycle. The mean number of days with secretions was 12.1, which is comparable with the standard days method *(24)*.

Symptothermal Technique

A more effective method of ovulation detection for NFP or FAM is the symptothermal technique, which combines at least two of the above techniques and may add other potential signs and symptoms to detect ovulation. Experienced patients may check the cervix for changes in texture, dilation, and position (at ovulation the cervix softens, moistens, dilates, and elevates in the vagina). In addition, clues about ovulation may come from changes in libido or the discomfort of Mittelschmerz. Effectiveness of this method has been 2–3% among perfect users and as high as 20% among typical users *(25)*.

Having used any of these methods to detect ovulation, couples may use different strategies to prevent pregnancy. Intercourse can be permitted only after all risk of ovulation has passed (i.e., the post-ovulatory approach) or it may also be permitted at times when the risk of impending ovulation is minimized (e.g., the dry, scant mucus days immediately after menses). Sperm have been noted to survive in the vagina for 7 days. None of the available methods can anticipate ovulation 1 week in advance.

Ovulation Detection Monitors

Hand-held ovulation detection monitors are in use in England, Ireland, Germany, Italy, and the Netherlands to provide ongoing analysis of a woman's vulnerability to pregnancy. Each day a woman opens the monitor to check her fertility status. The monitor has three colored lights. A green light indicates a safe day; the red light advises abstinence. A yellow light reflects uncertainty. When the yellow light appears, the user removes a test strip from the monitor, applies a sample of her urine and reinserts the strip into the monitor, which then rapidly analyzes the specimen for levels of luteinizing hormone and estrone-3-glucuronide. After a few minutes of analysis, a definitive red or green light will shine. With use, the monitor gathers a considerable amount of information about the woman's cycle. Based on information about her menses and records of her hormonal testing, progressively fewer days of yellow lights and less testing are needed with prolonged use.

The Clearplan Easy Fertility Monitor™ is a fertility monitor available in the United States. By measuring urinary metabolites, it provides the user with a daily indication of low, high, and peak fertility. Use of these monitors results in a period of abstinence shorter than those recommended with cervical mucus or calendar methods, which may result in higher failure rates because they may not provide enough time before ovulation to avoid intercourse. Alone, monitors are accurate for predicting ovulation 60% of the time. It has been postulated that, if used in conjunction with cervical mucus screening, they might be more effective at preventing pregnancy. However, studies of efficacy of home monitors in combination with other NFP methods have yet to be performed *(26)*.

Other devices used in assessing the fertile period include small hand-held microscopes (Lady Free Biotester®) used to check for cervical mucus and salivary ferning, which is indicative of fertility *(27)*. A comparison of microscopes and home fertility monitors found neither to be as effective as the symptothermal method; microscopes had a high false-negative rate for fertile days *(28)*.

Lactational Amenorrhea

During the postpartum period, the hypothalamic–pituitary–ovarian axis is temporarily suppressed. Lactation temporarily raises prolactin, which blocks activation of the axis. Amenorrhea induced by breastfeeding in the first 6 months postpartum is a relatively accurate clinical marker of ovulation suppression. During the first 6 months postpartum, the first menses a woman experiences (if she has a period) is usually anovulatory bleeding; menstrual bleeding usually precedes ovulation. Being forewarned, a woman can utilize other contraceptive methods to protect herself after such a menses against future, probably ovulatory, cycles. After 6 months of postpartum amenorrhea, however, the first cycle is usually ovulatory. This places the woman at risk for an unannounced return of fertility if she relies exclusively on the lactational amenorrhea method (LAM) beyond 6 months.

Over time, the requirements for this method have changed. Early World Health Organization studies included only women who were amenorrheic, fully breastfeeding on demand, and offered no other source of suckling to the infant. Uterine sloughing within 56 days postpartum did not count because this has been shown not to represent a return to ovulation *(29)*. Later studies abandoned the need to exclude pacifiers. Until recently, exclusive breastfeeding was defined by the fact that the infant received at least 90% caloric intake via breast milk. Most recently, studies have clarified the two most important predictors of pregnancy protection: amenorrhea and time since delivery. In amenorrheic women who were fully or partially breastfeeding, pregnancy rates were 1% in the first 6 months. However, pregnancy rates rose to 4–7% by 12 months. Interestingly, there was no difference in pregnancy rates between partially or fully breastfeeding women *(30)*.

All the studies demonstrated the need to provide added protection after 6 months, even if the woman remains amenorrheic while breastfeeding. A recent review of Finnish-American women who traditionally have used no birth control other than breastfeeding found a very high pregnancy rate. One couple was photographed with 99 grandchildren clustered around them; three of their daughters had 17 children each *(31)*.

Candidates for LAM

Women who remain amenorrheic and breastfeed may use LAM as their only method for up to 6 months postpartum. However, some women may not be able to breastfeed for medical or social reasons. An HIV-infected woman should avoid breastfeeding if other sources of nutrition are available to her infant. Similarly, women taking drugs that cross into the breast milk and may harm the baby should not breastfeed. Breastfeeding requires privacy and continuous accessibility of the mother to her child. Working mothers may not have that opportunity, although breast pumping and milk storage for later consumption is a possibility for some women.

Noncontraceptive Benefits of LAM

Breast milk is best suited to meet the nutritional requirements of the human infant. Breast-fed children have fewer gastrointestinal problems and decreased rates of allergies and asthma later in life. The mother–child bond reinforced by breastfeeding is also very important. The convenience of the temporary protection offered by LAM in women already dedicated to breastfeeding can be very attractive at this busy time in a woman's life. Epithelial ovarian cancer rates are reduced in women who breastfeed before age 30 years *(32)*. Breast cancer rates are not affected by lactation unless it is continuous for at least 2 years.

Side Effects/Drawbacks of LAM

Breastfeeding may be perceived as embarrassing or inconvenient by some women. Cracked nipples, mastitis, and even breast abscesses are possible complications of breastfeeding. The hypoestrogenic state induced by LAM may decrease vaginal lubrication and cause dyspareunia *(31)*. Most of these side effects, however, result from breastfeeding alone. The decision to use LAM for birth control can be viewed as an independent decision not adding any additional side effects. It must be remembered that LAM does not offer any protection against STIs. This is particularly important during the first weeks postpartum, when an STI could easily result in upper tract infection. The hypoestrogenated vagina may also be more vulnerable to HIV infection.

Coitus Interruptus

Coitus interruptus, or withdrawal, requires that the penis be removed from the vagina and directed away from the external genitalia of the woman before ejaculation to prevent sperm from entering the upper reproductive tract and fertilizing an ovum. Historically, *coitus interruptus* has been an important method. By the end of the 1800s, birth rates in France were significantly reduced by its widespread practice. In the United States, official estimates from the 1995 National Survey of Family Growth are that 2.9% of married women rely on this method. This estimate excludes single women (often adolescents) who utilize this method in even greater numbers. The Youth Risk Behavior Survey in 1997 reported that 13% of sexually active high school students used *coitus interruptus* to prevent pregnancy at their last sexual intercourse *(33)*.

Effectiveness of *Coitus Interruptus*

Coitus interruptus is much more effective than is generally perceived; it is roughly equivalent to some female barrier methods. Clinical trial data are not available to calculate the failure rates for consistent and correct use, although some experts have estimated that the failure rate should be approximately 4%. Typical use first-year rates have been measured to be 27%. There is considerable intercouple variation around that estimate *(2)*. The benefits of this method are obvious: it requires no drugs or devices; it does not interfere with foreplay or precoital spontaneity; and it is readily portable and available.

Candidates for *Coitus Interruptus*

A male partner who is able to sense impending ejaculation and to resist the involuntary urge for deeper thrusting is required for success of this method. He must be able to withdraw before ejaculation. Coital positioning is also important. Unless the couple is effectively able to communicate in time to permit the woman to move, the male superior position or at least a male-controlled coital position is necessary.

Noncontraceptive Benefits of *Coitus Interruptus*

Rates of HIV seroconversion of the uninfected woman in discordant stable relationships are reduced by at least 50% by *coitus interruptus* compared with unprotected intercourse *(34,35)*. In a 1994 study of HIV transmission between heterosexual partners, DeVincenzi showed that couples who practiced *coitus interruptus* with every intercourse had zero seroconversion of uninfected partners. This is compared with a 4.8 per 100 person-years conversion in couples inconsistently using condoms and a zero seroconversion rate in couples consistently using condoms *(36)*. It would be expected that the male-to-female transmission rate of gonorrhea, trichomonas, and chlamydia would be reduced, but that ulcerative lesions such as herpes, chancroid, and lymphogranuloma venereum would not be substantially altered by the use of *coitus interruptus* as a method of birth control.

Side Effects/Drawbacks of *Coitus Interruptus*

With *coitus interruptus*, the dynamics of intercourse are disrupted. Researchers have reported mild to extreme clouding of consciousness just before ejaculation; deep thrusting motions are involuntarily triggered in many men with impending ejaculation *(37)*. Interruption of penile vaginal contact at this phase of the sexual response curve may decrease the intensity of the male orgasm. Similarly, for the woman who may be at another phase of sexual arousal, complete cessation of all penile stimulation may not only diminish pleasure but also result in frustration.

Patient Education

Minimal instructions are necessary, but the man should know to urinate and wipe of the tip of his penis before intercourse to remove any sperm lingering from a recent ejaculation. Most importantly, he must learn how to completely withdraw his penis and direct it away from the woman's genitals before ejaculation.

As with any barrier or behavioral method, emergency contraception should be provided to the couple to have readily available should the woman have an accidental exposure to sperm.

Other Sexual Practices

Although they are not routinely discussed in traditional textbooks, many heterosexual couples use a wide variety of non-vaginal intercourse sexual practices to prevent pregnancy while still achieving sexual pleasure. In fact, recent publication of a 1994 America Medical Association survey revealed that many Americans do not classify these practices as sex *(38)*. However, it is important for physicians to be aware of these practices so that they can advise patients appropriately about possible health implications and can test more successfully for STIs. Heterosexual anal intercourse is not uncommonly practiced by teens for hymenal preservation and by older couples for penile stimulation before vaginal ejaculation *(39)*. In each instance, it is important to discuss the implications for rectal infection and sphincteric trauma and, in the latter case, to understand, perhaps, why the female partner may suffer recurrent vaginal infections, especially with bacterial vaginosis. The risk of pharyngeal infection with gonorrhea is appreciated in the medical community, but few physicians appreciate how very common oral–genital sexual practices are, especially among adolescents. Other practices, including mutual masturbation, may also protect a woman from pregnancy, but may not be volunteered by her unless she feels comfortable discussing the more intimate details of her relationship. Such information may be helpful to the physician to understand why she may now not need other forms of birth control.

SUMMARY

Total sexual abstinence is the most effective method of birth control, but incomplete commitment can result in high rates of unintended pregnancies. Periodic abstinence and fertility awareness methods rely on menstrual calendars, CycleBeads, BBT, the Billings method, or the symptothermal method to detect at-risk fertile days. *Coitus interruptus* has failure rates similar to the female barrier methods. LAM is very effective for up to 6 months postpartum. Other practices, which admittedly may not even be characterized as sex, also provide sexual pleasure without incurring the risk of pregnancy but do not protect against STIs.

REFERENCES

1. World Health Organization (WHO), Task Force on Methods for the Determination of the Fertile Period, Special Program of Research, Development and Research Training in Human Reproduction. (1981) A prospective multicentre trial of the Ovulation Method of natural family planning. II. The effectiveness phase. Fertil Steril 36:591–598.
2. Hatcher RA, Trussell J, Stewart F, et al. (2004) Contraceptive Technology, 18th rev ed. New York: Ardent Media.
3. World Health Organization (WHO), Task Force on Methods for the Determination of the Fertile Period, Special Programme of Research, Development and Research Training in Human Reproduction. (1981) A prospective multicentre trial of the Ovulation Method of natural family planning. I. The teaching phase. Fertil Steril 36:152–158.
4. Abma JC, Martinez GM, Mosher WD, Dawson BS. (2004) Teenagers in the United States: sexual activity, contraceptive use, and childbearing, 2002. Vital Health Stat 23:1–48.
5. Moore KA, Driscoll AK, Lindberg LD. (1998) A statistical portrait of adolescent sex, contraception, and childbearing. Washington, DC: National Campaign to Prevent Teen Pregnancy.
6. Centers for Disease Control and Prevention. (2004) Violence-related behaviors among high school students—United States, 1991–2003. MMWR Morb Mortal Wkly Rep 53:651–655.
7. Kirby D. (1997) No easy answers: research findings on programs to reduce teen pregnancy. Washington, DC: The National Campaign to Prevent Teen Pregnancy, p. 25.
8. Kirby D, Korpi M, Barth RP, Cagampang HH. (1997) The impact of the postponing sexual involvement curriculum among youths in California. Fam Plann Perspect 29:100–108.
9. Howard M, McCabe JB. (1988) Helping teenagers postpone sexual involvement. In: Bennett D, Williams M, eds. New Universals: Adolescent Health in a Time of Change. Curtin, Australia: Brolga Press.
10. Ellickson P, Robyn A. (1987) Toward more effective drug prevention programs. Santa Monica, CA: The Rand Publication Series, The Rand Corporation.
11. Kirby D. (1984) Sexuality education: an evaluation of programs and their effects, vol. 1. Atlanta, GA: Bureau of Health Education, Centers for Disease Control.
12. Haffner D. (1994) Facing facts: sexual health for America's adolescents. New York: Sexuality Information and Education Council of the United States.
13. Kirby D. (2001) Emerging answers: research findings on programs to reduce teen pregnancy. Washington, DC: National Campaign to Reduce Teen Pregnancy.
14. Koo HP, Dunteman GH, George Cet al. (1994) Reducing adolescent pregnancy through a school- and community-based intervention: Denmark, South Carolina, revisited. Fam Plann Perspect 26:206–211, 217.
15. Schuster MA, Bell RM, Petersen LP, Kanouse DE. (1996) Communication between adolescents and their physicians about sexual behavior and risk prevention. Arch Ped Adol Med 150:906–913.
16. Boekeloo BO, Schamus LA, Simmens SJ, Cheng TL, O'Connor K, D'Angelo LJ. (1999) A STD/HIV prevention trial among adolescents in managed care. Pediatrics 103:107–115.
17. United Nations. (2001) World contraceptive use 2001. New York: Department of Social and Economic Affairs.
18. Burkhart MC, de Mazariegos L, Salazar S, Hess T. (1999) Incidence of irregular cycles among Mayan women who reported having regular cycles: implications for fertility awareness methods. Contraception 59:271–275.
19. Lamprecht VM, Grummer-Strawn L. (1996) Development of new formulas to identify the fertile time of the menstrual cycle. Contraception 54:339–343.

20. Wilcox AJ, Dunson D, Baird DD. (2000) The timing of the "fertile window" in the menstrual cycle: day specific estimates from a prospective study. BMJ 321:1259–1262.
21. Arevalo M, Jennings V, Sinai I. (2002) Efficacy of a new method of family planning: the standard days method. Contraception 65:333–338.
22. Klaus H. (1995) Natural Family Planning: A Review, 2nd ed. Bethesda, MD: Natural Family Planning Center of Washington, DC.
23. World Health Organization (WHO), Task Force on Methods for the Determination of the Fertile Period, Special Programme of Research, Development and Research Training in Human Reproduction. (1983) A prospective multicentre trial of the Ovulation Method of natural family planning. III. Characteristics of the menstrual cycle and of the fertile phase. Fertil Steril 40:773–778.
24. Arevalo M, Jennings V, Nikula M, Sinai I. (2004) Efficacy of the new TwoDay Method of family planning. Fertil Steril 82:885–892.
25. Frank-Herrman P, Freundl G, Baur S, Bremme M, Doring GK, Godehardt EAJ, Sottong U. (1991) Effectiveness and acceptability of the symptothermal method of natural family planning in Germany. Am J Obstet Gynecol 165:2052–2054.
26. Fehring RJ, Raviele K, Schneider M. (2004) A comparison of the fertile phase as determined by the Clearplan Easy Fertility Monitor TM and self-assessment of cervical mucus. Contraception 69:9–14.
27. Fehring RJ, Gaska N. (1998) Evaluation of the Lady Free Biotester® in determining the fertile period. Contraception 57:325–328.
28. Freundl G, Godehardt E, Kern PA, Frank-Herrmann P, Koubenec HJ, Gnoth C. (2003) Estimated maximum failure rates of cycle monitors using daily conception probabilities in the menstrual cycle. Hum Reprod 18:2628–2633.
29. Visness CM, Kennedy KI, Gross BAet al. (1997) Fertility of fully breast-feeding women in the early postpartum period. Obstet Gynecol 89:164–167.
30. World Health Organization (WHO). (1999) The World Health Organization multinational study of breast-feeding and lactational amenorrhea. III. Pregnancy during breast-feeding. Fertil Steril 72:431–440.
31. Henderson P III. (1999) Bone mineral density analysis of grandmultiparas with extended lactation. Presented at Pacific Coast Obstetrical and Gynecological Society Annual Meeting Cancun, Mexico, October 22.
32. Riman T, Nilsson S, Persson IR. (2004) Review of epidemiological evidence for reproductive and hormonal factors in relation to the risk of epithelial ovarian malignancies. Acta Obstet Gynecol Scand 83:783–795.
33. Everett SA, Warren CW, Santelli JS, Kann L, Collins JL, Kolbe LJ. (2000) Use of birth control pills, condoms, and withdrawal among US high school students. J Adol Health 27:112–118.
34. Darrow WW. (1989) Condom use and use-effectiveness in high-risk populations. Sex Transm Dis 16:157–160.
35. Musicco M, Nicolosi A, Saracco A, Lazzarin A (for the Italian Study Group on HIV Heterosexual Transmission). (1994) The role of contraceptive practices in HIV sexual transmission form man to woman. In: Nicolosi A, ed. HIV Epidemiology: Models And Methods. New York: Raven Press, Ltd., pp. 121–135.
36. DeVincenzi, I. (1994) A longitudinal study of human immunodeficiency virus transmission by heterosexual partners. N Engl J Med 331:341–346.
37. Kinsey AC, Pomeroy WB, Martin CE, Gebhard PH. (1953) Sexual Behavior in the Human Female. Philadelphia, PA: WB Saunders.
38. Sanders SA, Reinisch JM. (1999) Would you say you "had sex" if…? JAMA 281:275–257.
39. Schuster MA, Bell RM, Kanouse DE. (1996) The sexual practices of adolescent virgins: genital sexual activities of high school students who have never had sexual intercourse. Am J Public Health 86:1570–1576.

12 Emergency Contraceptives

Donna Shoupe, MD

Contents

INTRODUCTION

Emergency contraceptives (ECs) offer a "second chance" to prevent an unintended pregnancy. It is estimated that if the general population had better knowledge and easier access to ECs, their use could potentially cut the number of abortions performed each year in the United States in half. There are three major options available for emergency contraception: progestin-only pills (POPs), combination oral contraceptives (OCs), and insertion of an intrauterine device (IUD). Currently, there are 2 POPs and 18 combination pills (estrogen plus progestin) available that must be taken within 72 hours of unprotected sex according to treatment protocols listed in Table 1. The third option is insertion of a copper IUD within 5 days of unprotected sex. The progestin-only products, Plan B® and Ovrette®, are associated with less nausea than combined estrogen plus progestin EC products. Plan B is the only product designated and packaged as an EC.

From: *Current Clinical Practice: The Handbook of Contraception: A Guide for Practical Management*
Edited by: D. Shoupe and S. L. Kjos © Humana Press, Totowa, NJ

Table 1
Hormonal Options for Emergency Contraception

	Content	Pills per dose (two doses 12 hours apart)	
Dedicated product (manufacturer)			
Plan B (Duramed)	0.75 mg LNG	1 + 1	No pretreatment necessary
Progestin-only pill			
Plan B (as above)	0.75 mg LNG	1 + 1	No pretreatment necessary
Ovrette® (Wyeth)	0.075 μg NOR	20 + 20	
Combination OCs (Yuzpe method)			
Ogestrel® (Watson)	50 μg EE plus 0.5 mg NOR	2 + 2	Pretreatment with anti-emetic recommended
Ovral® (Wyeth)			
Lo/Ovral® (Wyeth)	30 μg EE plus 0.3 mg NOR	4 + 4	Pretreatment with anti-emetic recommended
Low-Ogestrel® (Watson)			
Cryselle® (Barr)			
Levlen® (Berlex)	30 μg EE plus 0.15 mg LNG	4 + 4	Pretreatment with anti-emetic recommended
Levora® (Watson)			
Nordette® (Monarch)			
Portia®, Seasonale® (Barr)			
Alesse® (Wyeth)	20 μg EE plus 0.1 mg LNG	5 + 5	Pretreatment with anti-emetic recommended
Aviane® (Barr)			
Lessina® (Barr)			
Levlite® (Berlex)			
Lutera® (Watson)			

	Pill color (critical)	Content	Pills per dose (two doses 12 hours apart)	
Triphasic combination ECs				
Enpresse® (Barr)	Orange	Pill in triphasic pack that contains 30 μg EE plus 0.125 mg LNG	4 + 4	Pretreatment with anti-emetic recommended
Trivora® (Watson)	Pink			
Triphasil® (Wyeth)	Light yellow			
Tri-Levlen® (Berlex)	Light yellow			

LNG, levonorgestrel; NOR, norgestrel; EE, ethinyl estradiol; OC, oral contraceptive; EC, emergency contraceptive.

Although education and access are gradually improving, EC usage continues to be low *(1)*. Unfortunately, there continues to be controversy and confusion surrounding use and distribution of ECs. In 2001, more than 70 professional organizations, including American College of Obstetricians and Gynecologists, supported a petition requesting that the Food and Drug Administration (FDA) make EC pills available without prescription. In 2003, after reviewing the safety and efficacy data, an FDA advisory panel recommended making Plan B available without prescription. However, under political pressure *(2)*, the FDA issued a "Not Approvable Letter" citing a lack of information on the effect of Plan B on adolescent women *(3)*. A revised application for over-the-counter distribution of Plan B, placing restrictions on access of the medication to women under 16, was recently reviewed and deferred so that "legal issues could be examined." In protest, the head of the FDA's women's health office resigned.

Six states now allow pharmacists to dispense EC pills without a prescription including Alaska, California, Hawaii, Maine, New Mexico, and Washington. EC pills are available over the counter or through a pharmacist in France, Sweden, Canada, and the United Kingdom.

MECHANISM OF ACTION

Like other hormonal forms of contraception, both combined estrogen plus progestin and progestin-only EC pills prevent pregnancy by having several effects:

- Ovulation is inhibited or delayed *(4,5)*.
- Fertilization is impaired by altering tubal transport of sperm or ova *(6,7)*.
- Endometrial changes that prevent a fertilized egg from implantation *(8)*.
- Cervical mucus is thickened.

When being used as a routine method of contraception, the copper IUD primarily prevents fertilization by affecting sperm transport and function *(9,10)*. It is likely that use of the copper IUD for emergency contraception includes this action along with a variety of other anti-fertility effects, including disruption of the endometrium.

EFFECTIVENESS

> *Regardless of the time period a woman has unprotected sex, the sooner EC pills are taken the more effective they are (11). If Plan B is used properly within 72 hours of unprotected intercourse, the risk of pregnancy falls to 1%.*

The effectiveness of the method is measured by comparing the number of pregnancies expected in a sexually active population with the number of pregnancies actually occurring in that population following treatment. The expected pregnancy rates are highly dependent on the specific day of the menstrual cycle that each woman in the population had unprotected sex and a host of other factors affecting fecundity *(12)*.

- If EC pills containing estrogen–progestin are taken within 72 hours after unprotected sex, the risk of pregnancy is reduced by at least 75% *(13)* (this equates to an overall 1–2% failure rate because not all women with unprotected sex will become pregnant).
- If levonorgestrel-only pills (Plan B, Ovrette) are specifically taken, the risk of pregnancy is reduced by 89% *(14)*. This equates to a 1% failure rate.
- Insertion of a copper-releasing IUD reduces the risk of pregnancy by up to 99% *(15,16)*.
- Although controversial, emesis following treatment with combination EC pills does not appear to decrease efficacy.
  - It is thought that the high circulating levels of estrogen (acting on the central nervous system causing emesis) are evidence that the pills have already been absorbed *(7)*.

ADVANTAGES

Advantages of EC Pills

- EC pills are safe for most women.
- No serious side effects associated with Plan B.
- EC pills are available without prescription through some pharmacies in six states (Alaska, California, Hawaii, Maine, New Mexico, and Washington) *(17)* and approved for use in Canada for women over age 16 without a doctor's prescription.
- Progestin-only EC pills can be used by women who are not candidates for combination OCs.
- EC pills can be bought in advance and kept on hand for use in an emergency.
- In the event of a failure, no teratogenicity or other adverse outcomes are reported after exposure to EC pills *(7)*.

Advantages of Using a Copper IUD for EC

- The IUD provides an ongoing highly effective method of contraception.
- Can be inserted up to 5 days after unprotected sex.

DISADVANTAGES

- Combination EC pills are associated with a high rate of nausea (42%) and vomiting (16%) *(18)* and pretreatment with an anti-emetic is recommended.
  - Plan B is better tolerated.
- Not all women know about EC pills or know how to get access to them.
- Many women do not know that they can use some types of regular OCs.
- There is only a 72-hour window in which to start the first dose.
- There is no protection from sexually transmitted infections (STIs) or HIV.

- Opponents link emergency contraception to abortion or that it may encourage sexual activity among teenagers.
  - Research studies report that increased availability of EC pills does not result in increased unprotected sexual activity *(19,20)*. In some states where prescriptions are necessary, "conscience laws" allow pharmacists to refuse to fill prescriptions for EC pills.
- There is confusion between EC pills and the abortion pill RU-486 (mifepristone).
  - RU-486 is *not* an EC pill. It is taken *after* pregnancy is established (within 49 days of the last menstrual period).

INDICATIONS AND USAGE

Within 72 Hours of Unprotected Sex

Plan B is an EC that can be used to prevent pregnancy following unprotected intercourse or a known or suspected contraceptive failure. To obtain optimal efficacy, the first tablet should be taken as soon as possible, and within 72 hours of intercourse. The second tablet must be taken 12 hours later. Other protocols with various OC pills containing levonorgestrel or norgestrel are listed in Table 1. Note that for triphasic combination pills, the color of the tablet is critical.

Indications for EC include the following conditions:

- Unplanned, unprotected sexual relationship.
- Regardless of the time of the month when unprotected sex occurs, all women seeking EC should be evaluated for treatment.
- Condom breakage or improper use.
- Diaphragm, cap, or shield slippage.
- Missed OCs (especially missing the first week of OCs).
- Late in starting a new patch or vaginal ring.
- Late in getting depot medroxyprogesterone acetate (DMPA) or depo-subQ provera 104™ injection.
- Mistake in calculating "safe days" when practicing natural family planning.
- Rape *(21)*.

After 72 Hours of Unprotected Sex

Women presenting with the any of the above indications between 72 and 120 hours after unprotected sex may be best served by having a copper IUD inserted (that can be placed up to 5 days following unprotected sex). There are reports that EC pills have some, although limited, effectiveness when initiated this late *(22)*.

SIDE EFFECTS

Possible side effects of Plan B (or Ovrette) are shown in Table 2. Plan B has a lower rate of adverse events than the estrogen–progestin (Yuzpe) EC pill regimens:

Table 2
Common Side Effects Associated With Plan B (Adverse Events in ≥5% of Women, by % Frequency)

Most common adverse events in 977 users (Plan B, levonorgestrel)	*(%)*
Nausea	23.1
Abdominal pain	17.6
Fatigue	16.9
Headache	16.8
Heavier menstrual bleeding	13.8
Lighter menstrual bleeding	12.5
Dizziness	11.2
Breast tenderness	10.7
Other complaints	9.7
Vomiting	5.6
Diarrhea	5.0

- Nausea: 23% *(23)* in Plan B compared with 50% on estrogen–progestin EC pills.
- Vomiting: 6% in Plan B compared with 19% on estrogen–progestin EC pills.

Effect on Menses

After taking a hormonal EC, most women will start their next menses within 3 days of their expected time *(24)*.

After taking Plan B, some women may have spotting for a few days. At the time of the expected menses, about 75% of users have vaginal bleeding similar to their normal menses, 13% have heavier bleeding, and 12% bleed less. The onset of this next menses is within ±7 days of the expected date in 87% of users, whereas 13% experience a delay of more than 7 days. If there is a delay of more than 1 week, pregnancy should be considered.

Ectopic Pregnancy

Up to 10% of pregnancies that occur as method failures in women on POPs are ectopic (Chapter 4). This is higher than the approximately 2% rate normally reported. Therefore, although a history of ectopic pregnancy is not a contraindication to Plan B, health providers should keep in mind this possibility in women who become pregnant after taking Plan B or who complain of abdominal pain *(25,26)*.

METABOLIC EFFECTS

The acute metabolic effects of progestin-only EC pills (Plan B) are similar to the early metabolic effects seen with POPs, although these changes are only short term and quickly normalized (Chapter 4). Similarily, the acute effects of estrogen–progestin EC pills are similar to the early effects of combination OCs (Chapter 2).

WARNING: Plan B not recommended for routine use as a contraceptive. Plan B not effective in terminating an existing pregnancy.

CONTRAINDICATIONS

There are a very limited number of medical contraindications to treatment with EC pills.

- Women who are pregnant (EC pills cannot terminate an established pregnancy).
- Undiagnosed vaginal bleeding.
- Allergy to any component in medication.
- Not intended for geriatric (age 65 and older) or pediatric populations.
- Not recommended for routine use as a contraceptive.

Progestin-only EC pills are preferable to combination EC pills for women with the following conditions:

- History of thromboembolic disease.
- Vascular disease.
- Heart disease.
- Focal migraines.
- Liver disease.
- Some health care providers prefer to use progestin-only ECs in patients for whom combination OCs are contraindicated; however, because of the short duration of treatment, this is not routinely necessary.

Eligibility requirements for the copper IUD are the same as for insertion for routine use as listed in Chapter 9.

Of particular importance, however, is ruling out the presence of STIs or organisms associated with pelvic inflammatory disease, because women seeking emergency protection may have new partners and may be at greater risk.

- Women at high risk for STDs or victims of rape are not good candidates for IUD insertion and use.

FETAL EFFECTS

There is no evidence that exposure to EC pills will harm a fetus. Studies in women who have accidentally taken OCs containing levonorgestrel during early pregnancy report no adverse effect on the fetus.

COUNSELING TIPS BEFORE TREATMENT

It is not necessary for women to have a physical exam before prescribing Plan B.

- It is necessary to exclude the chance that the woman is already pregnant so consider the following:
  - Timing of most recent sexual relationships, establish 72 hours or less (or <120 hours for copper IUD) treatment window.
  - Last normal menstrual period.
  - Current use of a contraceptive method.
- Pregnancy test if indicated (should be negative to proceed), if positive, emergency contraception is *not* indicated.
- The most common side effects related to EC pill use are nausea, vomiting, menstrual irregularities, breast tenderness, headache, abdominal pain and cramps, and dizziness.
  - If prescribing an estrogen–progestin EC pill, consider adding an anti-nausea medication (meclizine 1 hour before first dose *[18]*).
  - There is limited data and no agreement on whether to repeat a dose if a user vomits within 2 hours of ingestion.
- Following treatment, users should be counseled to get a pregnancy test and seek medical care if her period does not start within 3 weeks.
- Counsel regarding regular use of a contraceptive method after EC use.
  - OCs, POPs, vaginal ring, DMPA, implant, or patch can be started immediately the day after EC pill treatment is completed, or alternatively started with onset of next menses (use barrier methods while waiting).
  - Insert IUD during the next menstrual period; consider using a copper IUD for EC treatment.
- Consider screening for STIs.
- It is very important to counsel the woman that use of ECs is not 100% effective.
- The progestin-only EC pills are more effective and have fewer side effects than the estrogen–progestin EC pills and are thus the preferred method.

COUNSELING AFTER TREATMENT

- A follow-up physical or pelvic exam is needed if there is concern about either the general health of the user or the pregnancy status after treatment.
- Although there is limited data, a rapid return to normal ovulation and fertility is typical.
- In 2001, an American College of Obstetricians and Gynecologists practice bulletin recommended that clinicians consider giving an advance prescription for EC pills at the time of a routine exam *(7)*.

OPTIONS

Product Prepackaged as Dedicated EC Pills

- Progestin-only (Plan B). Consists of two 0.75-mg levonorgestrel tablets. The first pill is taken as soon as possible within 72 hours of unprotected intercourse and a second tablet is taken 12 hours later (Table 1).

  - Both pills taken as a single dose of 1.5 mg levonorgestrel reported to be as effective *(22)* as traditional two-dose regimen.
- Preven™ Emergency Contraceptive Kit (containing four 0.25-mg levonorgestrel/50-μg ethinyl estradiol pills). The dosage is two doses of two pills, 12 hours apart.
  - Pretreatment with an anti-emetic is recommended.
  - The Preven Emergency Contraceptive Kit was removed from the market by the manufacturer in 2004.

Combination OCs Containing Levonorgestrel or Norgestrel

The FDA issued a summary statement in the *Federal Register* in 1997 *(27)*. This statement is reassuring to clinicians using OCs for this off-label indication.

> *The FDA is announcing that the Commissioner of Food and Drugs has concluded that certain combined oral contraceptives containing ethinyl estradiol and norgestrel or levonorgestrel are safe and effective for use as postcoital emergency contraception.*

- Combination OCs containing either levonorgestrel or norgestrel are used in specific regimens based on the Yuzpe method (Table 1).
  - The first dose of two to five pills is taken as soon as possible within 72 hours of unprotected intercourse and the second dose is taken 12 hours later.
  - Pretreatment with an anti-emetic is recommended.
    - Meclizine 1 hour before treatment.
- POPs (Table 1).
  - Plan B regimen is prepackaged as a dedicated OC pill.
  - Ovrette regimen is 20 pills taken as soon as possible after unprotected intercourse followed 12 hours later with another 20 pills.

Copper IUD (ParaGard®)

Insertion of the copper IUD is a highly effective method when inserted within 5 days of unprotected intercourse. The copper IUD can be left in place for long-term contraception.

REFERENCES

1. Salganicoff A, Wentworth B, Usha R. (2004) Emergency contraception in California. Kaiser Family Foundation report. Menlo Park, CA: Kaiser Family Foundation.
2. Drazen J, Greene M, Wood A. (2004) The FDA, politics, and Plan B. N Engl J Med 350:1561–1562.
3. Food and Drug Administration. FDA's decision regarding Plan B: questions and answers. Available from: www.fda.gov/cder/drug/infopage/planB/planBQandA.htm. Accessed March 10, 2006.
4. Croxatto HB, Devoto L, Durand M, et al. (2001) Mechanism of action of hormonal preparations used for emergency contraception: a review of the literature. Contraception 63:111–112.
5. Hapangama D, Glasier AF, Baird DT. (2001) The effects of peri-ovulatory administration of levonorgestrel on the menstrual cycle. Contraception 63:123–129.

6. Glasier A. (1997) Emergency postcoital contraception. N Engl J Med 337:1058–1064.
7. American College of Obstetricians and Gynecologists (ACOG). (2001) ACOG Committee on Practice Bulletins—gynecology. Emergency oral contraception. No. 25.
8. Ling WY, Robichaud A, Zayid I, Wrixon W, MacLeod SC. (1979) Mode of action of DL-norgestrel and ethinyl estradiol combination in postcoital contraception. Fertil Steril 32:297–302.
9. Alvarez F, Brache V, Fernandez E, et al. (1988) New insights on the mode of action of intrauterine contraceptive devices in women. Fertil Steril 49:768–773.
10. Rivera R, Yacobson I, Grimes D. (1999) The mechanism of action of hormonal contraceptives and intrauterine contraceptive devices. Am J Obstet Gynecol 181:1263–1269.
11. Piaggio G, von Hertzen H, Grimes DA, Van Look PF. (1999) Timing of emergency contraception with levonorgestrel or the Yuzpe regimen. Task Force on Postovulatory Methods of Fertility Regulation. Lancet 353:721.
12. Trussell J, Ellertson C, von Hertzen H, et al. (2003) Estimating the effectiveness of emergency contraceptive pills. Contraception 67:259–265.
13. Trussell J, Rodriquez G, Ellertson C. (1999) Updated estimates of the effectiveness of the Yuzpe regimen of emergency contraception. Contraception 59:147–151.
14. Women's Capital Corporation. (1999) Plan B package insert; information for providers and clients. Washington, DC: Women's Capital Corporation.
15. Zhou l, Xiao B. (2001) Emergency contraception with Multiload Cu-375 SL IUD: a multicenter clinical trial. Contraception 64:107–112.
16. Trussell J, Ellertson C. (1995) The efficacy of emergency contraception. Fertil Control Rev 4:8–11.
17. Pharmacy Access Partnership. Homepage. Available from: www.go2ec.org. Accessed March 10, 2006.
18. Raymond E, Creinin M, Barnhart K, Lovvorn A, Rountree R, Trussell J. (2000) Meclizine for prevention of nausea associated with use of emergency contraceptive pills: a randomized trial. Obstet Gynecol 95:271–277.
19. Glasier A, Baird D. (1998) The effects of self-administering emergency contraception. N Engl J Med 339:1–4.
20. Ellertson C, Ambardekar S, Hedley A, Coyaji K, Trussell J, Blanchard K. (2001) Emergency contraception: randomized comparison of advance provision and information only. Obstet Gynecol 98:570–575.
21. Stewart FH, Trussell J. (2000) Prevention of pregnancy resulting from rape; a neglected preventive health measure. Am J Prevent Med 19:228–229.
22. von Hertzen H, Piaggio G, Ding J, et al. (2002) Low dose mifepristone and two regimens of levonorgestrel for emergency contraception: a WHO multicentre randomized trial. Lancet 360:1803–1810.
23. Task Force on Postovulatory Methods of Fertility Regulation. (1998) Randomised controlled trial of levonorgestrel versus the Yuzpe regimen of combined oral contraceptives for emergenchy contraception. Lancet 352:428–433.
24. World Health Organization (WHO). (1998) Emergency contraception: a guide for service delivery. Geneva, Switzerland: WHO.
25. Nielsen CL, Miller L. (2000) Ectopic gestation following emergency contraceptive pill administration. Contraception 62:275–276.
26. Sheffer-Mimouni G. (2003) Ectopic pregnancies following emergency levonorgestrel contraception. Contraception 67:267–269.
27. Food and Drug Administration. (1997) Prescription drug products; certain combined oral contraceptives for use of postcoital emergency contraception. Federal Register: report no. 62:37.

13 Female Tubal Sterilization

Traditional and Research Methods

Charles M. March, MD

Contents

INTRODUCTION

Although the first tubal sterilization was performed more than 125 years ago, it took many years before it gained widespread acceptance. Today surgical sterilization is a simple, safe, and cost-effective method of achieving long-term contraception. It remains the second (behind oral contraceptives [OCs]) most widely used form of contraception in the United States (Chapter 1). The emergence of sterilization as a popular method of avoiding pregnancy paralleled the introduction of OCs. Both methods became readily acceptable at the time of the "sexual revolution."

The previous strict guidelines for performing sterilization that coupled age and parity were dramatically relaxed when the introduction of laparoscopy made female sterilization an outpatient procedure. Laparoscopy is safer and cheaper than laparotomy, provides a superior cosmetic result, and allows a woman to resume normal activities sooner. The increased safety of anesthesia coupled with concerns about the long-term safety of OCs and intrauterine devices (IUDs) continues to drive interest in permanent sterilization. Features of the "ideal method" of sterilization are listed in Table 1.

From: *Current Clinical Practice: The Handbook of Contraception: A Guide for Practical Management*
Edited by: D. Shoupe and S. L. Kjos © Humana Press, Totowa, NJ

Table 1
Attributes of the Ideal Method of Sterilization

Attributes
Minimal skill and training required
Performed by paramedical personnel
One-time procedure
Highly effective
Effective immediately
Office procedure
Local or no anesthesia
Minimal pain
Minimal morbidity
No mortality
Little equipment required
Reusable equipment
Equipment maintenance minimal
No visible scar
Performed during pregnancy, postpartum, or post-abortion
Inexpensive
Reduce/prevent STDs
Reversible

POPULARITY

The percentage of women who use sterilization as a method of contraception rises from about 5% between 20 and 24 years of age to almost 50% for those between 40 and 44 years of age. It is a safe (in both the long and short term), highly efficacious, cost-effective procedure that requires a single act of compliance, separates contraception from sexual activity, and does not rely on partner behavior.

Sterilization's ability to achieve long-term contraception with a single event is unique and is an important reason for its popularity. This feature makes sterilization an ideal method of permanent contraception in developing countries where access to health care providers is limited.

Although vasectomy is faster, safer, less complex, and less costly than those methods available to women and equally effective, more women than men undergo sterilizing procedures, the current ratio being approximately 3:2. Although many ill-founded concerns about the short- and long-term consequences of vasectomy have reduced the willingness of some men to undergo surgery, other important factors are likely to maintain the current ratio. Among these factors is the high rate of cesarean section driven by multiple factors, including an increasing number of older primiparas with multiple gestations, convenience, and the current litigious environment. The ready access to the oviducts at the time of cesarean section makes simultaneous sterilization a convenient option. Postpartum ster-

Table 2
Methods of Female Sterilization

Associated with pregnancy
Postpartum—with cesarean section or minilaparotomy
Pomeroy or modified Pomeroy partial salpingectomy
Uchida, Irving, Fimbriectomy
Post-abortal—minilaparotomy or laparoscopic
Interval
Laparotomy
Mini-laparotomy
Laparoscopy
Fulguration, clips, rings, loops
Vaginal
Blind transcervical, chemicals, tissue adhesives
Hysteroscopic
Endometrial ablation
Hysterectomy

ilization via a small periumbilical incision is also a convenient option because recovery from both the delivery and the extra surgery can occur at the same time, obviating the need to return for an interval surgery. The desire to remain in control of one's reproductive health is another critical reason for the popularity of female sterilization.

HEALTH BENEFITS OF STERILIZATION

The most widely touted and most significant health benefit of tubal sterilization appears to be a reduced risk of ovarian cancer. One large prospective study that followed 396,000 women for 9 years found that the risk of ovarian cancer was 30% less in the group who had undergone tubal ligation *(1)*. This finding has been confirmed by other investigators. Although the mechanism is unknown (some have suggested that tubal closure protects the ovary by preventing carcinogens from ascending into the upper reproductive tract), this is a most welcome benefit. Tubal closure does not prevent colonization of the lower female reproductive tract by sexually transmitted organisms, but it does reduce the risk of salpingitis and pelvic peritonitis.

TRADITIONAL STERILIZATION METHODS

Approaches to female sterilization are listed in Table 2. Sterilization may be performed in close proximity to a pregnancy or it may be an "interval" procedure. The techniques, along with the advantages and disadvantages of the different methods, are discussed in the subheadings below. Each of these methods should be evaluated against the backdrop of the "ideal method."

Postpartum Methods

Sterilization at the time of cesarian section or immediately following a vaginal delivery is popular and convenient, but there are some additional risks that deserve consideration. The postpartum pelvic viscera are more vascular and thus the risk of excessive bleeding is higher at this time. Generally, however, bleeding is usually recognized immediately and controlled. Bleeding is rarely of clinical significance and re-operation, transfusion, or anemia are very uncommon complications.

Instead, most concerns are related to the issue of regret. Tubal sterilization at the time of cesarean section presents a unique situation because the desire for no more children often rests on the assumption that the newly delivered infant will be viable and healthy. Unfortunately, this outcome is not a certainty and a re-evaluation of whether or not the procedure should be done may be necessary in some circumstances. A difficult pregnancy and/or the delivery of an infant whose health status is uncertain or grave are cause for concern. Is the request for sterilization emanating from a reaction to a physically, emotionally, or financially difficult pregnancy? Would a neonatal or infant death cause the couple to desire another pregnancy?

Often, the delivery of a very ill infant is not anticipated, and the topic is not discussed. In any case, delivery of a neonate with medical uncertainties or adverse outcome prompts a re-evaluation of the couple's wishes before performing the procedure. If the delivery is by elective cesarean section under regional anesthesia, a discussion with the mother is possible. After a vaginal delivery, the delay before minilaparotomy provides a time interval to more thoroughly re-evaluate the options. Avoidance and management of regret are covered more completely at the end of this chapter.

Partial Mid-Tubal Salpingectomy: Modified Pomeroy, Uchida, and Irving

Although there are many methods of interrupting the oviducts at the time of cesarean section, some modification of the Pomeroy partial salpingectomy procedure is the most common. The modified Pomeroy procedure is also a popular method used during postpartum and interval minilaparotomies. The postpartum minilaparotomy is performed through a small sub-umbilical incision because the uterus is enlarged and this approach allows easy access to the tubes.

Regardless of the approach, all modified Pomeroy procedures begin with a positive identification of the fallopian tube by following its course laterally to locate the fimbria. The mid-portion of the fallopian tube is then elevated with a Babcock clamp and the approximately 2-cm knuckle of tube that is created, is ligated with no. 1 plain catgut suture. After the suture has been tied and cut, the ends are grasped with a small Kelly clamp and used to steady the tube. The 2-cm knuckle of tube, still elevated with the Babcock clamp, is cut, one side at a time, about 3–5 mm above the suture tie. Generally, a small section of mesosalpinx is also removed, and the specimen is sent to pathology to provide histological confirmation. The cut ends of the tube should not be too close to the ligature because they may slip through and cause delayed hemorrhage. The rapidly dissolving plain catgut suture allows the ends to separate in the immediate postoperative period.

Many variations of the procedure are performed, including the use of different absorbable sutures, coagulation of the ends of the tubes, and repeat ligation of the cut ends. All of these procedures have similar success rates. In the Parkland modification, after a segment of the mid-tube is removed, both cut ends are religated. In the Madlener procedure, the tube is crushed and then tied with permanent suture. Because of its high failure rate and lack of a specimen for histological review, this procedure is rarely performed. The Uchida and Irving procedures were designed to reduce the risk of tuboperitoneal fistulae. Although the advocates claim that they are slightly more effective, the opponents insist they take longer to perform and have a slightly higher morbidity. The use of clips or bands is not recommended in the postpartum patient because the tubes are dilated, making the devices difficult to apply and resulting in a high failure rate.

Fimbriectomy and Salpingectomy

Fimbriectomy was developed as a single suture alternative to salpingectomy that would have a low risk of recanalization and failure. Unfortunately this procedure does not appear to be more effective and it has three important disadvantages. The first is that the procedure often leaves a substantial proximal segment ending with a small section of ampulla where fluid may collect and form hydrosalpinges. These can become quite large and may cause pain, undergo torsion, become infected, or may be interpreted as neoplasms. Any of these complications can lead to surgical intervention. Secondly, unless the fimbria-ovarica is incorporated in the suture, a tubo-peritoneal fistula and subsequent pregnancy, often ectopic, may occur. Finally, the intrauterine pregnancy rate after reversal of a bilateral fimbriectomy is significantly lower than that following mid-tubal sterilization *(2)*.

On occasion, significant tubal pathology is discovered and sterilization is best accomplished by salpingectomy. It is important that all clamps and sutures be placed as close as possible to the fallopian tube so that the mesosalpinx and collateral blood supply to the ovary is spared during excision.

Interval Methods

Sterilization at a time removed from pregnancy (at least 6 weeks after a term delivery or a few weeks following a spontaneous or induced abortion) is the most common in the United States. When requesting an interval tubal ligation, the patient is able to make the decision without the stress of pregnancy or any related complications, and with the knowledge of the health status of all of her children. Interval procedures are most safely performed in the follicular phase of the menstrual cycle because it is very unlikely that the patient is pregnant and it avoids bleeding from trauma to a recent corpus luteum.

Laparotomy

The same operations performed at the time of cesarean section (as discussed above) can be performed via interval laparotomy. Rings or clips may also be applied but are more often used during a laparoscopic procedure and are discussed below. Except for certain patients who have contraindications to laparoscopy (morbid obesity, multiple prior abdominal or pelvic laparotomies, severe cardiac or pulmonary disease), laparotomy is rarely performed for the sole indication of sterilization unless in conjunction with a laparotomy mandated by other pelvic or abdominal pathology. The tubal ligation procedure adds little cost or morbidity and affords the patient significant benefits. Educating general surgeons to inquire about a patient's desires for future childbearing during the counseling session for a non-emergent gallbladder or intestinal surgery is a valuable milestone.

Minilaparotomy

Minilaparotomy employs a small (2–3 cm) suprapubic incision and is performed under local, regional, or general anesthesia. Except for the very obese, access to the fallopian tubes is generally easy. This procedure is performed in the lithotomy position and a uterine elevator is employed to facilitate access to and identification of the oviducts. The introduction of a paracervical block before application of the uterine manipulator reduces significantly the discomfort for those who elect local anesthesia. Tubal occlusion may be obtained by a partial salpingectomy or by a variety of implants (bands or clips) that are discussed in the "Laparoscopic Approach" section. Minilaparotomy is often performed on an outpatient or overnight basis. If significant pelvic adhesions are present, the incision may have to be enlarged and/or general anesthesia used.

Vaginal Approach

Tubal sterilization via a colpotomy incision is performed infrequently despite the advantages of the approach. The procedure is usually performed in the follicular phase on an outpatient basis, and the problem of cul-de-sac infection has been virtually eliminated by the use of prophylactic antibiotics. After entering the peritoneal cavity through a colpotomy incision, a fimbriectomy or a partial salpingectomy are the most common techniques. If the latter is employed, tubal ligation is often accomplished using an Endoloop.

Even in the absence of clinical infection, adhesions of the oviducts and/or ovaries to the site of incision or vaginal scarring at that site may occur, resulting in dyspareunia. Perhaps the main reason for the fall in popularity of the vaginal approach to sterilization is the overall reduction in the amount of vaginal surgery. As average parity has fallen and the frequency of cesarean section has risen, prolapse of pelvic organs is less common. Surgery to treat urinary incontinence is commonly treated by a suprapubic approach, rather than a vaginal approach.

Laparoscopic Approach

The reintroduction of laparoscopy in the late 1960s (the first laparoscopic sterilization had been performed in 1936 by Bosch in Switzerland) had a most dramatic impact on interval sterilization. At that time, the prime indications for laparoscopy were diagnostic (to investigate the cause for pelvic pain or for infertility) or therapeutic (for sterilization). Laparoscopy offered a faster, safer, and cheaper method of sterilization than laparotomy or minilaparotomy with a shorter recovery period and a superior cosmetic result.

Before beginning surgery, all equipment should be checked to verify that all is in proper working order. Either closed or open laparoscopy is an acceptable approach and both can accomplish the same goal of safe placement of the primary trocar. Thus, the choice is driven primarily by operator preference. In closed laparoscopy, a Veress needle is introduced blindly into the peritoneal cavity followed by the insufflation of carbon dioxide, or direct primary trocar placement followed by insufflation. The latter permits more rapid insufflation, but if a vital structure is injured, the size of the wound is larger. After the primary trocar has been placed, a laparoscope is introduced and the pelvis visualized.

In open laparoscopy, a small (but larger than for closed laparoscopy) subumbilical incision is made and the peritoneum is entered under direct vision. A primary trocar is then placed and anchored to the fascia with sutures or secured in place by an inflatable base. It is important to obtain an airtight seal to prevent the soon-to-be-insufflated carbon dioxide from leaking from the peritoneal cavity. The benefit of open laparoscopy is that the peritoneum is entered under visualization, not blindly, thus making it a good approach for those with prior abdominal or pelvic surgery and/or known or suspected adhesive disease. Although the data demonstrate that the frequency of inadvertent damage to structures is identical between open and closed procedures, this may be biased because more high-risk patients may be selected for open laparoscopy. Another option for patients who are likely to have adhesions in the periumbilical region is closed laparoscopic entry into the left upper quadrant.

Many disposable closed laparoscopic trocars have a spring-loaded cover that retracts when meeting significant resistance, allowing the blade to be exposed during entry. After the peritoneum is entered and there is no further resistance, the blade is covered. This was designed as an added degree of safety and has become a popular choice.

A hybrid approach, blending open and closed laparoscopy techniques, is to introduce the Veress needle and then to enter the peritoneum with an optical trocar after the carbon dioxide has been introduced. This type of non-bladed optical trocar has a somewhat sharp and transparent tip. The telescope is passed into the trocar and with gentle pressure the preperitoneal layers are dissected under direct visualization until the peritoneum is reached and a "window" is identified through which the trocar and telescope are advanced. In short, this is another attempt to reduce the risk of major visceral or vascular injury.

The laparoscope may be of the operating type that has an accessory channel that can be used as a port for introduction of an operating instrument, or a diagnostic laparoscope with only the telescope. The latter laparoscope requires the introduction of the operating instrument via a secondary trocar. Although the use of an operating laparoscope permits the operation to be performed more rapidly and uses only one incision, its primary advantage is that (in carefully selected patients) it allows sterilization to be performed under local anesthesia. The goal is rapid identification and occlusion of the oviducts when a thorough pelvic inspection is not needed. For an obese woman, local anesthesia, minimal peritoneal distention, and minimal Trendelenberg positioning may not permit good visualization and safe surgery. For these patients, those with pelvic adhesions, or those with symptoms such as pelvic pain, the alternate choice of a diagnostic laparoscope with a secondary trocar permits a full visualization of the pelvis as well as appropriate surgical intervention.

Laparoscopic Electrocoagulation Methods

The original method of tubal sterilization was via monopolar coagulation. In this procedure, the mid-portion of the oviduct is grasped with a monopolar coagulator and elevated away from all other pelvic structures before coagulation. As electro-coagulation proceeds, the tube appears white. The desired "end point" of the procedure is the destruction of approximately 1.5 cm of the fallopian tube in both directions from the coagulator. Usually a small portion of mesosalpinx immediately below the site of application of the forceps is also coagulated. Commonly, the tube is cut and divided in the center of the burned area. This method is rapid and highly effective.

Three potential problems are associated with this method. The first is the formation of tubo-peritoneal fistulae and subsequent failures, especially ectopic pregnancies. This occurrence was surprising, especially because the white area of injury does not typically extend to the cornual portion of the uterus. To solve this problem, it is now recommened that tubal coagulation be done in the isthmic-ampullary junction, well away from the uterotubal junction. Overall, the frequency of ectopic pregnancies is not high but the proportion tends to rise as the interval from the time of surgery increases *(3,4)*. This fact suggests that failures occurring early in the postoperative period may be related to technique, whereas subsequent ones are likely related to self-repair of the oviducts.

The second problem is that there is often only a small amount of fallopian tube remaining, making tubal reversal difficult or impossible: the residual fallopian tubes may be represented solely by small cornual stumps and a few tufts of fimbria. Clearly, greater-than-expected tubal damage occurs during monopolar coagulation. Hulka demonstrated that lateral spread of monopolar energy is much greater than judged at the time of application and characterized a "burst" effect of monopolar energy.

The third problem of monopolar tubal sterilization is the occurrence of delayed bowel injuries. This complication has led to legal action and battles over whether these injuries resulted from an unrecognized "sparking" from the monopolar electrode to the bowel or from surgical error with direct touching of the electrode to the large and/or small bowel. If a very small serosal burn is detected, the patient may be observed. However, if the area is larger or if injury beyond the serosal layer is suspected, bowel resection including a 5-cm margin on each side should be performed. Attempts to oversew the area will usually fail because of the occult damage that occurs with the use of unipolar electrodes. In the postoperative period, the area of burn and suture placement may undergo necrosis and bowel perforation and peritonitis may ensue. Hybrid trocars, that permit some of the electrical charge to be transferred and stored in the telescope or in another instrument, are no longer used because it was demonstrated that injuries could come from "capacitive coupling" *(5)*.

These three problems led to a drop in the popularity of monopolar tubal sterilization and a move toward use of bipolar forceps. By 1980, bipolar forceps had replaced unipolar electrodes in most centers *(6)*. Because the electrical energy is transmitted only between the two jaws (electrodes) of the forceps, a number of the problems related to monopolar electrode use were solved immediately: neither capacitive coupling nor "sparking" can occur, and the lateral spread of the energy can be controlled. Truly "what you see is what you get" and provided the electrodes are placed 2 cm or more from the uterotubal junction, fistulae will almost never occur. Because the extent of the tubal damage is not extensive, reversal of sterilization is usually possible if only one area is coagulated. However, the greater spread of damage during the application of monopolar injury does have two important advantages: superior hemostasis and a very low failure rate. Even if the placement of the monopolar electrode is not perfect, the diffusion of the burn tends to compensate.

In an effort to minimize the risk of failure using bipolar forceps, double- and triple-burn techniques are commonly employed. Although this approach reduces the failure rate, the "promise" of possible reversal is mostly eliminated. The frequency of bowel injuries has fallen with bipolar sterilization, but whether this is related to inherent equipment differences, an overall improvement in surgical equipment, or the increased experience of current surgeons remains unclear. If a single-burn bipolar technique is used, many surgeons divide the tube in the center of the coagulated area. The area of coagulation and the incision should include a minimal amount of mesosalpinx, because further damage may compromise ovarian blood supply, lead to excessive bleeding necessitating further coagulation, or rarely, cause delayed hemorrhage and re-operation. If the oviduct is divided, coagulating the proximal and distal stumps again reduces the risk of both fistula formation and postoperative bleeding.

Some have challenged the reports indicating that the failure rate of bipolar sterilization is higher if only a single area is coagulated and claim that a single burn is adequate as long as it is done properly. Because blanching and swelling of the portions of the oviduct within and adjacent to the electrodes do not ensure that the innermost portion of the tube has been desiccated, it is advisable to use a generator with an ammeter. This device provides both visible and audible signals to the surgeon indicating when the area has been properly and thoroughly coagulated.

A new choice, the endocoagulator, was designed to reduce the risk of damaging internal structures such as bowel and ureter *(7)*. With an endocoagulator, heat (as opposed to electrical energy) is applied directly to the tubes. By avoiding the conversion of electrical energy to heat in the tubes, this procedure may offer added safety. Few surgeons, however, use an endocoagulator for any other laparoscopic or open procedure and thus its availability is limited. It is not expected that this instrument will gain widespread use for sterilization.

Laparoscopic Mechanical Methods

Tubal occlusion by mechanical means avoids the concerns of safety associated with electrosurgery but generally are not used in situations in which tubes are dilated, such as the postpartum period. Three devices are used commonly and each has its own idiosyncrasies. Each device is highly effective and has a unique applicator and a different mechanism of achieving tubal occlusion. Because each device is somewhat unique, it is advisable that each surgeon identifies his or her preferred method. Whether the decision is based on ease of use, perceived efficacy, cost, or other factors, the surgeon should ideally use this chosen method exclusively and use an electrosurgical method as back-up. Efficacy of a procedure is greatest when the nuances of each instrument are learned through prolonged experience.

Laparoscopic Silastic Rings (Yoon Band and Falope Ring)

The 3.6-mm silastic band is mounted on a 6-mm applicator that is inserted into the pelvis through an accessory trocar *(8)*. This band is impregnated with 5% barium sulfate to provide radio-opacity. Immediately before application to the oviduct, the band is stretched and advanced over the outer cylinder of the applicator. If the band remains on the applicator in a stretched condition for an extended time period, it may lose "memory" and thus some occluding capacity. The fallopian tube is grasped at the junction of its proximal and middle thirds and elevated. A portion (approximately 2.5 cm) of tube is drawn into the inner cylinder of the applicator. The surgeon must ensure that the tube is encircled completely by the jaws of the instrument so the band will seal the tube completely, not simply a tangential application. Next, the ring is advanced from the outer cylinder over the tubal segment. It is important to confirm that the ring is "seated" properly over the knuckle of tube. Improper placement may allow tubal motility to cause the ring to slide off the tube. Proper application of the jaws to the oviduct must be accurate to avoid incorporating any mesosalpingeal vessels. The placement process should be slow, deliberate, and controlled so minimal tension is placed on the oviduct and that no tearing of the tube or mesosalpinx occurs. Tearing of either of these structures may lead to early or delayed hemorrhage. Usually, the segment of tube within the band is not excised.

Intra-operative application of a local anesthetic to the site of ring application can alleviate some of the postoperative pain associated with this procedure. If one or both oviducts are large, bleeding occurs, or adhesions are present, conversion to an electrosurgical method of tubal sterilization is advised. Failure rates are approximately 1% after 2 years. Over time the bands become peritonealized. In most cases, the lack of an excessive inflammatory reaction, minimal adhesion formation, and the small amount of tube damage makes this method of sterilization highly reversible.

Laparoscopic Clips

Laparoscopic clips are associated with the least amount of tubal damage and thus are the most amenable to reversal. The Hulka spring-loaded clip has two Lexan plastic jaws with multiple teeth *(9)*. The lower jaw has a distal hook. The jaws are joined with a stainless steel hinge pin. After the isthmic portion of the oviduct is identified, the jaws are placed over this tubal segment perpendicular to its long axis. This right angle application of the clip is mandatory and may necessitate a double-puncture technique. After proper placement, the jaws of the clip are closed and a gold-plated stainless steel spring is advanced over the jaws, sealing the tube. The teeth of the clip must extend into the mesosalpinx, ensuring complete closure of the tube. Because the amount of damage to the tube is minimal (3 mm), this method of sterilization is very amenable to reversal. However, as is true for all tubal sterilization procedures, those that induce the least amount of damage are associated with the highest failure rate over time, again testimony to the tubes' regenerative powers *(10)*.

The Filshie clip uses a specially designed applicator that can be used with a diagnostic or operating laparoscope or during laparotomy *(11)*. The clip is made of titanium lined with silicone rubber and has a concavity on its antimesenteric side conforming to the shape of the oviduct. Application of the clip must be perpendicular to the tubal isthmus and is facilitated by the use of a secondary trocar. Initially, the clip occludes the tube by the pressure applied during application. However, as tubal necrosis ensues, the silicone rubber expands and maintains luminal obstruction. Only 4–5 mm of tube is damaged, facilitating reversal of sterilization.

Laparoscopic Salpingectomy

Salpingectomy, whether by laparoscopy or laparotomy, has a limited but important role to play among sterilizing procedures. Patients with hydrosalpinges should not undergo mid-tubal interruption because it is likely that the isolated segment(s) will become large, cause pain, and may be mistaken for a neoplasm. After extensive adhesiolysis, severely damage tube may have little, if any, normal-appearing portions and removal may be advised. If laparoscopic sterilization is done in conjunction with endometrial ablation, the small isthmic segment of oviduct may fill up with blood or secretory products from the uterine horns, and cause the "post-ablation tubal sterilization syndrome" *(12)*. Removal of the lateral intramural segment during salpingectomy, or leaving the lateral troughs of the endometrial cavity intact during the ablation, may reduce the risk of the post-ablation tubal sterilization syndrome. If salpingectomy is performed, the incision should be placed immediately below the oviduct to spare the collateral ovarian blood supply.

Laparoscopic Complications

Both morbidity and mortality of laparoscopic procedures remain low. A 1993 American Association of Gynecologic Laparoscopists report indicated a death rate of 1 in 22,966 procedures. In another report, the US mortality rate was 1.5 per 100,000 procedures *(13)* with many of the mortalities occurring in patients with pre-existing medical conditions. Although a significant number of deaths may be attributed to anesthetic complications, vascular and intestinal injuries also account for some of the mortality. Patient selection, intra-operative and postoperative vigilance, and operator experience and judgment influence the rate of serious complications and the success rate of the surgical procedure.

Overall, the rates of minor and major complications are approximately twice as high among women who undergo a minilaparotomy with a partial salpingectomy compared with those who have laparoscopic tubal coagulation. However, the types of complications tend to be different. With minilaparotomy, longer operating times, longer convalescence, higher rate of wound infections, and greater postoperative pain predominate, whereas vascular and bowel injuries, although rare, are the significant complications of laparoscopic procedures. Careful inspection of the pelvis immediately after entry and again before removing the instruments is necessary to reduce the frequency of "delayed" diagnosis. Delays can be associated with severe morbidity, multiple repeat operations, and even death.

A little-discussed "complication" is the inability to complete the procedure laparoscopically and a necessity to convert to a minilaparotomy procedure. Rather than a true complication from the procedure, these events are usually owing to technical issues related to adhesions, poor visualization, or difficult port placement. However, this possibility should be mentioned during the pre-operative discussion.

The low degree of complications coupled with the low risk of method failure makes sterilization one of the safest and most effective methods of preventing pregnancy. It is obviously the ideal choice for those in a stable, long-term rela-

Table 3
Cumulative 10-Year Failure Rates of Tubal Sterilization by Method

Method	*Failure rate (%)*
Postpartum partial salpingectomy	0.75
Unipolar coagulation	0.75
Silastic ring	1.77
Interval partial salpingectomy	2.01
Bipolar coagulation	2.48
Hulka clip	3.65

tionship. Methods that reduce the amount of tubal damage are preferable because they are less likely to interfere with ovarian blood supply and less likely to cause adhesion formation. Procedures that minimize tubal damage also facilitate reversal should circumstances change in the future. Sterilization does not affect the functioning of the ovaries or other endocrine organs, alter the age of menopause, change sexual function or desire, or increase the risk of hysterectomy *(14)*. Psychological problems and sexual dysfunction do not occur more often following sterilization. Although irregular menses and dysmenorrhea have been reported to occur more often after tubal sterilization, most of these reports include a large number of women who used oral contraceptives for painful menses and/ or cycle regulation before the surgery *(15–18)*.

Laparoscopic Failures

Failures can be either early or late: the former are usually related to technique and the latter related to tubal recanalization. Failures are more common in younger women, probably because there is more time for tubal recanalization and a greater likelihood that they will have a high proportion of quality oocytes if re-canalization occurs. For all of the procedures performed by laparotomy, failure rates of around 1–2% are reported. Failure rates vary according to the method used (Table 3) *(19)* but generally are between 0.1 and 0.8% during the first year.

In the US Collaborative Review of Sterilization (CREST) study, 10,685 women were enrolled. The 10-year cumulative probability of pregnancy was 18.5 per 1000 procedures. However, for postpartum and laparoscopic procedures using unipolar tubal coagulation, the rate was 7.5 pregnancies per 1000 compared with 36.5 after clip application. For bipolar tubal coagulation, the rate of failure was reduced if three or more sites were coagulated *(20)*. In the CREST study, luteal phase pregnancies, estimated to occur in 2 or 3 per 1000 procedures, were not reported as failures. Curettage at the time of sterilization does not completely insure that a procedure will not "fail" because of a pre-existing pregnancy *(21)*. A better approach is limiting surgery to the follicular phase of the cycle that will also reduce the risk of traumatizing a fresh corpus luteum.

Table 4
Advantages of Transcervical Sterilization

Office procedure
Less invasive
Local/no anesthesia
No incision
Safe
Effective
Inexpensive
Rapid recovery
Ideal for high-risk patient

The likelihood that a pregnancy will be extrauterine is greater if it occurs after a sterilizing operation. The proportion of ectopic pregnancies increases over time, being three times higher 4–10 years after surgery than in the first 3 years. If a pregnancy occurs after tubal sterilization, ectopics are most common after bipolar coagulation (65%) and interval partial salpingectomy (43%). Unipolar coagulation (17%) and spring clip application (15%) are associated with the lowest proportion of ectopic pregnancies.

TRANSCERVICAL APPROACH

Transcervical sterilization has a host of advantages (Table 4) and has been the dream of many dedicated to finding the ideal method of population control. The lack of an incision is an important advantage because it affords patient privacy and a quick recovery. The ready access to the tubal ostia and the proximal portions of the fallopian tubes makes this method most attractive. It has long been hoped that a simple transcervical sterilization technique be developed that could be easily performed by paramedical personnel.

However, the intramural oviduct has unique properties that, to date, have proven impossible for all candidates to overcome. The intramural oviduct is quite tortuous, often having convolutions in excess of 360° in a length of less than 2 cm, thereby preventing the introduction of long, rigid devices *(22)*. The uterine muscle enveloping the proximal portion of the tube undergoes contractions that can dislodge intraluminal plugs. The tube is somewhat compliant and it may dilate after a device is placed, thus preventing complete microscopic occlusion, essential to prevent sperm transport. Tubal secretory capability is known to prevent the adherence and tissue in-growth needed for some devices to be effective. Finally, as is true with the more distal oviduct, healing and regeneration may lead to failures.

Transcervical sterilization has a number of important disadvantages (Table 5). An important disadvantage is that transcervical sterilization must be performed

Table 5
Disadvantages of Transcervical Sterilization

Disadvantages of Transcervical Sterilization
Complex delivery systems
Expensive disposables
Long learning curve
Possible intraperitoneal injury
Not possible postpartum
Not possible post-abortion
Follicular phase timing required
Normal anatomy required
Delayed efficacy
Long-term effectiveness unknown
Long-term risks uncertain
Insurance coverage variable

in the proliferative phase of the cycle at a time well-removed from a pregnancy. Even more important, however, is that none of the methods in use today are effective immediately.

Essure® Micro-Insert

The Essure micro-insert, approved by the US Food and Drug Administration in 2002, has gained widespread acceptance. The insert is a 4-cm-long device consisting of a flexible, stainless steel inner coil, a very elastic expandable outer coil of a nickel titanium alloy (Nitinol), and a layer of polyethylene terephthalate running along and through the inner coil.

The insert is introduced into the intramural portion of the oviduct under hysteroscopic guidance. An operating hysteroscope with a 5F instrument channel is used. Surgery is performed under local anesthesia in the proliferative phase. Using a narrow-diameter release catheter, the device is maintained in a "wound-down" configuration (0.8 mm in diameter) to facilitate placement. After the ostium is identified, the insert is advanced into the ostium until only 5–10 mm remains visible. The device is disengaged from the release catheter and the outer coil expands to up to 2 mm, anchoring the device in place and spanning the distance between the intramural and proximal isthmic portions of the tube. The polyethylene terephthalate fibers induce a foreign body reaction that peaks 2–3 weeks after placement of the coil. Over the next 3 months, tissue in-growth occurs, completely occluding the tube and anchoring the device in place permanently. This in-growth begins at the periphery of the device and enters its interior. Overall approximately 5 cm of tube is affected. The reaction spares the uterine and tubal serosa as well as the tubal epithelium distal to the device *(23)*.

Successful placement can be achieved in more than 90% of women. The safety, efficacy, and patient satisfaction were demonstrated in prospective, multicenter trials involving more than 700 patients *(24)*. Adverse events were reported in 7% of patients. Almost all who had successful placement reported being happy with the method. Another method of contraception was used until an hysterosalpingogram (HSG) could demonstrate bilateral tubal obstruction. Proper device placement and bilateral tubal occlusion was demonstrated in 96% of women 3 months after surgery. Almost all others had occlusion documented after another 3 months.

After placement of the insert by experienced hysteroscopists, 87% relied on the method for permanent contraception. After 9620 women-months of exposure to intercourse, no pregnancies were reported *(25)*. Of 643 women followed for up to 5 years, there were no pregnancies in 29,357 women-months of follow-up *(26)*.

Endometrial Ablation

Any tubal sterilization procedure, including the Essure micro-insert, can be combined with one of the global methods of endometrial ablation in women who desire sterilization and treatment for menorrhagia. Irrespective of the method of endometrial ablation used, it cannot be considered as a method of sterilization. Although the number of reported pregnancies after endometrial ablation is quite low, perhaps 1 in 400, these data are difficult to interpret. Many women who undergo ablation are older and thus relatively infertile. Many others have had sterilizing operations or use contraception. Finally, in some of the pregnancies that have occurred after endometrial ablation, there have been serious complications. Simultaneous hysteroscopic sterilization adds little operating time to the ablation, avoids the risk of post-ablation tubal sterilization syndrome, and is an ideal combination for the high-risk patient.

Hysterectomy

Hysterectomy for sterilization is associated with a longer recovery period, more morbidity and mortality, and is more costly than tubal sterilization. Costs included are those related to surgery, anesthesia, medications, and hospitalization, as well as those related to lost time from work and childcare. Nevertheless, when associated conditions exist, hysterectomy may be considered. Associated conditions include menorrhagia, leiomyomata, pelvic relaxation, severe cervical dysplasia, endometriosis, and significant dysmenorrhea. If possible, hysterectomy should be vaginal because of the lower morbidity and faster recovery time. If the patient has significant pain mandating inspection of the pelvis and/or significant pelvic adhesions, laparoscopically assisted vaginal hysterectomy is appropriate.

AVOIDING AND MANAGING REGRET

In a study of 7000 women followed for at least 5 years after sterilization, the frequency of regret increased over time and was reported to be 6% overall *(27)*.

Table 6
Factors That Influence the Success of Tubal Sterilization Reversal

Method of sterilization
Amount of tubal damage
Patient age
Presence of other infertility factors
Surgeon experience

The overall frequency of regret within 14 years after surgery was 20.3% for women who were under 30 years at the time of surgery, and 5.9% in those above that age. Those under 30 indicated regret because of the desire to have for more children, whereas those over 30 attributed gynecological or medical disorders to the sterilizing procedure, a claim not supported by data.

Parous women and women in unstable relationships are more likely to regret having been sterilized than are nulliparous women. In some studies, regret is reported to be more common among those who had a postpartum sterilization *(28)*. The probability of regret decreases as the time from the last birth increases. After 8 years it falls to approximately 5%, not different from the rate of regret among all women.

Obviously, careful counseling by an experienced health care professional is critical to reducing the frequency of regret *(29)*. The physician is involved in this process, especially when the method of sterilization is discussed. Those candidates for sterilization requesting a "reversible" method are obviously going down the wrong path. The method of sterilization selected should be the one that the surgeon believes to be the most efficacious and the one with which he or she has the most experience and comfort. Performing a procedure that the surgeon has had little experience with is likely to have a lower success rate.

Reversal of Sterilization

Factors affecting the success of reversing tubal sterilization are listed in Table 6. Unlike vasectomy, the success rate of reversal does not appear to be related to the number of years during which the tube was occluded (when corrected for age and the presence of other infertility factors). The amount of damage induced by surgical sterilization (in decreasing order) is multiple-burn monopolar coagulation, fimbriectomy, multiple-burn bipolar coagulation (with or without tubal division), single-burn bipolar coagulation, partial salpingectomy, and falope rings and clips *(30,31)*. The chance of successful surgical reversal is inversely related to the amount of damage. Very little data are available to assess the likelihood of reversing hysteroscopic sterilization.

After a couple requests a reversal of sterilization, a referral should be made to a reproductive surgeon, experienced in tubal microsurgery. A review of the prior surgery and pathology reports (if available), and an HSG are helpful in determining the amount of remaining proximal and distal tubal length and predicts the chance of successful reanastomosis. If the HSG shows significant intrauterine pathology, a procedure such as hysteroscopic correction may be added.

After these data are gathered, an informed discussion of the two alternatives (in vitro fertilization [IVF] and reconstructive surgery) for restoring fertility follows. The couple may base their decision on multiple factors specific to the clinic or medical office that would be performing the procedure. For IVF, the live birth rate per cycle; cumulative live birth rate after a specific number of cycles; added success rate of subsequent frozen embryo transfer; and risk of multiple pregnancy, abortion, and extrauterine pregnancy are compared with the success rates and risk of extrauterine pregnancy rates associated with reconstructive surgery.

The advantages of IVF are that it avoids major surgery, has a low rate of ectopic pregnancy, and overcomes significant male factor infertility or various ovulatory defects. Cryopreservation of extra embryos may make embryos available for future attempts. However, IVF is expensive, usually not covered by health insurance carriers, associated with a high rate of multiple pregnancies and cesarean sections, and an increase in the rate of spontaneous abortion. Some patients may reject IVF for personal reasons.

Reconstructive surgery can provide years of menstrual cycles during which a couple can achieve one or more pregnancies. The risk of spontaneous abortion is not increased among those who conceive after tubal surgery compared with age-matched controls. With the exception of posterior or cornual tubal implantation, the need for cesarean section is not increased by tubal reparative surgery. The risk of an ectopic pregnancy is very low following mid-tubal reanastomosis. However, tubal reconstructive surgery is usually not covered by insurance and involves a surgical procedure (generally minilaparotomy but in some clinics laparoscopy) and associated minor and major morbidities.

If the chance of success from reconstructive surgery equals or exceeds the "threshold" selected by the patient, microsurgical repair is indicated. A diagnostic laparoscopy before the minilaparotomy allows assessment of the remaining distal and proximal tubal segment. Doing both procedures at the same time is safer and less expensive, and insures that reconstruction is possible. Under certain conditions, diagnositic laparoscopy is skipped and only minilaparotomy is performed.

During the diagnostic laparoscopy, the presence, location, extent, and density of adhesions; the presence and extent of endometriosis; the presence leiomyomata or ovarian pathology; and finally, the amount of proximal and distal oviduct(s) available are evaluated. Hydrochromopertubation confirms that the remaining proximal portion(s) of oviduct(s) are patent and free of salpingitis isthmica nodosa (that predisposes to ectopic pregnancy). If the HSG suggested obstruction at the tubocornual junction, the instillation of dye transcervically under anesthesia may determine that the cause was spasm. If obstruction is confirmed, attempts can be made to overcome the block by proximal tubal cannulation under hysteroscopic guidance *(32)*.

Table 7
Outcome of Tubal Reconstructive Surgery

Procedure	*IUP*	*Live birth*	*Ectopic*
Salpingostomy by laparotomy	20–40%	18–35%	10–40%
Salpingostomy by laparoscopy	10–40%	10–30%	10–35%
Reanastomosis by laparotomy	45–80%	30–80%	2–10%
Reanastomosis by laparoscopy	50–75%	50–60%	3–30%
Tubocornual anastomosis	50–60%	30–50%	5–15%

The types of procedures are multiple and their outcomes vary considerably (Table 7). A combination of one of these procedures with another microsurgical repair has a lower success rate. In addition to magnification, all the principles of microsurgery should be used, including gentle tissue handling and complete hemostasis. If surgery fails, a repeat operation may not be the best option and referral for IVF considered.

RESEARCH METHODS

With the exception of some recently developed methods and the newer versions of quinacrine administration, many of the following methods are of historical significance and included here to demonstrate the variety of problems encountered. The early attempts at developing an "easy" technique for tubal sterilization focused on finding a caustic agent that could be placed blindly into the uterus, find its way into the fallopian tubes, and cause tubal scarring. Most commonly, an acorn-type device surrounding the introducer was used to prevent reflux of the caustic agent into the vagina. Unfortunately, no such safety device has been designed to prevent intraperitoneal spillage. These early techniques required a number of applications of the caustic agent to the uterine cavity and the use of some other form of contraception until bilateral tubal obstruction could be documented (usually with an HSG).

The more recently developed techniques avoided the blind placement of material by using new steerable hysteroscopes. Direct hysteroscopic tubal coagulation is also now possible, although the complication rate has been higher than expected. The worldwide need for easy, affordable sterilization continues to stimulate research efforts along these lines.

Research Methods: Chemical Agents

When caustic agents, such as silver nitrate (in a paste), zinc chloride, formaldehyde, or 2% ethanol/formalin were tested, bilateral tubal closure rates of only 50–70% were reported after one application but up to 95% after six applications. Histological evidence of marked tubal necrosis was documented with most agents. Unfortunately, pregnancies occurred in patients that had HSG-documented bilateral tubal obstruction. It is likely that some HSGs documenting proximal obstruction did so because of tubal spasm rather than tubal damage, but regeneration of the epithelium and restoration of tubal patency may also explain these failures. The sclerosing agent sodium morrhuate had little effect on the tubal epithelium. When phenol was used alone as a liquid, mucilage, or in a paste with atabrine, closure rates of 78–94% were reported, but peritonitis also occurred. Although talc caused a very extensive intraperitoneal reaction, it did little damage to the oviducts.

Research Methods: Quinacrine

The cytotoxic agent quinacrine has been delivered to the proximal portion of the fallopian tubes in the form of a quinacrine hydrochloride solution, in quinacrine-impregnated IUDs and as quinacrine pellets. Quinacrine sterilization remains the safest, most effective, and the most widely used (>125,000 cases) non-surgical method. The ongoing interest in quinacrine is derived from the pioneering research of Jaime Zipper *(33)*. When the solution form of quinacrine hydrochloride at a concentration between 125 and 167 mg/mL was delivered to the proximal oviducts, bilateral closure rates of 55, 80, and 95% were achieved after one, two, and three instillations, respectively. However, possible intravascular administration and intraperitoneal spillage with attendant local damage have limited its general acceptance.

Quinacrine-impregnated IUDs of a "T" or "Y" configuration were developed to deliver quinacrine from their lateral arms, which would be maintained in close proximity to the tubal ostia. These devices solved the problems of multiple applications and intraperitoneal spillage. In addition, they provide a back-up method of contraception while the process of tubal closure is ongoing. However, they did not improve efficacy or eliminate the need for an HSG.

Cylindrical quinacrine pellets (3.2 mm in diameter) have been used also as a method of limiting peritoneal spread. The pellets are introduced via a sterile copper T IUD introducer. Seven 36 mg pellets (total dose of 252 mg) are delivered monthly to the top fundal portion of the uterus during the proliferative phase (between days 7 and 10) of the cycle for 2 months. The pellets dissolve within 30 minutes, releasing quinacrine, which causes necrosis of the endometrium and endosalpinx. The former recovers within two cycles but scar tissue forms within the intramural portion of the tubes within 12 weeks, during which time contraception is mandatory. Initial reports indicated that a bilateral tubal closure rate of 73% could be achieved *(34)*. This rate rose to 84% after a third insertion. Perhaps as testimony to the regenerative capabilities of the oviducts, the first year pregnancy rate of 0.7% rises to 3.8% at 24 months, but remains stable thereafter (4% at 36 months). In a 4-year follow-up study, Bhatt and Waszak reported a failure rate of 3.7% *(35)*.

With a newer insertion technique and the administration of oral papaverine as smooth muscle relaxer, Hieu et al. reported a major complication rate of 0.03%

and a failure rate of 2.7% after 4 years *(36)*. However, at 5 years the pregnancy rate was 12.9% with two insertions and 27.3% after one insertion *(37)*. These pregnancy rates are considerably higher than those from Chile in which the 10-year cumulative pregnancy rate was 10.7% among women who were under 35 years of age at the time of sterilization and only 3.1% for those who were older than 35 *(38)*. In an attempt to address the issue of relaxing both uterine and tubal musculature at the time of quinacrine administration, pellets of diclofenac or ibuprofen were placed in the uterus at the time of quinacrine pellet instillation. No improvement in tubal closure rates was detected.

Liquid quinacrine has been delivered hysteroscopically but may reflux into ampulla and peritoneum while the contralateral oviduct is cannulated *(39)*. A more practical approach is the use of quinacrine rods that are delivered into the intramural portions of the oviducts under hysteroscopic guidance. The ease of administration and very low cost of quinacrine is likely to maintain ongoing interest in the United States and elsewhere.

Research Methods: Tissue Adhesives

The tissue adhesives gelatin–resorcinol–formaldehyde and methylcyano-acrylate (MCA) deserve special attention. Their use recognized the importance to provide complete and permanent microscopic occlusion. Gelatin–resorcinol–formaldehyde was highly efficacious but required a special mixing device and had a complication of peritoneal spillage.

Bilateral closure rates were 66 and 89% after one and two instillations, respectively. MCA has a somewhat unique property compared with other agents in that as it flows from the proximal to more distal oviduct, the material changes from a monomer to a polymer. The polymerized form is on the outside of the advancing stream and protects the peritoneum from injury if any should spill into the cavity, a very rare event. Cell necrosis begins within 24 hours and proceeds rapidly. By 12 weeks, the tubes are scarred and the MCA has been cleared by macrophages.

To reduce the volume of solution instilled via a small, disposable device, MCA was applied via a unique delivery system, the Femcept™ device *(40)*. A volume of only 0.65 mL was instilled and the cannula was 4 mm in diameter. When "triggered," a balloon inflated beginning in the area of the lower uterine segment, preventing vaginal reflux. Milliseconds later the fluid containing the adhesive was released from the tip of the cannula. As the balloon became larger, the adhesive was "pushed" toward the cornual recesses of the uterus. With this technique, very small volumes could be instilled, thereby reducing the risk of peritoneal contamination. In preliminary studies, the device was introduced under fluoroscopic guidance and a radio-opaque dye was instilled to prove that peritoneal spillage did not occur. Subsequently, clinical trials began. Bilateral closure rates were 74–80% after one application but they rose to 90–98% after a repeat application. The cumulative pregnancy rate was 3.7% 24 months after discontinuing contraception *(41)*. With the addition of a radio-opaque material to the MCA, some flow and polymerization properties were improved and a plain X-ray could replace an HSG to verify intratubal placement.

Research Methods: Hysteroscopic Approach

Coagulation of the tubal ostia has been practiced for many decades beginning with a report by Kocks in 1878 *(42)*. Hysteroscopy was introduced by Pantaleoni in 1869 *(43)*. Under hysteroscopic guidance, electrocoagulation of the fallopian tubes was reported by Mikulicz-Radecki and Freundin in 1928 *(44)*. However, it was not until high-viscosity dextran was introduced as a uterine-distending medium that good, clear visualization became easy to achieve *(45)*. Researchers built on the pioneering work of Rodolfo Quinones who used glucose in water as a uterine-distending medium and Hans Lindemann who used carbon dioxide *(46,47)*.

Protocols for hysteroscopic tubal coagulation were simple. Early in the follicular phase, a hysteroscope was placed into the uterine cavity after a paracervical block had been introduced. Each tubal ostium was identified, a flexible 3-mm monopolar electrode was placed for a distance of 5 mm and the electrosurgical generator was activated using the coagulating mode. The distal end of the electrode was shielded to prevent lateral spread of the energy. Energy was delivered in 6-second intervals until the familiar white end point used in laparoscopic tubal coagulation had been achieved. Surgery time was usually less than 5 minutes. The patient returned to home or work within 30 minutes, continued contraception until having an HSG in 3 months. Investigators reported bilateral closure rates of almost 90%. Because the amount of periostial damage was easy to verify, perfect coaxial placement of the electrode was not necessary.

Regular inspection of the uterine cavity demonstrated the high incidence of congenital and acquired uterine abnormalities, perhaps explaining some of the failures of non-hysteroscopic methods *(48)*. New steerable hysteroscopes were developed so that access to eccentrically placed tubal ostia was possible *(49)*. Enthusiasm was high as it appeared the ideal method of female sterilization was at hand.

However, within a couple of years, many complications were reported *(50)*. Some of the serious peri-operative complications included peritonitis, bowel injury, and even death. Most complications were delayed and related to the occurrence of pregnancies months and even years after HSGs had documented bilateral tubal closure. Many of these pregnancies were extrauterine, commonly in the intramural segment of the tube, and associated with delayed diagnosis and profound hemorrhage. Trials in the United States were discontinued.

To investigate a possible etiology for these failures, we performed laparoscopy in 20 patients with successful hysteroscopic tubal coagulation procedures as documented by HSGs. *(51)*. To assess tubal occlusion and verify HSG findings, a dilute solution of indigo carmine was instilled transcervically. Tubal closure at the cornual portion was confirmed, but 16 of the 20 patients had developed sinus tracts and fistulae. Of the 16 patients, 11 involved only the cornual portion(s) of the uterus and 7 extended into the broad ligament(s). We concluded that the amount of monopolar energy delivered in the original hysteroscopic tubal coagulation far exceeded what was expected. Additionally, lateral spread and a "burst effect" (when the generator is set in the coagulating mode) caused excessive damage to the intramural portion of the fallopian tubes. Although the procedure had successfully interrupted the fallopian tubes, extensive damage had been done and the regenerative powers of the tubes resulted in channel and fistulae formation, and resultant extrauterine pregnancies.

Research Methods: The Brundin P-block

The Brundin P-block consists of a hydrogel of polyvinyl pyrrolidone and methylacrylate on a nylon skeleton. This combination allows both expansion of the device after placement and tissue in-growth. The device is small (1.4 mm in diameter × 4 mm long) and held in place after placement by two 2-mm anchoring wings. Unfortunately, only 49% of the patients achieved bilateral tubal closure *(52)*. Because no pregnancies occurred in the patients with patent tubes, the author theorized that the device acted as an intratubal contraceptive device and/or that distention of the intramural portion of the tube altered gamete transport. Without complete tubal obstruction, however, the device cannot be considered "sterilizing."

Investigational Procedures: Hosseinian Uterotubal Junction Device

The Hosseinian device is a 1-cm long polyethylene device *(53)*. It is 1 mm in diameter at its intramural side but 2 mm in diameter at its base where four 5.2-mm spines are attached by a screw. These spines were designed to anchor the device in place. Nonreactive materials were used in the hope that removal would restore fertility. However, neither high levels of tubal occlusion nor reversibility could be demonstrated and trials were discontinued.

Research Methods: Hamou Intratubal Thread

Hamou intratubal thread was designed to be reversible and minimize or avoid damage to the tubes *(54)*. The device consisted of a 28- to 30-mm-long- × 1-mm-in-diameter nylon thread. At each end of the thread was a loop that prevented migration of the device in either direction (into the uterus and the peritoneum). The loop on the uterine side also could be used for removal via hysteroscopy. Of 166 patients, 156 (94%) had successful placement. After 1 month there were four expulsions proven by hysteroscopy and after 1471 cycles, there was one intrauterine pregnancy.

Research Methods: Rigid Plugs

The rigid 7 × 2-mm 3-M ceramic plug was designed to provide complete tubal occlusion via a reaction to the porous α alumina *(55)*. Expulsion was common and only two-thirds of the subjects had bilateral tubal closure. Premolded silicone devices were provided with or without a central metal core. The rates of expulsion and of perforation were high. For reversible sterilization, a 10- × 1.5-mm notched device was developed but neither the promise of efficacy nor that of reversibility was realized *(56)*.

Research Methods: Formed-in-Place Silicone Plugs

Formed-in-place silicone plugs were another novel concept and appeared to have a bright future *(57,58)*. As with other hysteroscopic approaches, follicular phase timing and normal anatomy were prerequisites. Procedures were completed in less than 30 minutes under paracervical block anesthesia. Unlike the rigid silicone plugs used in previous trials, the shape of these plugs was customized to the anatomy of each individual oviduct. After a tubal ostium was identified, a catheter with an obturator tip was passed through the operating channel of the hysteroscope. The obturator tips were hollow and of varying shapes to conform to different ostial configurations. Liquid silicone and its catalyst, stannous octoate, were removed from the freezer, mixed, and then instilled into the catheter. This mixture flowed through the center of the obturator tip and bonded to it. The flow of silicone continued and an exact mold of the oviduct was created from the proximal oviduct to the ampulla. Tiny amounts of elemental silver within the liquid silicone allowed the operator to monitor flow of the silicone-catalyst mixture and made the plugs radio-opaque. An immediate postoperative X-ray and another in 3 months could assure proper placement, configuration, and that the distal plug remained bonded to the obturator tip. Because these plugs were larger at both ends, a properly configured plug should be larger at both ends than in the middle and thus would be "locked" into place.

Placement of plugs on both sides was successful in 90% of patients and in 90% of these patients the plugs were normal providing an overall 81% success rate *(59)*. For those whose placement of normal was successful, the procedure was both satisfying and efficacious. However, among all patients who underwent hysteroscopy, an overall success rate was just above 81%, a not very acceptable result.

Because the obturator tip had a small nylon thread at the end, it could be identified and grasped under hysteroscopic guidance. With traction, the plug could be retrieved and an HSG could confirm tubal patency. Had a method of sterilization been found that was readily reversible? No, significant tubal damage occurred, perhaps as a reaction to the silver. When the plugs migrated into the peritoneum or were placed there at the time of the original hysteroscopic procedure, adhesion formation occurred.

Research Methods: Adiana

The Adiana device accomplishes sterilization using a two-step procedure that has been evaluated in the EASE (*E*valuation of the *A*diana System for Transcervical *S*terilization Using *E*lectrothermal Energy) trial that was completed in mid-2005. Although the protocol had many similarities to the Essure trials, this device and its method of achieving sterility is considerably different.

Under hysteroscopic guidance and in the proliferative phase of the menstrual cycle, a catheter is placed into the intramural portion of the tube. The electrode at the distal end of this catheter delivers low level (<5 W) of radiofrequency energy, causing superficial destruction of the epithelial layer. The radiofrequency generator output is automatically regulated to maintain a desired tissue temperature during lesion formation. This approach limits the amount of damage induced but also individualizes treatment to compensate for variations in patient anatomy. Exact placement of the catheter in the center of intramural portion with 360° contact is critical to the induction of a symmetrical circumferential injury. After the lesion is created, a porous nonbiodegradable matrix implant of medical-grade silicone is deposited into the area. The process of tubal repair induces tissue in-growth into the matrix and complete tubal occlusion. Proper placement is documented visually and by ultrasound in the immediate postoperative period. An HSG and follow-up ultrasound are performed 3 months after surgery.

Research Methods: Intratubal Ligation Device

The intratubal ligation device is still in an early stage of development. The overall approach involves placement of the catheter system into the lumen of the fallopian tube, invagination of a portion of the endosalpinx, and ligation of the resulting pedicle with an elastomeric band. Sterility is achieved immediately via band placement over the tubal lumen and thus it differs from all other hysteroscopic methods in a most important way.

This device consists of a triple layer of coaxial catheters made of extruded nylon. The retracted tip of the inner catheter forms a deflated balloon, the middle lumen has an expanded tip that houses an O-ring, and the outer catheter pushes the O-ring over an invaginated tissue pedicle of endosalpinx. During insertion, the leading tip of the device is approximately 1 cm of double-hulled silastic tubing that reduces the risk of perforation during insertion and serves as the inflatable balloon during device deployment. The device is advanced into the tubal ostium and tubal lumen until the isthmic-ampullary junction has been reached. The balloon is inflated and a minimal amount of methylcyanoacrylate is delivered through the pores in the outer balloon. Adherence occurs on contact. The balloon is deflated and the adhered tissue is withdrawn slowly toward the second lumen. Further retraction of the expanded tip envelopes the invaginated tissue and the O-ring is deployed over the tissue, sealing the oviduct. Following tissue necrosis and sloughing, long-term contraception is achieved by means of localized scarring.

Although work with this procedure is in preliminary stages, it is an exciting concept and its unique property of immediate effectiveness is a most important milestone for hysteroscopic sterilization.

Table 8
Today's Methods of Sterilization Versus the Ideal Method

Parameter	*Ideal*	*PS*	*LTC*	*LTB*	*BTC*	*HSC*
Skill/training	Minimal				+	
Paramedic procedure	Yes				+	
One treatment	Yes	+	+	+		+
Effectiveness	High	+	+	+		+
Effective immediately	Yes	+	+	+		
Office procedure	Yes				+	+
No anesthesia	Yes				+	+/–
Pain	Minimal		+	+	+	+
Morbidity	Minimal	+	+	+	+	+
Mortality	None	+/–	+/–	+/–		
Equipment needed	Little	+			+	
Reusable equipment	Yes	+	+	+/–		+/–
Equipment maintenance	Minimal	+			+	
Visible scar	None				+	+
Possible during pregnancy	Yes	+				
Possible postpartum or post-abortion	Yes	+	+	+/–		
Inexpensive	Yes				+	
Reduce/prevent STDs	Yes					
Reversible	Yes	+	+/–	+		

PS, partial salpingectomy (at cesarean section, interval, abdominal or vaginal); LTC, laparoscopic tubal coagulation (monopolar or bipolar); LTB, laparoscopic application of band or clip; BTC, transcervical blind; HSC, hysteroscopic.

Research Methods: Microwave Sterilization

The same approach to endometrial destruction by means of microwaves may be applied to the intramural oviduct. If trials demonstrate safety, studies may begin perhaps with delivery of the energy under ultrasound guidance.

Research Methods: Reversible Tubal Occlusion

Varieties of inert devices have been and are in very preliminary stages of development. To date, none has demonstrated the sufficient promise needed to attract significant amounts of private or governmental funding.

CONCLUSION

Table 8 compares various methods of sterilization available today in the United States and a number of other countries. Although we are still somewhat removed from the ideal, transcervical approaches remain the most attractive because of ready access to the fallopian tubes, safety, and the fact that they can be performed with minimal anesthesia.

REFERENCES

1. Miracle-McMahill HE, Calle EE, Kosinski AS, et al. (1997) Tubal ligation and fatal ovarian cancer in a large prospective cohort study. Am J Epidemiol 145:349–357.
2. Tourgeman DE, Bhaumik M, Cook GC, et al. (2001) Pregnancy rates following fimbriectomy reversal via neosalpingostomy: a 10-year retrospective analysis. Fertil Steril 76:1041–1044.
3. Peterson HB, Xia Z, Hughes JM, et al. (1997) The risk of ectopic pregnancy after tubal sterilization. New Engl J Med 336:762–763.
4. Chi I-c, Laufe LE, Atwed R. (1981) Ectopic pregnancy following female sterilization. Adv Plann Parenthood 16:52–55.
5. Centers for Disease Control and Prevention. (1980) Deaths following female sterilization with unipolar electrocoagulation. MMWR Morb Mortal Wkly Rep 30:150.
6. Soderstrom R. (1978) Electrical safety in laparoscopy. In: Phillips JM, ed. Endoscopy in Gynecology. Downey, CA: American Association of Gynecologic Laparoscopists, pp. 306.
7. Semm K. (1976) Thermocoagulation by endocoagulator. A new method for pelviscopic sterilization. Gynecologie 27:279–282.
8. Yoon IB, Wheeless CR, King TM. (1974) A preliminary report on a new laparoscopic sterilization approach: the silicone rubber band technique. Am J Obstet Gynecol 120:132.
9. Hulka JF, Omran K, Phillips JM, et al. (1973) Sterilization by spring clip: a report of 1,000 cases with a 6 month follow-up. Fertil Steril 26:1122–1125.
10. Chi C, Laufe LE, Garner SD, Tolbert MA. (1980) An epidemiologic study of risk factors associated with pregnancy following female sterilizations. Am J Obstet Gynecol 136:768–773.
11. Filshie GM, Casey D, Pogmore JR, et al. (1981) The titanium/silicone rubber clip for female sterilization. Br J Obstet Gynaecol 88:655–657.
12. Townsend DE, McCausland V, McCausland A, et al. (1993) Post-ablation-tubal sterilization syndrome. Obstet Gynecol 82:422–424.
13. Escobedo LG, Peterson HB, Grubb GS, et al. (1989) Case-fatality rates for tubal sterilization in U.S. Hospitals. Am J Obstet Gynecol 160:147–149.
14. Goldhaber MK, Armstrong MA, Golditch IM, et al. (1993) Long term risk of hysterectomy among 80,007 sterilized and comparison women at Kaiser Permanente, 1971–1987. Am J Epidemiol 138:508–511.
15. DeStefano F, Perlman JA, Peterson HB, Diamond EL. (1985) Long term risks of menstrual disturbances after tubal sterilization. Am J Obstet Gynecol 152:835–841.
16. Rulin MC, Davidson AR, Philliber SG, et al. (1993) Long term effect of tubal sterilization on menstrual indices and pelvic pain. Obstet Gynecol 82:118–121.
17. Gentile GP, Kaufman SC, Helbig DW. (1998) Is there evidence for a post-tubal sterilization syndrome? Fertil Steril 69:179–186.
18. Kjer JJ. (1990) Sexual adjustment to tubal sterilization. Eur J Obstet Gynecol Reprod 35:211–214.
19. Peterson HB, Xia Z, Hughes JM, et al. for the U.S. Collaborative Review of Sterilization Working Group. (1996) The risk of pregnancy after tubal sterilization from the U.S. Collaborative Review of Sterilization. Am J Obstet Gynecol 174:1161–1170.
20. Soderstrom RM, Levy BS, Engel T. (1989) Reducing bipolar sterilization failures. Obstet Gynecol 74:60–65.
21. Lichter ED, Laff SP, Friedman EA. (1986) Value of routine dilation and curettage at the time of interval sterilization. Obstet Gynecol 67:763–765.
22. Sweeney W III. (1962) The interstitial portion of the uterine tube—its gross anatomy, course and length. Obstet Gynecol 19:3–10.
23. Valle RF, Carignan CS, Wright, TC, et al. (2001) Tissue response to the STOP microcoil transcervical permanent contraceptive device: results from a prehysterectomy study. Fertil Steril 76:976–980.
24. Kerin JF, Carignan CS, Cher D. (2001) The safety and effectiveness of a new hysteroscopic method for permanent birth control: results of the first Essure pbc clinical study. Aust N Z J Obstet Gynaecol 41:364–370.

25. Cooper JM, Carignan CS, Cher D, et al. (2003) Microinsert nonincisional hysteroscopic sterilization. Obstet Gynecol 102:59–67.
26. Kerin J. (2005) Hysteroscopic sterilization, long-term safety and efficacy. Presented at the 53rd Annual Clinical Meeting of the American College of Obstetricians & Gynecologists, May 8, San Francisco, CA.
27. Hillis SD, Marchbanks PA, Tylor LR, et al. (1999) Poststerilization regret: findings from the United States Collaborative Review of Sterilization. Obstet Gynecol 93:889–898.
28. Chi I-c, Gates D, Thapa S. (1992) Performing sterilizations during a woman's postpartum hospitalization: a review of the United States and international experiences. Obstet Gynecol Surv 47:71–79.
29. Allyn DP, Leton DA, Westcott NA, et al. (1986) Presterilization counseling and women's regret about having been sterilized. J Reprod Med 31:1027–1029.
30. Siegler AM, Hulka J, Peretz A. (1985) Reversibility of female sterilization Fertil Steril 43:499–505.
31. Dubuisson JB, Chapron C, Nos Z, et al. (1995) Sterilization reversal: fertility results. Hum Reprod 10:1145–1151.
32. Novy MJ, Thurmond AS, Patton P, Uchida BT, Rosch J. (1988) Diagnosis of cornual obstruction by transcervical fallopian tube cannulation. Fertil Steril 50:434–440.
33. Zipper J, Strachetti E, Medel M. (1970) Human fertility control by transvaginal application of quinacrine on the fallopian tube. Fertil Steril 21:581–589.
34. El Kady AA, Nagib HS, Kessel E. (1993) Efficacy and safety of repeated transcervical quinacrine pellet insertions for female sterilization. Fertil Steril 59:301–304.
35. Bhatt R, Waszak CS. (1985) Four year follow-up of insertion of quinacrine hydrochloride pellets as a means of nonsurgical female sterilization. Fertil Steril 44:303–306.
36. Hieu DT, Tan TT, Tan DN, et al. (1993) 31,781 cases of non-surgical female sterilization with quinacrine pellets in Vietnam. Lancet 342:213–217.
37. Sokal D, Zipper J, King T. (1995) Transcervical quinacrine sterilization: clinical experience. Intl J Gynecol Obstet 51:S57–S69.
38. Feldblum P, Hays M, Zipper J, et al. (2000) Pregnancy rates among Chilean women who had non-surgical sterilization with quinacrine pellets between 1977 and 1989. Contraception 61:379–384.
39. Alvarado A, Quinones R, Aznar R. (1974) Tubal instillation of quinacrine under hysteroscopic control. In: Sciarra JJ, Butler JC Jr, Speidel JJ, eds. Hysteroscopic Sterilization. New York: Intercontinental Medical Book Corporation, pp. 85–94.
40. Richart RM, Neuwirth RS, Bolduc L. (1977) Single application fertility regulating device: Description of a new instrument. Am J Obstet Gynecol 127:86–90.
41. Moyer DL, Neuwirth RS, Rioux JE. (1983) Discussion: research and clinical experience with MCA. In: Zatuchni GI, Shelton JD, Goldsmith A, Sciarra JJ, eds. Female Transcervical Sterilization. Philadelphia: Harper & Row, pp. 223–233.
42. Kocks J. (1878) Eine neue methode der sterilization der frauen. Zentralblatt fur Gynakologie 2:617–619.
43. Pantaleoni DC. (1869) On endoscopic examination of the cavity of the womb. Med Press Circ 8:26–29.
44. Mikulicz-Radecki F von, Freund A. (1928) Ein neue hysteroskop und seine anwendung in der Gynakologie. Zschr Gebertsh 92:13–21.
45. Edstrom K, Fernstrom I. (1970) The diagnostic possibilities of a modified hysteroscopic technique. Acta Obstet Gynecol Scand 49:327–331.
46. Quinones GR, Alvarado DA, Anzar AA. (1973) Tubal electrocauterization under hysteroscopic control. Contraception 7:195–199.
47. Lindemann HJ. (1973) Transuterine tubensterilisation per hysteroskop. Gerburtsh u Frauenheilk 33:709–713.

48. Cooper JM, Houck RM, Rigberg HS. (1983) The incidence of intrauterine abnormalities in patients undergoing elective hysteroscopic sterilization. J Reprod Med 10:659–661.
49. March CM, Israel R. (1976) A comparison of steerable and rigid hysteroscopy for uterine visualization and cannulation of tubal ostia. Contraception 14:269–274.
50. Richart RM. (1974) Complications of hysteroscopic sterilization. Contraception 10:230–235.
51. March CM, Israel R. (1975) A critical appraisal of hysteroscopic tubal fulguration for sterilization. Contraception 11:261–269.
52. Brundin J. (1987) Observations on the mode of action of an intratubal device, the P-block. Am J Obstet Gynecol 156:997–1000.
53. Hosseinian AH, Morales WA. (1983) Clinical application of hysteroscopic sterilization using uterotubal junction blocking devices. In: Zatuchni GI, Shelton, JD, Goldsmith, Sciarra JJ, eds. Female Transcervical Sterilization. Philadelphia: Harper & Row, pp. 234–239.
54. Hamou J, Gasparri F, Scarselli GF, et al. (1984) Hysteroscopic reversible tubal sterilization. Acta Eur Fertil 15:123–129.
55. Craft I. (1976) Uterotubal ceramic plugs. In: Sciarra JJ, Droegmueller W, Speidel JJ, eds. Advances in Female Sterilization Techniques. Hagerstown, MD: Harper & Row, pp. 176–181.
56. Sugimoto O, ed. (1978) Hysteroscopic reversible sterilization. In: Diagnostic and Therapeutic Hysteroscopy. Tokyo: Igahu-Shoin, pp. 196–207.
57. Reed TP III, Erb R. (1983) Hysteroscopic tubal occlusion with silicone rubber. Obstet Gynecol 61:388–392.
58. Loffer FD. (1984) Hysteroscopic sterilization with the use of formed-in-place silicone plugs. Am J Obstet Gynecol 149:261–269.
59. Cooper JM. (1992) Hysteroscopic sterilization. Clin Obstet Gynecol 35:282–298.

14 Contraceptives for Special Populations

Adolescents and Perimenopausal Women Following Pregnancy and During Lactation

Donna Shoupe, MD

CONTENTS

ADOLESCENTS

Delaying sexual activity is the goal until responsible sexual, contraceptive, and protective behaviors for sexually transmitted infections are established.

Introduction

In 2004, the Department of Health and Human Services estimated that about 47% of female and 46% of male teenagers had had sexual intercourse at least once *(1)*. Sexually active teenagers report that they use a contraceptive method only 75 to 90% of the time. Among the developed countries, the United States continues to have one of the highest adolescent pregnancy rates (up to 90 per 1000).

A 1994 report claimed that 20% of sexually active girls 15–19 years of age in the United States become pregnant *(2,3)*. About 33% of these pregnancies end in abortion, about 14% end in miscarriage, and 54% end in live births. In 1999, 12% of all births in United States were to women younger than 20 years of age *(4)*. Unfortunately, teenage pregnancy is associated with high rates of welfare dependency, poverty, lack of education, and inadequate workforce training.

It is also of serious concern that of the18.9 million new cases of STIs each year in the United States, 9.1 million occur in adolescents and young adults *(5)*. Long-term problems associated with early sexual activity include pelvic inflammatory disease, infertility, cervical dysplasia, emotional disturbances, as well as criminal prosecution (Table 1) *(6)*.

From: *Current Clinical Practice: The Handbook of Contraception: A Guide for Practical Management*
Edited by: D. Shoupe and S. L. Kjos © Humana Press, Totowa, NJ

Table 1
Statistics on Risk of STIs and HIV in Young People

- Of all STIs occurring each year, 50% are in young people ages 15–24 *(5)*.
  - HPV is the highest STI incidence in ages 15–24 with 4.6 million new cases per year.
  - In one study of inner city sexually active teenagers, 90% had HPV on the cervix *(68)*.
  - The highest risk for cervical cancer is among those who are sexually active during adolescence and have multiple sexual partners *(69)*.
- About 25% of newly diagnosed HIV cases are in young people under age 22 years *(41)*.

STI, sexually transmitted infection.

Table 2
Adolescent Counseling

- Abstinence information.
  - Benefits of delaying.
  - Negotiation and refusal skills.
    - Address peer pressure.
  - Realistic expectations on condoms and other contraceptives.
    - Limits on contraceptive effectiveness.
    - Limits on STI protection.
- Accurate contraceptive information.
  - Options and proper use.
  - Emphasis that contraceptive and STI protection most reliable when method used consistently and correctly.

STI, sexually transmitted infection.

Counseling the Teenager

In the ideal case, the health care provider can reach the adolescents before their sexual debut and convey to them the associated personal, social, economic, and health consequences they should consider (Table 2). Delaying sexual activity is clearly the goal until responsible sexual, contraceptive, and sexually transmitted infection (STI) protective behaviors are developed. Multiple studies demonstrate the value and need for parental guidance as well as appropriate teenager counseling.

- A national research study conducted in 1468 teenagers addressed several aspects of contraceptive use among teenagers and identified some important trends *(7)*. In both females and males, the odds of consistent use of a contraceptive method increased with the duration of a relationship. Discussion of contraceptive use with a partner before a sexual experience was associated with a higher and more consistent use of a method. Increased number of dates before sexual activity resulted in higher contraceptive use.

- In a Zogby International survey done in 2003, 93% of the parents of adolescents felt it was important to encourage teenagers to abstain from sex until they were, at least, out of high school *(8)*.

Appropriate adolescent counseling includes an emphasis on the benefits of abstaining or delaying sexual activity, the fact that no contraceptive insures absolute protection, and the potential negative consequences of sexual contact. Providing accurate, pertinent information regarding the limits of contraceptive and STI protection from currently available methods is important. Although condoms offer the best protection, no method offers complete protection from pregnancy or STI transmission. Abstinence is the only a sure way to be protected.

Adolescents choosing to begin or to continue engaging in sexual activity should be given up-to-date information regarding condom and other contraceptive choices. Counseling includes a brief but clear description of female anatomy and the reproductive cycle and how birth control methods work *(9)*. Many adolescents resist contraceptive or condom use for a variety of reasons, including a denial that they could become pregnant, fear or embarrassment to ask for contraceptives, lack of access, concerns about cost, fear of partner rejection, worry about parental discovery, ignorance, desire to have a child, or lack of planning. Selecting the best contraceptive method for a teen includes an assessment of psychosocial and physical development, motivation, level of understanding, and financial ability. To improve compliance, delaying the pelvic exam in an overly reluctant patient may be appropriate.

Choosing the Correct Contraceptive Method

When choosing the type of birth control, the following factors are important to consider.

- Does the method address the teen's risk of STI exposure?
- Will the patient be able to easily obtain the method?
- Does the teen have any medical contraindications to the chosen method?
- Is the teen informed on how to use and motivated to use the chosen method?
- Does the teen understand the side effects associated with the method?
- Is the level of protection against pregnancy appropriate for the teen?

Options for Adolescents: Male and Female Condom

Counseling for most teenagers should include the short- and long-term risks associated with STIs and a realistic assessment of prevention strategies.

Most sexually active teenagers are at risk for STI exposure. A male or female condom used alone or in conjunction with another contraceptive method is often the best choice. If used correctly and consistently, male (and probably female) condoms substantially reduce the risk of HIV transmission *(10)*. Condoms are not 100% effective, but in 1986, the US Surgeon General's report advised use of latex condoms to prevent AIDS.

There are not yet studies showing strong reductions in STI transmission with use of condoms. However, the World Health Organization (WHO), along with many other health care providers, advises that their use can help reduce the spread of STI infections *(11)*.

Options for Adolescents: Oral Contraceptives, Patch, or Ring

> *Generally, oral contraceptives are first-line options for contraceptive protection in this age group. Adding a condom for STI protection may be appropriate and highly beneficial. Teens like the bleeding control and decline in menstrual cramps and acne.*

There is no evidence of any adverse effect on growth or maturation of the hypothalamic–pituitary axis by taking hormonal contraceptives in healthy, menstruating adolescents. As long as a girl has had at least three regular, presumably ovulatory menstrual cycles, it is safe to prescribe oral contraceptives (OCs), contraceptive ring, or patches.

In choosing the correct contraceptive method for a sexually active, healthy adolescent, the clinician should be particularly concerned about the ability of the teen to use the method correctly. OCs are relatively easy to use, regulate and reduce menstrual bleeding, as well as reduce menstrual cramps and acne. These are good reasons for teenagers to keep taking OCs.

The contraceptive patch offers these same benefits and adds the additional benefit of a once-a-week rather than daily dosing (Chapter 5). Some studies show that compliance with the patch may be particularly good in adolescents. In a recent study in adolescents, consistent and proper use of the transdermal patch was significantly better than the inconsistent performance seen with OC use *(12)*. Side effects of breast tenderness, nausea, and headache may occur. Development of a second-generation low-dose patch would be a particularly good option for this age group.

The following suggestions may improve OC compliance among adolescents.

- Cue use of method to a daily activity, e.g., near sink in morning.
- Explain protocol for missed dose.
- Establish liberal prescription renewal.
  - Advise regarding necessary yearly follow-up visits.
- Emphasize other benefits, including less acne, less hirsutism, less dysmenorrhea, less bleeding, and more regular menses.
- Emphasize safety and effectiveness of the method.

  - A nonsmoker aged 15–19 years using OCs has a method-related mortality rate of 0.3 per 100,000 women per year. Compare this with a mortality rate for motor vehicle accidents of 19.6 per 100,000 in the general population or with 7 per 100,000 pregnancy-related death in this age group (Table 1).
- Prepare the adolescent for breakthrough spotting or bleeding that may occur during the first few months of use.
- Discuss concerns regarding weight gain.
  - Although some cyclic fluctuations may occur, OCs and patches are generally not associated with a weight gain of more than 0.5 lb.

Options for Adolescents: DepoProvera (DMPA) and depo-subQ provera 104™

According to the US Department of Health and Human Services' *Health, United States, 2004: With Chartbook on Trends in the Health of Americans* report, nearly 10% of adolescent girls ages 15–19 chose depot medroxy-progesterone acetate (DMPA) as their method of contraception, as compared with only 3% in the overall contraceptive market (ages 15–44). In all age groups, use of DMPA should be accompanied with promotion of adequate daily calcium and exercise (Chapter 7). The newly released depo-subQ provera 104 (depo-subQ) is a lower dose than DMPA and is injected subcutaneously rather than intramuscularly. It is also approved for treatment of pelvic pain associated with endometriosis.

DMPA and depo-subQ are highly effective methods that may be particularly good in teens that do not want to take a pill every day. Other good candidates include teens that have become pregnant on OCs, those that forget to take their pills every day, or those who have discontinued use of OCs because of side effects. DMPA and depo-subQ are administered every 3 months and may be more cost-effective compared with other methods. The irregular bleeding, weight gain, or amenorrhea *(13)* that may occur during DMPA use are not popular, particularly in this age group, and may lead to discontinuation. Adequate counseling regarding the early bleeding changes and later amenorrhea, and potentially a better side effect profile with the use of the lower-dose depo-subQ may improve user satisfaction.

Questions remain whether or not adolescents using DMPA or depo-subQ will achieve normal peak levels of bone density or whether long-term use will result in significant bone loss. A black-box warning in the package insert warns that use of DMPA or depo-subQ should be limited to 2 years of use or less, unless other methods are inadequate. Although it is important to counsel adolescents about this warning, it is important to keep this risk balanced with the social, psychological, and medical risks of unintended pregnancy. WHO guidelines suggest that the benefits of use in adolescents under 18 outweigh the risks.

Some very reassuring papers concerning the long-term safety of DMPA have been published. Use of DMPA does not appear to increase the risk of osteoporosis later in life. In a cohort study of 170 adolescents, bone mineral density (BMD) was completely recovered 12 months post-DMPA discontinuation *(14)*. In fact, the adjusted mean BMD values at all anatomic sites at 12 months after discontinuation of DMPA was as high or higher than those of nonusers. In a randomized, double-blind controlled trial of 123 adolescents, low-dose estradiol supplementation to DMPA use resulted in no decline in BMD *(15)*.

These findings are similar to the findings associated with lactation showing that bone losses associated with lactation are reversible and do not lead to long-term skeletal changes *(16)*. The bone loss occurring in both teenage and adult DMPA users is probably the result of the contraceptive-induced reduction in ovarian estradiol production *(17)*. For health care providers, this is reassuring information. Although it is rarely necessary to monitor bone loss with bone imaging studies, calcium supplementation is recommended for most teenagers, regardless of contraceptive choice. Calcium supplementation plus adequate exercise may substantially reduce the risk of bone loss when on DMPA therapy. Estrogen supplementation is generally unnecessary because full recovery of bone density is expected after discontinuation.

Options for Adolescents: Subdermal Progestin Implant

It is anticipated that the etonorgestrel implant system (Implanon®), currently approved in Europe, will shortly get final Food and Drug Administration (FDA) approval. This method has many advantages in adolescents. After insertion, the user need do nothing else and will continue to have very effective contraceptive protection for 3 years. Progestin-only methods are associated with irregular bleeding.

Options for Adolescents: Intrauterine Device

The intrauterine device (IUD) is usually not a good choice for adolescents, although it may be appropriate for a parous or certain monogamous adolescents. The risk of sexually transmitted infection (STI) transmission is often high in this age group because of high-risk sexual activities, often making the IUD a poor option. Health care providers may hesitate to insert an IUD in a nulliparous patient because it is more difficult and is off-label. WHO recommendations:

- From menarche to younger than 20 years old, there is concern about the risk of STIs and the increased risk of explusion owing to nulliparity, however, the benefits of either the copper IUD or levonorgestrel intrauterine system (LNG-IUS) may outweigh the risks.

Options for Adolescents: Diaphragm and Cervical Caps or Shields

The diaphragm and cervical caps have not been popular methods for this age group because many adolescents are reluctant to be fitted for a diaphragm, prefer not to touch their genitals, and dislike having interrupt sexually activity. Correct and consistent use on every sexual contact is a difficult challenge for many adolescents.

Although the diaphragm can be a very effective method in highly motivated users, the typical failure rate with the diaphragm is higher than for the male condom, OCs, patch, or injectable contraceptives. Diaphragms and cervical caps may provide only limited STI protection.

Options for Adolescents: Emergency Contraception

Appropriate counseling for sexually active adolescents includes information regarding the availability of emergency contraception and how to get it. All states have laws that address the medical treatment of minors, including a minor's ability to consent to a least some form of specific health care, such as contraceptives (Chapter 12). The FDA is currently considering approval of over-the-counter availability of emergency contraception. However, the concern for misuse in the under-16-year-old age group has been a major obstacle and restrictions on adolescents are likely.

PERIMENOPAUSAL WOMEN

Introduction

Women in perimenopause are entering a final phase of reproductive life that is associated with lowered risk of pregnancy, changes in menstrual bleeding patterns, and "roller-coaster" changes in ovarian hormone production. In many patients, their long-standing poor health habits may be associated with early physical changes that may eventually lead to serious health problems, including cancer, osteoporosis, and cardiovascular disease (CVD). Consideration of these risk factors can help to lead to proper selection of a contraceptive method, as well as to intervention strategies.

Many women in perimenopause, especially those with irregular menses, believe they are no longer fertile and therefore tend not to use contraceptive protection *(18)*. Although fertility is decreased and pregnancy rates are low in this age group, sexually active perimenopausal women may still be at risk. Even with menstrual irregularities, some women may have sporadic ovulation *(19)* and thus some risk of pregnancy. If pregnancy occurs in this age group, it is often unintended and unwanted. Pregnant women over age 40 have one of the highest induced abortion rates, surpassed only by pregnant teenagers *(20)*.

Women ages 35–44 now constitute the largest single group of reproductive-age women in the United States. As these older women seek contraceptive counseling, many non-contraceptive benefits of hormonal contraceptives become increasingly more relevant. Many of these benefits are discussed in detail in the remaining Subheadings and in Chapter 2.

Concerns of the Perimenopausal Woman: Cancer Risk

The reported effect of various contraceptive methods in reducing the risk of endometrial, ovarian, and colorectal cancer is shown in Table 3.

Table 3
Reported Reductions in Cancer Risks With Use of Specific Contraceptive Methods Compared With Nonusers

	Use duration	*Risk reduction*
Endometrial cancer		
Combination OCs *(70,71)*	1 year	40%
	12 years	72%
	20 years after stopping	50%
DMPA *(51)*	Ever-use	79% (protection persists ≥8 years after stopping)
Progestin IUDs *(48,49,72)*	Limited data	40–60%
Ovarian Cancer		
Combination OCs *(73–75)*	3–6 months	40%
	>5 years	50% (protection persists ≥30 years after stopping)
Colorectal Cancer		
Combination OCs *(62,76)*	Ever-use	16–18%
	96 months	40%

Adapted from ref. *36*.
OC, oral contraceptive; DMPA, depot medroxyprogesterone acetate; IUD, intrauterine device.

Concerns of the Perimenopausal Woman: Perimenopausal Bleeding Problems

Perimenopausal women can experience shorter or longer cycles, heavier or lighter periods, or irregular or skipped periods. Sexually active transitional women with irregular cycles or heavy periods are particularly good candidates for progestin-containing hormonal contraceptive methods including combination low-dose OCs, rings, DMPA or depo-subQ injection *(21)*, or the progestin-containing IUD *(22)*.

Concerns of the Perimenopausal Woman: Perimenopausal Symptoms

Many women during the transition to menopause experience at least one of the common perimenopausal symptoms. These symptoms include sleep disturbances, hot flashes, mood changes, vaginal dryness, and dyspareunia *(23)*. In a population-based prospective cohort study, 31% of African American and Caucasian women 35–47 years of age at entry reported having hot flashes *(24)*. Sexually active, symptomatic transitional women are good candidates to consider hormonal methods of contraception, including combination low-dose OCs, rings, or progestin-only injections *(25)*. Combination OCs are the best studied of the methods, and they have been shown by numerous trials to reduce hot flashes, improve vaginal dryness, and decrease sleep disturbances in symptomatic transitional women *(26)*.

Concerns of the Perimenopausal Woman: Decline of BMD

From age 30, there is a steady decline in BMD in women that generally accelerates during the final years of the transition and early menopause. Use of hormonal contraceptives is expected to prevent this loss, or at least the loss related to the hypoestrogenism. In an analysis of 13 studies reporting on BMD and low-dose OCs, 9 showed a positive effect and 4 showed a neutral effect *(27)*. In a 2-year randomized study of women aged 40–48, calcium only was associated with a 3.4% decrease in BMD, whereas low-dose OCs had a 1.71% significant increase *(28)*. In a case-controlled study, postmenopausal women who used OCs at age 40 or older had a significantly decreased risk of postmenopausal hip fracture (odds ratio 0.69, confidence interval 0.51, 0.94) compared with never-users *(29)*.

Concerns of the Perimenopausal Woman: Cardiovascular Risks

The major two concerns, especially of older reproductive-aged women, are risk of myocardial infarction and risk of breast cancer. There is a substantial body of evidence that although current use of low-dose OCs increase the risk of venous thromboembolism, the risk of myocardial infarction and stroke is not increased in nonsmoking, non-hypertensive current or past users *(30–32)*. This data is reassuring that with careful selection of healthy, nonsmoking perimenopausal women with routine screening for hypertension, low-dose OCs can be continued until menopause or until age 55 *(33,34)*. Although there is no long-term data, the safety profile associated with the ring is thought to be similar to low-dose OCs *(35)*.

Progestin-only contraceptives do not have effects on thromboembolism and can be used safely in women of any age who smoke or have other vascular risk factors *(36)*. The progestin-only contraceptive methods include DMPA, progestin-only OCs, and a progestin-only implant using etonogestrel. (Implanon is expected to be available in the United States shortly.)

Concerns of the Perimenopausal Woman: Breast Cancer Risk

A recent analysis of breast cancer risk and OC use among women 35–60 years of age reported no increased risk associated with current or past OC use *(37)*. However, a worldwide analysis of all reproductive-aged women found a slightly increased risk among current or recent OC users. This increased risk disappeared after 10 years of discontinuation and was identical to never-users after age 65 *(38)*. Use of DMPA also does not increase the overall breast cancer risk *(39)*, although a small transient increase during use is also reported *(40)*.

Contraceptive Options

Contraceptive Options for Perimenopausal Women: Sterilization

For perimenopausal women who have finished their childbearing and do not want to use any of the highly effective reversible methods available, a tubal ligation is a good option. A newer form of tubal sterilization that does not require abdominal incision is the hysteroscopic placement of microinserts into the fallopian tubes (Essure®; Chapter 13). For women who have a stable relationship, male vasectomy is an option.

Contraceptive Options for Perimenopausal Women: Barrier Methods

Perimenopausal women seeking contraceptive protection who have recently undergone lifestyle changes, such as widowhood or divorce, may be at risk of having multiple sexual partners and may want to consider male or female condom use. Notably, between 1998 and 2002, there was an increased incidence of AIDS in US women aged 45–65 years or older *(41)*. For a transitional-aged woman who is in a stable relationship and does not have significant uterine or vaginal prolapse owing to multiple childbirths, the diaphragm or cervical cap are good options. Chapter 10 discusses barrier methods in more detail. As in any age group, selecting the method the patient is most likely to use correctly and consistently is the goal.

Contraceptive Options for Perimenopausal Women: IUDs

The IUD is a good contraceptive choice for selected parous perimenopausal women. The potential user should be in a mutually monogamous relationship and have a normal endometrial cavity. For older smoking women, or those women with cardiovascular risk factors or known disease, the IUD is a good option. The two currently available IUD in the United States, the copper T 380A (ParaGard®) and the LNG-IUS (Mirena®), provide 5 years (LNG-IUS) or 10 years (copper T 380A) of contraceptive protection. The LNG-IUS adds an important non-contraceptive advantage for this age group: it decreases menstrual blood loss and dysmenorrhea *(42,43)* and may avoid the need for hysterectomy or endometrial ablation *(44,45)*. The copper IUD is generally associated with heavier menses.

In addition to decreasing menstrual blood loss, the local administration of LNG to the endometrium protects it from development of estrogen-induced endometrial hyperplasia. This is of benefit for transitional women with irregular bleeding and for women on tamoxifen *(46)* therapy following breast cancer. Use of the LNG-IUS is reported to reduce the risk of endometrial cancer by 40–60% (Table 3) *(47,48)*. Continuous estrogen-only therapy can be added to symptomatic women with hot flashes, sleeping problems, or mood changes without the need to add additional progestin therapy *(49)*.

Contraceptive Options for the Perimenopausal Women: Progestin-Only Methods: DepoProvera (DMPA), depo-subQ, Mini-Pills, and Implanon Implant

The progestin-only methods are generally safe in women of any age, regardless of whether or not the patient smokes or has CVD. Progestin-only methods do not have significant effects on clotting factors and are associated with decreased menstrual blood loss. Although overall blood loss is less, progestin-only methods are associated with unpredictable bleeding patterns and this may not be acceptable. However, transitional women with heavy blood loss may welcome the reduction in overall blood or possibility that they may have amenorrhea, a finding in 55% of DMPA users after 1 year of use *(21)*. In addition, ever-use of DMPA is associated with a 79% reduction in the risk of endometrial cancer (Table 3) *(50)*.

Symptomatic women with hot flashes may want to consider DMPA because it is associated with a reduction in hot flashes, even in women on tamoxiphen following breast cancer. There is always a concern about bone density after long-term use of DMPA and the black-box warning suggests a limit of 2 years. However, the overall risk–benefit profile should be carefully considered. Of positive note is one study reporting that the use of DMPA from age 25 to menopause reduced early menopausal bone loss in the spine and hip compared with controls *(51)*. On the negative side, use of DMPA may be associated with a tendency for weight gain (Chapter 7).

Contraceptive Options for Perimenopausal Women: Emergency Contraception

Regardless of the method chosen, it is important to offer counseling regarding availability and how to access emergency contraception (Chapter 12).

Contraceptive Options for Perimenopausal Women: Natural Family Planning

Irregular menstrual cycles may make this method more difficult for the perimenopausal patient (Chapter 11).

Contraceptive Options for Perimenopausal Women: Low-Dose Combination Hormonal Methods—OCs and Vaginal Ring

The low-dose OCs and rings are options for healthy, sexually active perimenopausal women who are nonsmokers, normotensive, and have no significant risk factors for CVD because they improve bleeding control and may lessen perimenopausal symptoms. The prescribing choice should be formulations containing the lowest amount of estrogen and progestin (preferably 20-μg estrogen OCs or rings).

Combination OCs may reduce perimenopausal symptoms, such as hot flashes, sleep disturbances, and vaginal dryness *(26,52)*. Some perimenopausal women may develop hot flashes or other perimenopausal symptoms during the pill-free interval and switching to an OC with a shortened pill-free interval may alleviate these problems. The 20-μg OCs that have a shortened pill-free interval are:

- Kariva® and Mircette®: only 2 days of hormone-free days. Twenty-one days of 20 μg ethinyl estradiol (EE) + 150 mg desogestrel plus 5 days of only 10 μg EE.

- Two new low-dose pills, Yaz® and Loestrin® 24 Fe, have a 4-day hormone-free interval (four placebo or iron pills) and 24 days of active pills with 20 μg EE and 3 mg drosperinone, or 1 mg norethinedrone acetate.
- New 20-μg extended-cycle and continuous-use OCs will soon be available.

Because of a lowered fecundity and better adherence *(53)*, older women using OCs tend to have very low rates of unintended pregnancies *(54)*. Use of OCs also regulate bleeding patterns *(55–57)*, an important benefit for many women in transition in which dysfunctional uterine bleeding is common *(58)*. Combination OCs may reduce the amount of blood loss by 44% *(59)* and protect from the development of endometrial cancer.

Patient Screening and Choosing a Combination Hormonal Method for Perimenopausal Women

In normotensive, nonsmoking, healthy perimenopausal women without significant risk factors for CVD or thrombosis, the lowest dose OCs and rings can be used into the early menopause. Evaluating a perimenopausal woman includes investigating the following:

- Health conditions, especially CVD.
- Significant risk factors for CVD.
- Clotting problems, previous thromboembotic events.
- Gynecological issues.
  - Sexual activity: need for contraception.
  - Bleeding problems and need for bleeding control.
  - Degree of perimenopausal symptoms.
  - Other gynecological problems, such as fibroids and endometriosis.

Contraindications for use in this older population (>35 years of age) include the following:

- Known CVD.
- A significant risk factor for vascular disease.
  - Hypertension.
  - Cigarette smoking.
  - Diabetes, long-standing insulin resistance.
  - Long-standing lipid abnormalities, statin therapy.
  - Long-standing obesity.
  - Systemic disease that affects the vascular system, such as lupus erythematosus.
- History of significant clotting problems.
  - Thromboembolism, thrombophlebitis, known thrombogenic mutation, deep vein thrombosis, pulmonary embolism.
- Cancer of the breast.
- Pregnancy.

- Migraine headaches.
- Current gallbladder disease.
- Active liver disease.
- Prolonged immobilization, impending minor surgery.

Non-Contraceptive Benefits of Low-Dose OCs in Perimenopausal Women

OCs, and presumably other combination products, offer a number of important non-contraceptive benefits and some women who have undergone sterilization or who are not at risk for pregnancy may choose to take OCs for these benefits. As discussed previously, these benefits may include:

- Controlled bleeding.
- Lowered risk for anemia.
- Lowering the risk of ovarian, endometrial cancer, and possibly colorectal cancer (Table 3) *(60)*.
- Decreasing the loss of bone density.
- Decreasing symptoms of perimenopause: less hot flashes, vaginal dryness, and atrophy.
- Lowered risk for ectopic pregnancy.

When It Is Safe to Discontinuing OCs or Switch to Hormone Therapy

Women now continue OCs into their 40s and 50s and there is unfortunately no "fail-safe" method in determining when it is safe to discontinue OCs or switch to hormone therapy. However, the following protocols are suggested:

- Begin checking follicle-stimulating hormone (FSH) annually after age 45 on day 6 of placebo pills; discontinue OCs when FSH 30 mIU/mL or higher.
- Arbitrarily choose age 50–52 years to discontinue OCs.
- After 2 weeks off OCs, an increased FSH and/or no change in basal estradiol levels is strong evidence that it is now safe to discontinue OCs *(61)*.

FOLLOWING PREGNANCY AND DURING LACTATION

Introduction

Choosing the right contraceptive method following pregnancy has a lot to do with whether a full-term pregnancy has occurred and whether or not a potential user plans to breastfeed. A major issue regarding contraception use following pregnancy is when to begin.

Timing of Initiation

The return of ovulation is different in women following a full-term pregnancy compared with a first-trimester pregnancy loss and the recommendations are different (Table 4). Following a term delivery, the suppression of ovulation is prolonged and the first bleeding episode is usually, but not always, anovulatory. In a non-breastfeeding woman, ovulation is usually delayed until 6 weeks postpartum, but it can occur as early as 4 weeks.

Table 4
Recommendations for Sexually Active, Postpartum Women

	Timing of initiation	
Condition	*Start date*	*Contaceptive method*
Postpartum		
Non-breastfeeding	3–4 weeks postpartum	Combination OCs, ring, DMPA, progestin-only OCs, barrier methods, progestin implant IUD
Fully breastfeeding	6 weeks postpartum	Progestin-only OCs, DMPA, progestin implant IUD, barrier methods
Partially breastfeeding	6 months postpartum	Progestin-only OCs, DMPA, progestin implant IUD, barrier methods, ring, combination OCs
After first- or second-trimester pregnancy loss or ectopic pregnancy	Immediately	Combination OCs, ring, DMPA, IUD, implant, progestin-only OCs, barrier methods

OC, oral contraceptive; DMPA, depot medroxyprogesterone acetate; IUD, intrauterine device.

Based on 2004 World Health Organization medical eligibility criteria for low-dose combination OCs, patches, rings, DMPA, and progestin-only pill.

Women who are breastfeeding every 4 hours, including during the night, will not ovulate until at least 10 weeks postpartum, and often as long as 6 months postpartum.

- Delaying starting a combination hormonal contraceptive avoids any further enhancement of thrombophilic risk during the postpartum period in which the risk is already increased.
    - It is also important to insure that a hormonal method will be safe and not adversely affect infant health and growth when used in breastfeeding users.
- Delaying placement of an IUD in the immediate postpartum period allows the uterus to return to normal size and reduces the risk of IUD expulsion.
- Delaying use of a diaphragm or cervical cap until after bleeding and lochia abates is recommended.

Following a spontaneous or induced first-trimester abortion, ovulation usually occurs within 2–4 weeks. The first month following a first-trimester pregnancy loss is usually an ovulatory cycle and pregnancy can occur. Beginning a contraceptive immediately is recommended following a first- or second-trimester pregnancy loss.

Options

Contraceptive Options for Postpartum: Progestin-Only Pill

Because estrogens inhibit the action of prolactin on breast tissues, the use of combination OCs may diminish the amount of milk production. The introduction of lower-dose OCs has presumably reduced this impact, but very few studies have been done *(62)*. Generally, it is best not to use combination OCs in women who are nursing unless the infant is receiving supplemental feedings. Progestins do not diminish the amount of breast milk and are good option for these women if started after the natural postpartum decline in progesterone that stimulates initiation of milk production *(63)*. No adverse effects on lactation or infant growth were demonstrated in reports in which breastfeeding women started progestin-only pills (POPs) early in the postpartum period *(64)*. WHO recommends starting POPs at 6 weeks in postpartum breastfeeding women, immediately following a first- or second-trimester abortion, or as early as 21 days in postpartum non-breastfeeding women *(65)*. For women with a past ectopic pregnancy, POPs may be used because the benefits outweigh the risks.

Only a small number of women will ovulate as long as they continue full nursing and remain amenorrheic. Therefore, a POP or barrier method can be used until menses resume. Once supplemental feeding is introduced, a switch can be made if desired to a method that provides less disruption of bleeding.

Contraceptive Options in Postpartum: DMPA or depo-subQ

Most women are happy to space their pregnancies and are not concerned that the return to fertility following DMPA or depo-subQ may be prolonged. No adverse effects on lactation or on growth of the infant are reported when DMPA is initiated within 7 days *(66)* or 6 weeks postpartum *(67)*. WHO recommends starting DMPA at 6 weeks postpartum in breastfeeding women, immediately following a first- or second-trimester abortion and as early as 21 days in non-breastfeeding postpartum women.

Contraceptive Options in Postpartum: Low-Dose OCs and the Vaginal Ring

For breastfeeding women who are introducing supplemental feeding, have had return of menses, and who need effective contraception, low-dose OCs and the ring are easy to use options. The ring is a particularly good option because it releases a very low daily dose of 15 μg EE, the lowest estrogen dose in any combination hormonal product. WHO recommends starting OCs after 21 days in non-breastfeeding postpartum women and immediately following first- or second-trimester abortions, and states that the benefits of starting combination OCs after 6 months in breastfeeding postpartum women outweigh the risks.

Contraceptive Options in the Postpartum: IUD

Either the copper-containing or LNG-releasing IUD is a good option as long as the woman is in a mutually monogamous relationship and would like to space pregnancies by a few years. Caution should be used if women have had a history of STDs or pelvic inflammatory disease. Heavier periods following insertion of the copper-containing device and lighter periods following insertion of the LNG-releasing IUD can be expected. WHO recommendations regarding timing of IUD insertions in postpartum patients are found in Table 5.

Table 5
WHO Recommendations for IUD Insertion in Postpartum Patients

	Copper IUD	*LNG-IUS*
Postpartum non-breastfeeding		
<48 hours	Increased risk of explusion but benefits outweigh risks	Increased risk of explusion but risks outweigh benefits
48 hours to <4 weeks	Risks outweigh benefits	Risks outweigh benefits
≥4 weeks	Recommended	Recommended
Puerperal sepsis	Do not use	Do not use
Postpartum breastfeeding		
<6 weeks	Recommended (after 4 weeks)	Risks outweigh benefits
Post-abortion		
Immediately after first trimester	Recommended	Recommended
Immediately after second trimester	Increased risk of expulsion but benefits outweigh risks	Increased risk of expulsion but benefits outweigh risks
Immediately post-septic abortion	Do not use	Do not use
Past ectopic pregnancy	Recommended	Recommended

Contraceptive Options in the Postpartum: Barriers

In the postpartum period, sexual activity may be less frequent and the on-hand protection provided by barriers may be sufficient. Some women particularly like the idea of a noninvasive, non-hormonal method. The female and male condoms offer protection from STDs and are recommended in women who are at risk. Women in the immediate postpartum period or those who are breastfeeding may have vaginal dryness and appreciate the lubrication of vaginal spermicides. Use of a diaphragm or cap is not recommended until bleeding and lochia has stopped.

Contraceptive Options in the Postpartum: Implant

FDA approval of Implanon, a contraceptive implant containing the progestin etonogestrel is expected shortly. Unlike the non-marketed Norplant®, this new implant is a single rod and it comes with its own inserter. The rod offers effective, easy contraceptive protection for up to 3 years (Chapter 8).

Contraceptive Options in the Postpartum: Tubal Ligation and Fallopian Tube Micro-Insert

It only takes about 35 minutes to place a 4-cm long micro-insert into the fallopian tube. The micro-insert then stimulates the body to form a tissue barrier and prevent pregnancy. Like a traditional tubal ligation, it should be considered as permanent sterilization. This procedure does not require incisions or punctures to the body and there is no burning or cutting. It is necessary to use a back-up method for 3 months following the procedure (Chapter 13).

REFERENCES

1. Abma JC, Martinez GM, Mosher WD, Dawson BS. (2004) Teenagers in the United States: sexual activity, contraceptive use, and childbearing, 2002. Vital Health Stat 24:1–48.
2. Alan Guttmacher Institute. (1994) Sex and America's Teenagers. New York, NY: Alan Guttmacher Institute.
3. Ventura SJ, Martin JA, Curtin SC, Mathews TJ. (1999) Births: final data for 1997. Nat Vital Stat Rep 47:1–96.
4. Ventura SJ, Martin JA, Curtin SC, Menacker F, Hamilton BE. (2001) Births: final data for 1999. Nat Vital Stat Rep 49:1–100.
5. Weinstock H, Berman S, Cates W. (2004) Sexually transmitted diseases among American youth: incidence and prevalence estimates, 2000. Perspect Sex Reprod Health 36:6–10.
6. Sulak PJ, Herbelin S. (2005) Teenagers and sex: delaying sexual debut. Female Patient 30:29–38.
7. Manlove J, Ryan S, Franzetta K. (2004) Contraceptive use and consistency in US teenagers' most recent sexual relationship. Persp Sex Reprod Health 36:265–275.
8. Zobby International. (2004) 2004 survey on parental opinions of character- or relationship-based abstinence education vs comprehensive (or "abstinence-first," then condoms) sex education: graphs of major findings.
9. American College of Obstetrics and Gynecology (ACOG). (2005) ACOG patient education pamphlet, especially for teens birth control. ACOG Patient Education.
10. National Institutes of Health. (2001) Workshop summary: scientific evidence on condom effectiveness for sexually transmitted disease (STD) prevention.
11. Holmes KK, Levein R, Weaver M. (2004) Effectiveness of condoms in preventing sexually transmitted infections. Bull World Health Organ 82:454–461.
12. Archer DF, Cullinhs V, Creasy GW, Fisher AC. (2004) The impact of improved compliance with a weekly contraceptive transdermal system (Ortho Evra™) on contraceptive efficacy. Contraception 69:189–195.
13. Cromer VE, Smith RD, Blair JM, Dwyer J, Brown RT. (1994) A prospective study of adolescents who choose among levonorgestrel implants, medroxyprogeserone acetate , or the combined oral contraceptive pill as contraception. Pediatrics 94:687–694.
14. Scholes D, LaCroix, AZ, Ichikawa LF, Barlow WE, Ott SM. (2004) Change in bone mineral density among adolescent women using and discontinuing depot medroxyprogesterone acetate contraception. Arch Pediatr Adolesc Med 159:139–144.
15. Cromer BA, Lazebnik R, Rome E, et al. (2005) Double-blinded randomized controlled trial of estrogen supplementation in adolescent girls who receive depot medroxyprogesterone acetate for contraception. Am J Obstet Gynecol 192:42–47.
16. Sowers M, Corton G, Shapiro B, et al. (1993) Changes in bone density with lactation. JAMA 269:3130–3135.
17. Kaunitz AM. (2001) Injectable long-acting contraceptives. Clin Obstet Gynecol 44:73–91.
18. Kaunitz AM. (2001) Oral contraceptive use in perimenopause. Am J Obstet Gynecol 1859:S32–S37.
19. Santoro N, Brown JR, Adel T, Skjurnick JH. (1996) Characterization of reproductive hormonal dynamics in the perimenopause. J Clin Endocrinol Metab 81:1495–1501.
20. Strauss LT, Herndon J, Chang J, et al. (2004) Abortion surveillance—United States, 2001. MMWR Surveill Summ 53:1–32.
21. Pharmaci and Upjohn Company. (2004) Depo-Provera contraception injection (product information). Kalamazoo, MI: Pharmaci and Upjohn Company.

22. Barrington JW, Bowen-Simpkins P. (1997) The levonorgestrel intrauterine system in the management of menorrhagia. Br J Obstet Gynaecol 104:614–616.
23. Gold EB, Block G, Crawford S, et al. (2004) Lifestyle and demographic factors in relation to vasomotor symptoms; baseline results from the Study of Women's Health Across the Nation. Am J Epidemiol 159:1189–1199.
24. Freeman EW, Sammel MD, Grisso JA, Battistini M, Garcia-Espagna B, Hollander L. (2001) Hot flashes in the late reproductive years: risk factors for African American and Caucasian women. J Womens Health Gend Based Med 10:67–76.
25. Lobo RA, McCormick W, Singer F, Roy S. (1984) Depo-medroxyprogesterone acetate compared with conjugated estrogens for the treatment of postmenopausal women. Obstet Gynecol 63:1–5.
26. Casper R, Dodin S, Reid RL, and study investigators. (1997) The effect of a 20 μg ethinyl estradiol/1 mg norethinedrone acetate (Minestrin®), a low-dose contraceptive, on vaginal bleeding patterns, hot flashes, and quality of life in synmptomatic perimenopausal women. Menopause 4:139–147.
27. Kuohung W, Borgatta L, Stubblefield P. (2000) Low-dose oral contraceptives and bone mineral density an evidence-based analysis. Contraception 61:77–82.
28. Gambacciani M, Spinetti A, Cappagli B, et al. (1994) Hormone replacement therapy in perimenopausal women with a low dose oral contraceptive preparation: effects on bone mineral density and metabolism. Maturitas 19:125–76.
29. Michaelsson K, Baron JA, Farahmand BY, Persson I, Ljunghall S. (1999) Oral-contraceptive use and risk of hip fracture: a case–control study. Lancet 353:1481–1484.
30. Pettiti DB, Sidney S, Bernstein A, Wolf S, Quesenberry C, Ziel HK. (1996) Stroke in users of low-dose oral contraceptives. N Engl J Med 335:8–15.
31. Sidney S, Siscovick DS, Petitti DB, et al. (1998) Myocardial infarction and use of low-dose oral contraceptive: a pooled analysis of 2 US studies. Circulation 98:1058–1063.
32. Hannaford PC, Kay CR. (1998) The risk of serious illness among oral contraceptive users: evidence from the RCGP's oral contraceptive study. Br J Gen Pract 48:1657–1662.
33. Gebbie A. (2003) Contraception in the perimenopause. J Br Menopause Soc 9:123–128.
34. American College of Obstetricians and Gynecologists (ACOG). (1995) ACOG technical bulletin. Health maintenance for perimenopausal women. Number 210—August 1995. American College of Obstetricians and Gynecologists. Int J Gynaecol Obstet 51:171–181.
35. Sibai BM, Odlind V, Meador ML, Shangold GA, Fisher AC, Creasy GW. (2002) A comparative and pooled analysis of the safety and tolerability of the contraceptive patch (Ortho EVRA/EVRa.) Fertil Steril 77:S19–S26.
36. Kaunitz A, Speroff L. (2005) Contraception in the perimenopausal woman. Dialogues Contracept 9:1–4.
37. Marchbanks PA, McDonald JA, Wilson HG, et al. (2002) Oral contraceptives and risk of breast cancer. N Engl J Med 346:2025–2032.
38. Collaborative Group on Hormonal Factors in Breast Cancer. (1996) Breast cancer and hormonal contraceptives: collaborative breast cancer reanalysis of individual data on 53,297 women with breast cancer and 100,239 women without breast cancer from 54 epidemiological studies. Lancet 347:1713–1727.
39. Strom BL, Berlin JA, Weber AL, et al. (2004) Absence of an effect of injectable and implantable progestin-only contraceptives on subsequent risk of breast cancer. Contraception 69:353–360.
40. Skegg DC, Noonan EA, Paul C, et al. (1995) Depot medroxyprogesterone and breast cancer: A pooled analysis of the World Health Organization and New Zealand studies. JAMA 273:799–804.
41. Centers of Disease Control and Prevention. (2002) HIV/AIDS surveillance report. 14:1–48. www.cdc.gov/hiv/stats/hasr1402.htm. Accessed March 11, 2006.

42. Andersson J, Rybo G. (1990) Levonorgestrel-releasing intrauterine device in the treatment of menorrhagia. Br J Obstet Gynaecol 97:690–694.
43. Sivin I, Stern J. (1994) Health during prolonged use of levonorgestrel 20μg/d and the Copper CU 380Ag intrauterine contraceptive devices: a multicenter study. Fertil Steril 61:70–77.
44. Crosignani PG, Vercellini P, Mosconi P, Oldani S, Cortesi I, De Giorgi O. (1997) Levonorgestrel-releasing intrauterine device verus hysteroscopic endometrial resection in the treatment of dysfunctional uterine bleeding. Obstet Gynecol 90:257–263.
45. Hurskainen R, Teperi J, Rissanen P, et al. (2001) Quality of life and cost-effectiveness of levonorgestrel-releasing intrauterine system versus hysterectomy for treatment of menorrhagia: a randomised trial. Lancet 357:273–277.
46. Gardner FJ, Konje JC, Abrams KR, et al. (2000) Endometrial protection from tamoxifen-stimulated changes by a levonorgestrel-releasing intrauterine system: a randomised controlled trial. Lancet 356:1711–1717.
47. Parazzini F, La Vecchia C, Moroni S. (1994) Intrauterine device use and risk of endometrial cancer. Br J Cancer 70:672–673.
48. Hill DA, Weiss NS, Voigt LF, Beresford SA. (1997) Endometrial cancer in relation to intrauterine device use. Int J Cancer 70:278–281.
49. Suvanto-Luukkonen E, Kauppila A. (1999) The levonorgestrel intrauterine system in menopausal hormone replacement therapy; five-year experience. Fertil Steril 72:161–163.
50. World Health Organization. (1991) Collaborative study of neoplasia and steroid contraceptives. Depot-medroxyporgesterone acetate (DMPA) and risk of endometrial cancer. Int J Cancer 49:186–190.
51. Cundy T, Cornish J, Roberts H, Reid IR. (2002) Menopausal bone loss in long-term users of depot medroxyprogesterone acetate contraception. Am J Obstet Gynecol 186:978–983.
52. Shargil AA. (1985) Hormone replacement therapy in perimenopausal women with a triphasic contraceptive compound: a three-year prospective study. Int J Fertil 30:15–28.
53. Trussel J. (2004) Contraceptive failure in the United States. Contraception 70:89–96.
54. Fu H, Darroch JE, Haas T, Ranjit N. (1999) Contraceptive failure rates: new estimates from the 1995 National Survey of family Growth. Fam Plann Perspect 31:56–63.
55. Andolsek KM. (1992) Cycle control with triphasic norgestimate and ethinyl estradiol, a new oral contraceptive agent. Acta Obstet Gynecol Scan Suppl 71:S13–S18.
56. Audet M-C, Moreau M, Koltun WD, et al, for the ORTHO EVRA/EVRA 004 study group. (2001) Evaluation of contraceptive efficacy and cycle control of a transdermal patch vs an oral contraceptive: a randomized controlled trial. JAMA 285:2347–2354.
57. Bjarnadottir RI, Tuppurainen M, Killick SR. (2002) Comparison of cycle control with a combined contraceptive vaginal ring and oral levonorgestrel/ethinyl estradiol. Am J Obstet Gynecol 186:389–395.
58. Awwad JT, Toth TL, Schiff I. (1993) Abnormal uterine bleeding in the perimenopause. In J Fertil 38:261–269.
59. Larsson G, Milsom I, Lindstedt G, Rybo G. (1992) The influence of a low-dose combined oral contraceptive on menstrual blood loss and iron status. Contraception 46:327–334.
60. Fernandez E, La Vecchia C, Balducci A, Chatenoud L, Franceschi S, Negri E. (2001) Oral contraceptives and colorectal cancer risk; a meta-analysis. Br J Cancer 84:722–727.
61. Castracane VD, Gimpel T, Goldzieher JW. (1995) When is it safe to switch from oral contraceptives to hormonal replacement therapy? Contraception 52:371–376.
62. Lonnerdel IB, Forsum E, Hambraeus L. (1980) Effect of oral contraceptives on composition and volume of breast milk. Am J Clin Nutr 33:816–824.
63. Moggia AV, Harris GS, Dunson TR, et al. (1991) A comparative study of a progestin-only oral contraceptive versus non-hormonal methods in lactating women in Buenos Aires, Argentina. Contraception 44:31–43.

64. McCann MF, Moggia AV, Higgins JE, Potts M, Becker C. (1989) The effects of a progestin-only oral contraceptive (levonorgestrel 0.03 mg) on breast-feeding. Contraception 40:635–648.
65. World Health Organization (WHO). (2000) Improving access to quality care in family planning medical eligibility criteria for contracetpvie use. Geneva, Switzerland: WHO. Available from: www.who.int/reproductive-health/publications.
66. McCann MF, Liskin LS, Piotrow PT, Rinehart W, Fox G. (1984) Breast-feeding, fertility and family planning. Popul Reports Nov–Dec:J525–J575.
67. Koetsawang S, Boonyaprakob V, Suvanichati S, Paipeekul S. (1983) Long term study of growth and development of children breast-fed by mothers receiving Depo-Provera during lactation. In: Zatuchni GI, Goldsmith A, Shelton JD, Sciarra JJ, eds. Long-Acting Contraceptive Delivery Systems; Proceedings From an International Workshop on Long-Acting Contraceptive Delivery Systems. May 31–June 3, 1983, New Orleans, LA. Philadelphia PA: Harper and Row, pp. 378–387.
68. Jacobson DL, Womack SD, Peralta L, et al. (2000) Concordance of human pappillomavirus in the cervix and urine among inner city adolescents. Pediatr Infect Dis J 19:423–428.
69. Disaia PJ, Creasman WT. (1997) Clinical Gynecologic Oncology, 5th ed. St Louis, MO: Mosby-Year.
70. Schlesselman JJ. (1997) Risk of endometrial cancer in relation to use of combined oral contraceptives: a practitioner's guide to meta-analysis. Hum Reprod 12:1851–1863.
71. Cancer and Steroid Hormone Study of the Centers for Disease Control and the National Institute of Child Health and Human Development. (1987) Combination oral contraceptive use and the risk of endometrial cancer. JAMA 257:796–800.
72. Castellsague X, Thompson WD, Dubrow R. (1993) Intra-uterine contraception and the risk of endometrial cancer. Int J Cancer 54:911–916.
73. Cancer and Steroid Hormone Study of the Centers for Disease Control and the National Institute of Child Health and Human Development. (1987) The reduction in risk of ovarian cancer associated with oral-contraceptive use. N Engl J Med 316:650–655.
74. Ness RB, Grisso JA, Klapper J, and the SHARE study group. (2000) Risk of ovarian cancer in relation to estrogen and progestin dose and use characteristics of oral contraceptives. Am J Epidemiol 152:233–241.
75. Hankinson SE, Colditz GA, Hunter DJ, Spencer TL, Rosner B, Stampfer MJ. (1992) A quantitative assessment of oral contraceptive use and risk of ovarian cancer. Obstet Gynecol 80:708–714.
76. Martinez ME, Grodstein F, Giovannucci E, et al. (1997) A prospective study of reproductive factors, oral contraceptive use, and risk of colorectal cancer. Cancer Epidemiol Biomarkers Prev 6:1–5.

15 Choosing the Optimal Contraceptive Method in Women With Medical Disease

Siri L. Kjos, MD

CONTENTS

INTRODUCTION

The risk of pregnancy in many women with a chronic medical disease generally far exceeds the risks associated with use of an appropriately selected contraceptive method. The primary goal of prescribing a contraceptive method in women with medical conditions is to select the method with the least risk relating to her specific disease process, the one with the greatest efficacy, and the one that is tailored to her lifestyle and reproductive history. Although the selected method may not be risk-free, individualized counseling, lifestyle interventions, and adequate control of her disease process generally can minimize these risks to an acceptable level.

This chapter addresses use of hormonal methods of contraception and intrauterine devices (IUDs). Barrier methods, including spermicides, diaphragm, condoms, cervical caps, and the contraceptive sponge will not be considered because there are very few, if any, medical contraindications for their use. The barrier methods generally have higher failure rates and are best used in highly motivated patients who will use them consistently and properly.

Goals for the Heath Care Practitioner

- Be able to provide individualized counseling for women with specific medical conditions who desire pregnancy planning and contraception.

From: *Current Clinical Practice: The Handbook of Contraception: A Guide for Practical Management*
Edited by: D. Shoupe and S. L. Kjos © Humana Press, Totowa, NJ

- Identify the level of risk and potential benefit of various contraceptive methods specific to each disease process.
- Utilize a step-wise approach to decide which contraceptive method is best suited for each patient based on disease and lifestyle issues.

GENERAL COUNSELING AND ASSESSING RISK

Deciding on the proper contraception prescription for a woman with medical disease is often a collaborative process involving the patient, her internist or medical specialists, and her obstetrician/gynecologist or perinatalogist. Depending on her medical condition, this decision may involve several physicians. By working together, the team can select a contraceptive method and an overall plan to optimize her contraceptive protection, keep her risk to a minimum, and plan for future pregnancies if desired (Table 1).

General Health and Lifestyle Counseling

Harmful lifestyle factors need to be addressed in the discussion of pregnancy planning and contraceptive choice (Table 2). Not only do they influence contraceptive choice, but more importantly adversely affect most medical conditions. Cigarette smoking is not only a significant independent risk factor for myocardial infarction and hypertension, it is also an absolute contraindication for combination oral contraceptive (OC) use in women older than 35 years of age. Even light cigarette smoking in women under 35, especially in those with a medical condition, needs special consideration and evaluation.

> *Changing lifestyle to engage in exercise, weight loss, and proper nutrition is the cornerstone of therapy for many disease processes.*

Women who are sedentary and obese are also prone to diabetes, hypertension, thrombotic events, lipid abnormalities, and the associated long-term sequelae. Similarly, women who abuse drugs or alcohol, engage in high-risk sexual behavior, or who are not reliable in taking their daily prescription drugs are adding risk factors that also have long-term health consequences. Correcting these lifestyle choices may be the single most important step in improving their chances for a healthy future and it may also make selecting a safe contraceptive method much easier.

Counseling Regarding the Disease Process and the Risk of Pregnancy to Mother and Fetus

The practitioner prescribing contraceptives for women with serious medical diseases must have a working knowledge of both the disease process and the risks of pregnancy to counsel these women and develop a reproductive health plan. Highlights of risks to the woman during pregnancy as well as risks to the fetus or neonate are summarized in Table 3.

Table 1
Contraceptive Counseling Guidelines

Contraceptive counseling for women with medical disease should:

- Discuss how to preserve and optimize current health.
- Identify the risks associated with pregnancy related to her medical condition.
  - Maternal morbidity/mortality associated with pregnancy (e.g., complications from or acceleration of disease state).
  - Obstetrical risks (e.g., prematurity, stillbirth, miscarriage, growth disturbances).
  - Possible teratogenic risks from medication or uncontrolled disease.
- Identify an optimal time to plan pregnancy with respect to her medical condition.
  - What therapeutic goals should be reached before conception?
  - What surgical procedures should be completed before conception?
- Review the risks of an unwanted pregnancy (e.g., termination).
- Identify any risks of possible disease interactions with contraceptive selection.
  - Complications resulting from interaction of method and disease process.
  - Changes in medication efficacy because of drug interaction, either contraceptive method or medical therapy.
  - Interactions with other risk factors or comorbidities that may influence disease.
  - Beneficial interactions or changes from specific contraceptive methods that may positively influence her medical disease.
- Recognize that there may not be a risk-free and highly effective contraceptive choice, and that successful contraception and avoidance of pregnancy may be the preferable and lower net risk option.
- Individualize of contraceptive options to select the safest choice that is acceptable to the patient and her lifestyle.
- Identify lifestyle factors she could positively alter to improve her general health and prepare her for pregnancy.
  - *All* women of reproductive age *capable* of becoming pregnant should consume 0.4 mg folic acid per day (US Public Health Service Recommendation, 1992) to reduce the risk of neural tube defect.

Table 2
General Health Counseling to Modify Lifestyle Factors That Adversely Affect Medical Disease and Contraceptive Options

Cigarette smoking
Obesity, excess caloric intake
Poor nutrition: high in saturated fats, salt, simple carbohydrates
Inactivity, lack of exercise
Drug abuse: illicit, alcohol, and prescription
High-risk sexual behavior: multiple partners, unprotected intercourse
Recurrent STIs
Low level of maturity and reliability

Table 3
Counseling Women With Medical Disease Regarding Risk of Pregnancy to Her and to Fetus/Neonate, Ongoing Health Risks and Surveillance, and Possible Risks and Benefits Related to Specific HC or IUD Use

Disease	*Risk of pregnancy and risk to fetus/neonate*	*Ongoing health risks and surveillance, risks and benefits of contraceptive options*
Cardiac and vascular disease states		
Cardiac lesions Complicated lesions Congenital Acquired valvular	Pregnancy: risk dependent on lesion and severity with possible significant mortality, hospitalization. Pregnancy not advised with Eisenmenger's syndrome, pulmonary hypertension, prior peripartum cardiomyopathy, or Marfan's syndrome with aortic involvement (mortality rates around 50%). Fetal/neonate: if anti-coagulated, teratogenic potential of Coumadin during embryogenesis, increased risk of intrauterine growth retardation, and prematurity. Exposure to medical therapy.	Risks: if not anti-coagulated: increased risk of thromboembolism, stroke, myocardial infarction with HC, especially those containing estrogen. Increased risk of hypertension and fluid retention (HC) and anemia (Copper IUD) on cardiac function. Increased risk of subacute bacterial endocarditis (IUD) Interaction with medications (HC) Health surveillance: monitor BP, weight, and cardiac review of systems each visit Monitor hemoglobin (Copper IUD)
Cardiac lesions Uncomplicated valvular disease Mitral valve prolapse	Pregnancy: minimal. Fetal/neonate: exposure to medical therapy (if any).	Risks: minimal risk of thromboembolism (HC). Possible increased risk of subacute bacterial endocarditis (IUD). Health surveillance: monitor BP, weight and cardiac review of systems each visit
Hypercoagulable states associated with: Cardiac valvular disease Valve replacement	Pregnancy: if not anti-coagulated, increased risk of thromboembolism. If anti-coagulated, increased risk of hemorrhage.	Risks: if not anti-coagulated, increased risk of thromboembolism with estrogen-containing HC. If anti-coagulated, increased risk of ruptured functional cysts and menorrhagia (progestin-IUD or progestin-only HC may be beneficial).

Native valve Mechanical Hx of venous or arterial thrombus Thrombogenic mutations: Factor V Leiden Prothrombin mutation Protein S deficiency Protein C deficiency Antithrombin deficiency	Fetal/neonate: teratogenic potential of Coumadin during embrogenesis. Switch to heparin or low-molecular-weight heparin during pregnancy. (Mechanical valves may require Coumadin anti-coagulation during the 12th–35th week secondary to high risk of thrombosis.)	Health surveillance: monitor for symptoms of excess bleeding 2° to anti-coagulation. Monitor hemoglobin if using Copper IUD.
Diabetes mellitus Type 1 diabetes mellitus Type 2 diabetes mellitus Type 1 or 2 diabetes with vascular sequelae	Pregnancy: risk dependent on presence of micro- or macrovascular complications. Decreased risk if institute lifestyle changes. Fetal/neonate: preconception glycemic control crucial to decreased risk of major congenital malformation in type 1 and 2 diabetes; overall rate: 6–10%. If poor glucose control, rate increases to 25%. Increased risk of fetal loss, stillbirth, and newborn morbidities.	Risks: exacerbation of glucose intolerance (progestins in HC may have some negative effect). Exacerbation of diabetic sequelae (weight gain, hyperlipidemia, hypertension) with some HC. Control of hypertension, lipid abnormalities, and glucose minimizes retinal and renal damage and cardiovascular complications. Increased risk of life-threatening infection. Health surveillance: monitor BP, weight, and glycosylated hemoglobin every 4–6 months. Diet, weight, and exercise counseling. Estrogen-containing HCs not an option with vascular disease.

(continued)

Table 3 *(Continued)*

Disease	*Risk of pregnancy and risk to fetus/neonate*	*Ongoing health risks and surveillance, risks and benefits of contraceptive options*
Pre-diabetes (prior gestational diabetes)	Pregnancy: high risk of recurrent GDM during subsequent pregnancy or of having developed undiagnosed diabetes after pregnancy. Fetal/neonate: If fasting hyperglycemia, fetus with same increased risk of malformation as type 2 diabetes. Increased risk of fetal loss, stillbirth, and newborn morbidities.	Risk: ≥60% risk of developing type 2 diabetes within 5–15 years after pregnancy. Increased risk of metabolic syndrome. Characteristics of metabolic syndrome (any three): triglycerides >150 mg/dL, HDL cholesterol <50 mg/dL, systolic BP ≥130 mmHg, diastolic BP ≥85 mmHg, fasting glucose ≥110 mg/dL, waist circumference >35 in. Health surveillance: need annual screening for diabetes: fasting serum glucose. ≥100 mg/dL: impaired, proceed to 2H oGTT. Fasting serum glucose >126 mg/dL: diabetes. Confirm with second fasting serum glucose. Screen for metabolic syndrome: diet, weight, and exercise counseling.
Coronary artery disease (current and history of)	Pregnancy not advised: with congestive heart failure or recent myocardial infarction mortality rates of up to 50%. Increased maternal morbidity and mortality, hospitalization. Fetal/neonate: intrauterine growth retardation, prematurity; exposure to medical therapy.	Risk: increased risk of thromboembolism, stroke, myocardial infarction (estrogen-containing HCs are contraindicated). Exacerbation of CVD risk factors: weight gain, hypertension, hyperlipidemia. Interaction with medical therapy (HC). Health surveillance: monitor BP, weight, and cardiac review of systems each visit. Screen for metabolic syndrome (see above). Diet, weight, and exercise counseling (in consultation).

History of cerebro-vascular accident	Pregnancy: risk dependent on etiology of stroke, whether can be surgically repaired (aneurysm). Increased maternal morbidity and mortality, hospitalization. Fetal/neonate: related to etiology, cofactors, and maternal course.	Risk: increased risk of thrombosis, hypertension, lipid abnormalities, and underlying disease (estrogen-containing HCs are contraindicated). Health surveillance: monitor BP, weight and cardiac review of systems each visit. Screen for metabolic syndrome (*see* above). Diet, weight, and exercise counseling.
Hypertension During pregnancy—now <140/90 mmHg Controlled with therapy Elevated on therapy	Pregnancy: risk dependent on severity and medical control, presence of other co-existing disease or morbidity. Possible significant morbidity, hospitalization. Lowered risk if institute lifestyle changes. Fetal/neonate: Increased intrauterine growth retardation, prematurity, fetal loss, placental abruption, and low birth weight.	Risk: increased risk of thromboembolism, stroke, myocardial infarction (progestin-only HC or IUD often the better choice; only option with current hypertension). Health surveillance: monitor BP, weight and cardiac review of systems each visit. Screen for metabolic syndrome (*see* above). Diet, weight, and exercise counseling.
Other CVD risk factors Hyperlipidemia Obesity: BMI >30 kg/m^2 Older (>35 years) Smoking <35 years ≥35 years Hypertension	Pregnancy: risk dependent on severity and medical control of condition, number of risk factors, presence of other co-existing disease or morbidity. Possible significant morbidity. Decreased risk if institute lifestyle changes. Fetal/neonate: intrauterine growth retardation, prematurity, fetal loss, placental abruption, low birth weight, risk of aneuploidy. Exposure to medical therapy (Lovastatin, ACE inhibitors).	Risk: increased risk of thromboembolism, thrombosis, stroke, myocardial infarction, exacerbation of medical condition (hypertension, hyperlipidemia, fluid retention, weight gain). Interaction with medication (HC). Health surveillance: monitor BP, weight, and cardiac review of systems each visit; metabolic syndrome screening (*see* above); diet, weight, and exercise counseling; smoking cessation program. Estrogen-containing HC contraindicated with hypertension, smoking > age 35, or multiple risk factors.

(continued)

Table 3 *(Continued)*

Disease	*Risk of pregnancy and risk to fetus/neonate*	*Ongoing health risks and surveillance, risks and benefits of contraceptive options*
Thyroid disease Hyperthyroid Hypothyroid	Pregnancy: Increased risk of preeclampsia, preterm delivery, and complications (thyroid storm) related to uncontrolled thyroid disease. Fetal/neonate: Increased risk of prematurity, symptoms of thyroid dysfunction in newborn 2° to crossing of maternal antibodies or medication; lower childhood development scores related to hypothyroidism.	Risk: drug interactions (HC). Health surveillance: monitor TSH and monitor for symptoms of thyroid dysfunction. Amenorrhea 2° to hypothyroidism (pregnancy test)
Systemic lupus erythematosus	Pregnancy: increased risk if active disease, lower risk if in remission. Increased risk if co-existing disease: renal failure, hypertension. Possible significant morbidity, hospitalization. Fetal/neonate: intrauterine growth retardation, fetal loss, placental abruption, prematurity, possible congenital neonatal lupus from autoantibodies	Risk: increased risk of thromboembolism (progestin-only methods or IUD an option). Increased risk to develop diabetes 2° to steroid Rx. Increased risk of infection from chronic immunosuppression and anemia (Copper IUD may increase anemia risk). Increased risk renal failure, 2° hypertension. Health surveillance: monitor BP, weight, and review of systems each visit.
Hemophilias Sickle cell disease Thalassemia Iron deficiency anemia	Pregnancy: risk related to frequency of sickle crisis, anemia, end-organ damage from sickling (kidneys, lungs, heart). Increased risk significant maternal morbidity and mortality, hospitalization. Fetal/neonate: inherited disease (sickle disease and thalassaemia): genetic counseling.	Risk: increased risk of sickle crisis 2° to infection, dehydration, deoxygenation, anemia. Health surveillance: monitor BP, review of systems (infection, crisis) each visit. Monitor hemoglobin (Copper IUD may cause further iron deficiency).

Seizure disorders requiring AEDs	Pregnancy: pregnancy does not increase seizure frequency. Fetal/neonate: teratogenic potential of AEDs: use lowest possible dose and monotherapy possible.	Risk: possible drug interactions with AED that may decrease contraceptive efficacy and increase breakthrough bleeding of HCs. Documented lower efficacy with progestin implant (Norplant®). Health surveillance: monitor seizure frequency, current AED medications. DMPA may decrease sequence frequency.
Migraine headaches Without aura With aura (classic)	Pregnancy: pregnancy has no dominant effect on migraine frequency. Fetal/neonate: possible exposure to medical therapy.	Risk: increased risk stroke in women with classic migraines independent of contraceptive method. Health surveillance: monitor migraine frequency, BP. (Estrogen containing HC contraindicated in those with aura or those older than 35 years without aura.)
Liver disease History cholestasis Of pregnancy COC related Symptomatic gallbladder disease	Pregnancy: increased risk: recurrent cholestasis. Increased severity of symptomatic gallbladder disease: may require surgery during pregnancy, hospitalization. Fetal/neonate: increased risk prematurity depending on maternal disease course.	Risk: recurrent cholestasis (HC). Health surveillance: baseline liver function and monitor for symptoms of liver dysfunction. Palpate liver edge for enlargement. Progestin-only HC or IUD options.
Active liver disease: Hepatitis Cirrhosis Liver tumor: adenomas, focal nodular hyperplasia	Pregnancy: increased risk metabolic and liver dysfunction. Fetal/neonate: Increased risk prematurity depending on maternal disease course, risk of transmission of hepatitis to newborn.	Risk: worsening liver function. (HC cannot be used in active/current liver disease.) Health surveillance: baseline liver function and monitor for symptoms of liver dysfunction.
Malignancy and pre-invasive disease	Pregnancy: dependent on type and stage of CA, and current therapy. Pregnancy may interfere	Risk: avoid hormonal contraception in estrogen-/progesterone-sensitive tumors.

(continued)

Table 3 *(Continued)*

Disease	*Risk of pregnancy and risk to fetus/neonate*	*Ongoing health risks and surveillance, risks and benefits of contraceptive options*
Breast cancer Gestational trophoblast disease Cervical cancer Cervical intra-epithileal neoplasia	or limit course of therapy. Fetal/neonate: fetal exposure to therapy (chemotherapy, radiation, surgery).	Medication interaction with HC. Immunocompromise, risk of pelvic infection (IUD). Health surveillance: routine, monitor PAPs, weight, appropriate follow-up.
HIV Infected AIDS	Pregnancy: morbidity dependent on viral load, immune status, possible significant morbidity. Fetal/neonate: vertical transmission of HIV. Fetal risk of exposure to combination retroviral therapy.	Risk: exacerbation of immunosuppression, susceptible to infection (IUD). Interaction with medication (HC). Transmission to partner (HC and IUD). Health surveillance: routine, monitor hemoglobin, weight. Condom use plus contraceptive good option. Monitor disease progress, development of ARC, viral load (with internist). Surveillance for abnormal cytology.
Mental disorders: Depression, bipolar disorder, schizophrenia Mental Retardation	Pregnancy: compliance with care, ability to care for oneself. Fetal/neonate: fetal risk from medication (Teratogenic exposure—lithium); ability to care for infant.	Risk: compliance with method (HC). Associated risk of drug abuse, rape, promiscuity. Medication interactions (HC). Health surveillance: routine.

Gynecological conditions: Benign breast disease Endometriosis Severe dysmenorrhea PID	Pregnancy: generally none, fertility may be affected by endometriosis, PID. Fetal/neonate: generally none	Risk: routine. Health surveillance: routine. HC or progestin-IUD may be beneficial.
Leiomyomas	Pregnancy: pain/enlargement of myoma; increased pregnancy loss and preterm delivery 2° to implantation over myoma. Fetal/neonate: prematurity.	Risk: menorrhagia, anemia (HC or progestin–IUD may be beneficial). Health surveillance: monitor hemoglobin and symptoms of menorrhagia, pain.
Polycystic ovarian syndrome	Pregnancy: increased spontaneous abortion, gestational diabetes 2° to insulin resistance.	Risk: amenorrhea, endometrial hyperplasia (HC or progestin–IUD beneficial). Hirsuitism, weight gain (HC may be beneficial). Health surveillance: screen for metabolic syndrome (*see* above). Diet, weight, and exercise counseling.
Prolactinoma	Pregnancy: loss of visual fields (enlarging macroadenoma)	Risk: amenorrhea, endometrial hyperplasia (progestin or HC may be beneficial). Health surveillance: follow status of adenoma, therapy as needed.

HC, hormone contraception; IUD, intrauterine device; BP, blood pressure; Hx, history; GDM, gestational diabetes mellitus; HDL, high-density lipoprotein; CVD, cardiocascular disease; BMI, body mass index; 2H GTT, 2-hour glucose tolerance test; ACE, angiotensin-converting enzyme; FSH, follicle-stimulating hormone; TSH, thyroid-stimulating hormone; AED, anti-epileptic drug; COC, combination oral contraceptive; CA, cancer; HIV, human immunodeficiency virus; AIDS, acquired immune deficiency virus; ARC, AIDS-related complex; PID, pelvic inflammatory disease.

Assessing Risk Factors of Contraceptive Methods

Selection of a safe hormonal contraception (HC) for women with various disease states requires knowledge of the metabolic effects of the currently available contraceptive methods. Table 4 lists some of the metabolic changes specific to oral estrogen and progestin, non-orally administered progestin, and IUDs *(1–15)*.

Many of the newer hormonal methods lack long-term epidemiological data regarding safety or detailed metabolic studies transferable to women with medical disease. In addition to OCs, various estrogen and progestin combinations are available in a weekly transdermal contraceptive patch or in a monthly contraceptive intravaginal ring. The risks and benefits of these non-oral methods are considered to be similar to those associated with combination oral contraceptives (COCs), but there is very little specific data on their metabolic effects and interactions with disease processes. Short-term studies appear to support a neutral effect on blood pressure, coagulation factors, and lipid metabolism with the combination injectable contraceptive (CIC) that is no longer marketed in the United States *(16,17)*. Less information is available regarding the patch *(18)* or vaginal ring.

There is a lack of data on the new progestin implant (etonogestrel), and therefore it is generally considered to be similar to the levonorgestrel (LNG) implant that is well studied but no longer marketed in the United States. In some instances, data is available to distinguish depot medroxyprogesterone acetate (DMPA) side effects from progestin implants and these are noted in Table 5.

Overall, the use of contraceptives in women with medical disease is poorly studied. Most studies are retrospective reviews and many are uncontrolled. Prospective studies are rare and, to date, no randomized trials have been published. Thus most of the recommendations are based on extrapolation from results of clinical trials and epidemiological studies in healthy women combined with an understanding of the pathophysiology of the individual disease process. The World Health Organization (WHO)'s *Medical Eligibility Criteria for Contraceptive Use (19)* provides a detailed summary of an international collaboration of agencies and organizations addressing this topic. The risk assessment criteria presented in Table 5 is adapted from the WHO classification categories of risk and their overall recommendations.

STEP-WISE QUESTIONS TO CONSIDER IN CHOOSING A BIRTH CONTROL METHOD FOR A WOMAN WITH A MEDICAL DISEASE

Question 1: Is She a Candidate for a Contraceptive Method That Contains Any Hormone?

Reproductive-aged women produce estrogen and progesterone and it is not surprising that most women can safely use some form of HC. Exceptions in which any HC is contraindicated include women with liver disease, which interferes with liver metabolism of steroids (e.g., active hepatitis, cirrhosis);

Table 4
Metabolic Effects of Contraceptive Methods and Components

	Oral estrogen	*Oral progestin*	*Intramuscular and implants of progestin*	*Intrauterine device*
Glucose tolerance	Neutral	Increased insulin resistance and glucose tolerance	Increased insulin resistance and glucose tolerance	Neutral
Lipids	Increased HDL cholesterol, decreased LDL cholesterol and increased triglycerides	Decreased HDL cholesterol, increased LDL cholesterol	Decreased triglyceride variable on HDL and total cholesterol	Neutral
Blood Pressure	Slight increase or neutral	Neutral	Neutral	Neutral
Coagulation	Increased globulins: dose-dependent increase	Neutral	Neutral	Neutral

Combination contraceptives delivered intramuscularly, transdermally, and transvaginally are relatively new and have effects similar to those of estrogen and progestin oral contraceptives.

HDL, high-density lipoprotein; LDL, low-density lipoprotein.

Table 5

Specific Considerations for Contraceptive Prescription in Women With Medical Conditions

Medical condition	*Specific considerations for combination estrogen/progestin contraceptives (oral, injectable, transdermal, and transvaginal)*	*Specific considerations for progestin-only oral contraceptives*	*Specific considerations for injectable or implanted progestin contraception*
Cardiac and vascular disease states			
Cardiac lesions Complicated cardiac lesions Congenital Acquired valvular	Contraindicated: all estrogen containing methods 2° to increased risk of thrombosis. Exception: if anti-coagulated: consider COC, to decrease menses and lower risk of bleeding corpus luteal cysts.	No restrictions.	No restrictions.
Cardiac lesions Uncomplicated valvular disease Mitral valve prolapse	Acceptable with risk: use lowest dose estrogen formulation.	No restrictions: preferred oral contraceptive.	No restrictions.
Hypercoagulable states associated with: Cardiac valvular disease	Contraindicated: all estrogen containing methods: increased risk of thrombosis, high blood pressure, and fluid retention.	No restrictions: valvular disease.	No restrictions: valvular disease.
Current or Hx of venous or arterial thrombus	If chronic anti-coagulated: can consider COC if heavy menses or Hx of ruptured corpus luteal cysts.	Acceptable with risk: Hx of DVT/PE. Avoid: Current DVT/PE.	Acceptable with risk: Hx of DVT/PE. Avoid: Current DVT/PE.

Known thrombogenic mutations: Factor V Leiden, Prothrombin mutation, Protein S deficiency, Protein C deficiency, Antithrombin deficiency	Contraindicated.	Acceptable with risk.	Acceptable with risk.
Coronary artery disease (current or history of)	Contraindicated.	Acceptable with risk.	Acceptable with risk.
History of cerebrovascular accident	Contraindicated.	Acceptable with risk.	Acceptable with risk.
Hypertension			
during pregnancy—now <140/90 mmHg	Acceptable with risk: small absolute but higher risk of myocardial infarction and thromboembolism with COC.	No restrictions.	No restrictions.
Controlled with therapy —<140/90 mmHg	Avoid: treated hypertension still at increased risk of myocardial infarction and stroke. No studies in treated hypertension and COC.	Acceptable with risk: may have small increased risk with POP and cardiovascular events.	Acceptable with risk: may have small increased risk of cardiovascular events with injectable progestins.

(continued)

Table 5 *(Continued)*

Medical condition	*Specific considerations for combination estrogen/progestin contraceptives (oral, injectable, transdermal, and transvaginal)*	*Specific considerations for progestin-only oral contraceptives*	*Specific considerations for injectable or implanted progestin contraception*
Elevated on therapy	Contraindicated: COC users at increased risk myocardial infarction, stroke, and thrombo-embolism.	Acceptable with risk. Avoid: in severe hypertension.	Acceptable with risk.
Diabetes mellitus			
Type 1 diabetes Type 2 diabetes	Acceptable with risk: choose the lowest dose/potency progestin to decrease effect on insulin resistance and lipid metabolism.	Acceptable with risk: short-term use of POP in type 1 found no deterioration in diabetes control or indicators.	Acceptable with risk: no data available.
Type 1 or 2 diabetes with vascular sequelae	Contraindicated with macro-vascular disease.	Acceptable with risk: no data available.	Acceptable with risk: No data available. Avoid: DMPA.
Pre-diabetes (prior gestational diabetes)	Acceptable: choose lowest dose estrogen/progestin formulation	No restriction: if not breastfeeding. Contraindicated: in prior GDM while breastfeeding (approximately threefold increase in diabetes).	No restrictions.
Other CVD risk factors			
Hyperlipidemia	Avoid: Multiple risk factors significantly increases risk for CVD. Can consider use in women with one risk factor with close monitoring and implementing lifestyle changes and/or therapy.	Acceptable with risk: multiple risk factors significantly increase risk for CVD. Monitor lipids, BP, diabetes screening.	Acceptable with risk: multiple risk factors significantly increase risk for CVD. Monitor lipids, BP, diabetes screening.

Obesity: BMI >30 kg/m²	Avoid in longstanding obesity.	No restrictions.	No restrictions.
Older	Acceptable with no other risk factors.	No restrictions.	No restrictions.
Smoking <35 years >35 years	Acceptable with risk: <35 years. Avoid: light smokers >35 years. Contraindicated: heavy smokers >35 years.	No restrictions.	No restrictions.
Thyroid disease Hyperthyroid Hypothyroid	No restriction.	No restriction.	No restriction.
Systemic lupus erythematosus	Contraindicated.	Acceptable with risks: retrospective controlled study showed no increase in lupus flares or morbidity	Acceptable with risks: no data.
Hemophilias Sickle cell disease Thalassaemia Iron deficiency anemia	Acceptable with risks.	No restrictions: POC has no adverse affect on sickling. Some studies show decreased sickling crisis, improved hematological parameters with POC.	No restrictions: preferred method. Some studies show decreased sickling crisis, improved hematological parameters with DMPA
Seizure disorders requiring AEDs	No restrictions: potential drug interactions, monitor AED levels, may require higher estrogen/progestin dose COC—may have decreased pregnancy protection.	No restrictions: potential drug interactions, monitor AED levels—may have decreased pregnancy protection.	No restrictions: DMPA may decreased seizure frequency. Potential drug interactions: monitor AED levels—may have decreased pregnancy protection.

(continued)

Table 5 *(Continued)*

Medical condition	*Specific considerations for combination estrogen/progestin contraceptives (oral, injectable, transdermal, and transvaginal)*	*Specific considerations for progestin-only oral contraceptives*	*Specific considerations for injectable or implanted progestin contraception*
Migraine headaches			
Without aura	Acceptable with risk. Risk of stroke increases with age, hypertension, smoking.	Acceptable with risk.	Acceptable with risk.
With aura (classic)	Contraindicated: increased risk of stroke with migraine with aura	Acceptable with risk.	Acceptable with risk.
Liver disease			
History cholestasis			
Of pregnancy	Acceptable with risk.	No restrictions.	No restrictions.
COC-related	Avoid: COC-related.	Acceptable with risk.	Acceptable with risk.
Symptomatic gallbladder disease	Avoid	Acceptable with risk.	Acceptable with risk.
Active liver disease: hepatitis, cirrhosis, liver tumor	Contraindicated.	Avoid	Avoid.
Malignancy and pre-invasive disease			
Breast cancer			
Current	Contraindicated.	Contraindicated.	Contraindicated.
Past (>5 years), no evidence of recurrence	Avoid.	Avoid.	Avoid.

Gestational trophoblast disease Benign Malignant	No restriction: no evidence of COC effect on course of benign or malignant trophoblastic disease.	No restriction.	No restriction.
Cervical cancer	Acceptable with risk.	No restriction.	Acceptable with risk.
Cervical intraepithileal neoplasia	Acceptable with risk: long-term COC use may increase risk of carcinoma with persistent HPV infection	No restriction.	Acceptable with risk: long-term DMPA use may increase risk of carcinoma with persistent HPV infection.
<u>HIV</u>			
Infected	No restriction: HIV-infected; limited evidence showing no increased RNA levels of HIV with COC use. Potential drug interactions.	No restriction: HIV-infected. Potential drug interactions.	No restriction: HIV-infected; potential drug interactions.
AIDS	Acceptable with risks: AIDS.	Acceptable with risks: AIDS.	Acceptable with risks: AIDS.
<u>Mental disorders</u> Depression, bipolar disorder, schizophrenia Mental Retardation	No restriction. COC use does not increase depressive symptoms. Compliance and STI protection may be an issue. Potential for drug interactions.	No restriction: POC does not increase depressive symptoms. Compliance and STI protection may be an issue. Potential for drug interactions.	No restriction: preferable 2° to longer duration, not user-dependent. STI protection may be an issue. Potential for drug interactions.
<u>Gynecological conditions</u>			
Benign breast disease	No restriction.	No restriction.	No restriction.
Endometriosis, severe dysmenorrhea	No restriction: may decrease pain and bleeding	No restriction: may decrease symptoms.	No restriction: may decrease symptoms.
PID			
Past—no current STI risk	No restriction: encourage concurrent condom use.	No restriction: encourage concurrent condom use.	No restriction: encourage concurrent condom use.

(continued)

Table 5 *(Continued)*

Medical condition	*Specific considerations for combination estrogen/progestin contraceptives (oral, injectable, transdermal, and transvaginal)*	*Specific considerations for progestin-only oral contraceptives*	*Specific considerations for injectable or implanted progestin contraception*
Current PID or STI	No restriction: COCs may increase chlamydial cervicitis.	No restriction: encourage concurrent condom use.	No restriction: encourage concurrent condom use.
Polycystic ovarian syndrome	No restriction: hirsutism: choose estrogen-dominant COC. Monthly menses decreases risk of hyperplasia	No restriction: second choice if unable to use COC (hirsuitism)	No restriction: second choice. . DMPA associated with weight gain, increased hirsuitism.
Benign ovarian tumors	No restriction.	No restriction.	No restriction.
Leiomyomas Without distortion of uterine cavity With distortion	No restriction: COCs may inhibit growth; use progestin-dominant COC.	No restriction.	No restriction.
Prolactinoma	No restriction: low-dose COCs do not accelerate growth of microadenoma, do promote regular menses and decreased risk of endometrial hyperplasia.	No restriction.	No restriction.

All combination estrogen/progestin methods are considered together as are injectable and implanted progestin methods, lacking study data from newer combination methods (injectable, transdermal, transvaginal, implants). Level of safety and conditions are indicated as (1) no restrictions: no known contraindications, possible benefits; (2) acceptable with risk: possible or theoretical risks that can often be reduced by additional monitoring; (3) avoid: not recommended unless special indications outweigh risks; and (4) contraindicated: method with definite risks that contraindicate its use.

IUD, intrauterine device; LNG, levonorgestrel; COC, combination oral contraceptive; Hx, history; DVT, deep vein thrombosis; PE, pulmonary embolism; DMPA, depot medroxyprogesterone acetate; POP, progestin-only pill; GDM, gestational diabetes mellitus; PID, pelvic inflammatory disease; CVD, cardiovascular disease; BMI, body mass index; BP, blood pressure; POC, progestin-only contraceptive; AED, anti-epileptic drug; GTD, gestational trophoblast disease; HPV, human papillomavirus; HIV, human immunodeficiency virus; AIDS, acquired immune deficiency syndrome; STD, sexually transmitted disease.

cholestasis associated with prior HC use; and malignant or benign liver tumors (e.g., focal nodular hyperplasia and adenomas that may enlarge and rupture with HC use). Another exclusionary category is women with estrogen- or progesterone-sensitive malignancies, such as breast cancer (Table 5).

If the answer to this question is "no," appropriate options for contraception include the copper-containing IUD (Cu-IUD), barrier methods, and tubal sterilization.

Question 2: If She is a Candidate for an HC in General, is She a Candidate for an Estrogen-Containing Contraceptive?

When given with a progestin, estrogen generally plays only a small role in providing contraceptive protection, but it does increase contraceptive efficacy and provide cycle control. For these reasons, COCs tend to be slightly more effective than progestin-only OCs (PO-OCs) and have far superior bleeding control. However, the estrogen component produces a dose-dependent increase in globulins resulting in increased coagulation factors and angiotensin II. These increases are associated with an increased risk for a thrombotic events and hypertension. Estrogen has a desirable effect on serum lipid levels and no has or little effect on insulin resistance (Table 4 *[2–4]*).

The use of low-dose COCs, those containing less than 35 µg of ethinyl estradiol, has been associated with reduced incidences of estrogen-related serious side effects (Chapter 2) compared with the older high-dose COCs. There continues to be trend toward use of COCs with the lowest dose of estrogen possible and currently there are a large number of COCs containing 20 and 25 µg of ethinyl estradiol.

The current recommendations exclude women from using COCs if they have a medical condition associated with vascular disease or with an increased risk of thrombosis. This includes women with cardiac lesions, cardiovascular disease, diabetes with vascular sequelae, hypertension, systemic lupus erythematosus, migraine headaches with localizing neurological signs, heavy smoking, or thrombogenic mutations (Table 5 [20]). In women with systemic lupus erythematosus, COC use has been linked to an increase in lupus flares (21–24), whereas the use of PO-OCs have not (25,26).

Several studies have demonstrated that COC use among women with hypertension is associated with an increase risk of myocardial infarction, stroke, and peripheral arterial disease compared with nonusers *(27–31)*. Similarly, it is prudent to avoid COC prescriptions in women with multiple cardiovascular risk factors, including those with metabolic syndrome *(32)*. The presence of a single risk factor in young woman may not override her need for an effective contraceptive, but she should be carefully monitored and encouraged to implement changes in her lifestyle (Table 3).

One exception exists in women who are chronically anti-coagulated to reduce their risk of thromboembolic disease (e.g., mechanical cardiac valves, thrombogenic mutations). Anti-coagulation places cycling women at increased risk of a ruptured corpus luteum cysts and intraperitoneal hemorrhage, requiring emergency surgery. In this case, COC use may be considered because it will reduce the risk of functional ovarian cysts, ruptured cysts, and bleeding complications. Adverse effect on clotting factors can be monitored and controlled with the use of anti-coagulants.

Currently, it is unclear whether monthly CICs, transdermal patches, or vaginal rings offer a metabolic advantage over orally administered COCs. Thus the route of combination contraceptives should be based on patient preference, expected reliability in administration of method (daily, weekly, or monthly), and reversibility (greater delay in return of fertility with CICs).

Question 3: If She is a Candidate for COCs, What Is the Best Dose and Formulation of the OC Pill? Does the Progestin Matter?

> *Generally, formulations with the lowest possible dose/potency of both estrogen and progestin should be selected for women with medical conditions who are candidates for COCs.*

Consideration of which COC formulation to prescribe is especially important in women in whom increased insulin resistance, unfavorable lipid profiles, and hirsutism should be minimized (e.g., diabetes, prior gestational diabetes, metabolic syndrome, and polycystic ovarian syndrome). COCs contain a wide variety of progestin formulations and doses. Most progestins are testosterone derivatives and have varying degrees of androgenic effects (e.g., decreasing sex-binding globulin, increasing insulin resistance, and adverse changes in serum lipids *[3]*). Newer formulations of COCs that contain either a more selective progestin (desogestrel, gestodene, norgestimate, drospirenone *[8,11]*) or contain a low dose of older progestins (norethindrone, LNG), have minimal androgenic side effects and are generally preferred. The exceptions, in whom higher progestin potency COCs may be preferred, include patients with symptomatic endometriosis or large fibroids or when better bleeding control is needed (Chapters 13 and 14).

Choosing an COC with a low-dose progestin for women with insulin resistance has been supported in several short-term, prospective studies. In women with type 1 diabetes who were followed for up to 1 year, use of lower doses of the older progestins, norethindrone ($\leq$0.75 mg mean daily dose) or triphasic LNG preparation, or the newer progestins (gestodene, desogestrel) were found to found to have minimal effect on diabetic control, lipid metabolism *(33–35)*, and cardiovascular risk factors *(36,37)*. COC formulations generally are not recommended in diabetic women with microvascular disease, however, retrospective, cross-sectional studies *(26)* and case–control trials *(38)* in women with type 1 diabetes have not found any increase risk or progression of diabetic sequelae (retinopathy, renal disease, or hypertension) with past or current use of OCs.

Question 4: For Women Who Cannot Take Estrogen and Are Therefore Not Candidates for COCs, What Is the Ideal Route of Administration of Progestin-Only Contraception?

Most women who are not able to use estrogen but desire a hormonal method will be candidates for progestin-only methods. Women with hypertension, cardiovascular disease, or high risk of thrombosis are able to use progestin-only formulations because progestin-only contraceptives are not associated with adverse effects on liver globulin production. Progestin-only methods are not associated with increased blood pressure or adverse changes in coagulation factors *(13,39)*. If a woman is a candidate for a progestin-only methods, she has the option of daily PO-OCs, an injection every 3 months (Depo-Provera® [DMPA] or depo-subQ provera 104™), an implant containing etonogestrel that lasts for 3 years, or an intrauterine system (IUS) containing LNG that lasts for 5 years. Unfortunately, there is a limited amount of literature comparing the metabolic effects of the various progestin-only contraceptives in either healthy or high-risk women.

Oral progestins are the best studied of all progestin methods and have the most documented safety profile. There are only two formulations of PO-OCs, one containing norethindrone (0.35 mg daily) and the other norgestrel (0.75 mg daily). Women must take a pill daily and should expect changes in bleeding patterns. PO-OC users are able to rapidly discontinue therapy if side effects occur and fertility usually returns within a few weeks. Occasionally, PO-OCs are given as a trial therapy before administering a longer acting (injectable or implant) progestin to see if a user is sensitive to progestin side effects.

Injectable progestins (DMPA and depo-subQ provera 104) have some particular advantages and disadvantages to consider. In several studies, DMPA was reported to have more adverse effects on lipids and insulin resistance *(4,5)* compared with Norplant® *(6,7)*. DMPA also has a longer return of fertility after discontinuation and has been associated with weight gain. Because of the adverse lipid effects and potential weight gain, DMPA may not a first-line choice for women with cardiovascular disease, including coronary artery disease, history of stroke, and diabetes with vascular disease, or for women with obesity.

The use of DMPA may provide a therapeutic advantage in epilepsy and sickle disease. In small study of women with uncontrolled seizures on antiepileptic medication, the administration of DMPA resulted in a significant decrease in seizure frequency in half of the women *(40)*. In women with sickle disease, intramuscular progesterone (10 mg) *(41)* and DMPA in a blinded, crossover study *(42)* decreased the severity and duration of sickle pain, sickle crisis, bone pain, and improved fetal and total hemoglobin indices. Another recent randomized trial comparing DMPA and COC with a sterilized control group found a modest improvement in the DMPA users. Of the DMPA users, 70% were pain-free, compared with 45.5% of the COC users and 50.5% of the controls *(43)*.

In conclusion, progestin-only contraceptives are often a good choice for women who cannot take estrogen-containing products because of cardiovascular- and thrombosis-related issues. There are some clear differences in timing and route of administration and some identifiable differences in side effects and metabolic profiles that may influence the selection of a particular method.

Question 5: Is She a Candidate for an IUD?

In general, guidelines for use of IUDs in women with medical disease follow the same guidelines as those for healthy women. Most parous women in mutually monogamous relationships and at low risk for sexaually transmitted infections (STIs) with no recent history of pelvic inflammatory disease (PID) or STI infection are good candidates for IUDs. In some instances, an IUD is the best option in nulliparous women.

Question 6: Should She Receive Antibiotic Prophylaxis at Time of IUD Insertion or Removal?

Although antibiotic prophylaxis at time of IUD insertion has not been shown to benefit healthy, STI culture-negative women *(44)*, prophylaxis may be appropriate for women with certain medical conditions. Women on steroids or chemotherapy or who have medical conditions that make them chronically immunosuppressed are at high risk of infection and good candidates for antibiotic prophylaxis. Antibiotic prophylaxis with ampicilin and gentamycin is recommended at the time of insertion to prevent subacute bacterial endocarditis in women with cardiac lesions or valve replacements *(45)*. The safety of this regimen was demonstrated in a large study of women with surgically treated cardiac lesions using a Cu-IUDs who all received prophylaxis and none developed bacterial endocarditis *(46)*.

Recently, the American Heart Association *(47)* changed their recommendations regarding antibiotic prophylaxis for subacute bacterial endocarditis and no longer requires prophylaxis at time of routine IUD insertion and removal. No studies have examined this issue in women with specific cardiac lesions or valve replacements.

Question 7: What are the Advantages/Disadvantages of the Cu-IUD Versus the LNG-Containing IUD?

The Cu-IUD is metabolically neutral, highly efficacious, and has minimal risks when patients are properly selected as low risk for STDs and an aseptic insertion technique is followed. In a large meta-analysis of several prospective WHO trials, the overall incidence of PID associated with Cu-IUD use was 1.6 per 1000 women-years of IUD use *(48)*. The one drawback is increased menstrual blood loss that may need to be counteracted by daily iron supplementation or multivitamin. In several high-risk populations, such as women with type 1 *(49,50)* or type 2 *(51)* diabetes, cardiac lesions *(46)*, or systemic lupus *(52)*, no IUD-associated increase in PID has been found.

The great advantage of the Cu-IUD is its 10-year duration, high efficacy, and its metabolic neutrality, permitting use in nearly all women with medical disease, especially those at increase risk of thrombosis, cardiovascular disease, and drug interactions (Table 5).

The LNG-IUS releases approximately 10% of the dose and reaches 5% of the plasma level of a typical OC pill containing 105 μg LNG. Although this small amount of LNG has a minimal systemic metabolic effect, it does exert a considerable local progestin effect on the endometrium and insertion of a LNG-IUS significantly decreases menstrual blood loss *(53)*. This feature makes it a very desirable option in conditions in which heavy blood loss or anemia occurs (e.g., sickle disease, thalassemia, anti-coagulated states, or menorrhagia [Table 5]). Because of a lack of studies examining the LNG-IUS in women with medical disease, its use is considered "acceptable with risk" or "avoid" in women in which HC is considered a poor choice.

REFERENCES

1. Spellacy WN, Buhi WC, Birk SA. (1971) The effect of estrogens on carbohydrate metabolism: glucose, insulin and growth hormone studies on one hundred seventy-one women ingesting premarin, mestranol and ethinyl estradiol for six months. Am J Obstet Gynecol 114:388–392.
2. Perlman JA, Russell-Briefel R, Ezzati T, Lieberknecht. (1985) Oral glucose tolerance and the potency of contraceptive progestins. J Chronic Dis 338:857–864.
3. Godsland IF, Crook D, Simpson R, et al. (1990) The effects of different formulations of oral contraceptive agents on lipid and carbohydrate metabolism. N Engl J Med 323:1375–1381.
4. Fahmy K, Abdel-Razik, Shaaraway M, et al. (1991) Effect of long-acting progestagen-only injectable contraceptives on carbohydrate metabolism and its hormonal profile. Contraception 44:419–429.
5. Liew DF, Ng CSA, Yong YM, et al. (1985) Long term effects of depo-provera on carbohydrate and lipid metabolism. Contraception 31:51–64.
6. Singh K, Viegas OA, Koh SC, Ratnam SS. (1992) The effect of long-term use of Norplant implants on haemostatic function. Contraception 45:141–153.
7. Konje JC, Otolorin EO, Ladipo AO. (1992) The effect of continuous subdermal levonorgestrel (Norplant) on carbohydrate metabolism. Am J Obstet Gynecol 166:15–19.
8. Speroff L, DeCherney A. (1993) Evaluation of a new generation of oral contraceptives. The Advisory Board of the New Progestins. Obstet Gynecol 81:1034–1047.
9. Fahraeus L, Sydsjo A, Wallentin L. (1986) Lipoprotien changes during treatment of pelvic endometriosis with medroxyprogesterone acetate. Fert Steril 45:501–506.
10. Deslypere JP, Thiery N, Vermeulen A. (1985) Effect of long-term hormonal contraception in plasma lipids. Contraception 31:633–642.
11. Fajumi JO. (1983) Alerations in blood lipids and side effects induced by depo-provera in Nigerian women. Contraception 27:161–175.
12. Shaaban MM, Elwan SI, Abdalla SA, Darwish HA. (1984) Effect of subdermal levonorgestrel contraceptive implants, Norplant, on serum lipids. Contraception 30:413–419.
13. Wilson ES, Cruickshank J, McMaster M, et al. (1984) A prospective controlled study of the effect on blood pressure of contraceptive preparations containing different types of dosages and progestogen. Br J Obstet Gynaecol 91:1254–1260.

14. Meade TW. (1982) Oral contraceptives, clotting factors and thrombosis. Am J Obstet Gynecol 142:758–761.
15. Shaaban M, Elwan SI, el-Kabsh MY, Farghaly SA, Thabet N. (1984) Effect of levonorgestrel contraceptive implants, Norplant, on blood coagulation. Contraception 30:421–430.
16. Haiba NA, el-Habashy MA, Said SA, Darwish EA, Abdel-Sayed WS, Nayel SE. (1989) Clinical evaluation of two monthly injectable contraceptives and their effects on some metabolic parameters. Contraception 39:619–632.
17. von Kessereau E, Aydinlink S, Etchepareborda JJ. (1991) A multicentered, two-year, phase III clinical trial of norethisterone enanthate 50 mg plus estradiol valerate 5 mg as a monthly injectable contraceptive. Contraception 44:589–598.
18. Smallwood GH, Meador ML, Lenihan JP, et al. (2001) Efficacy and safety of a transdermal contraceptive system. Obstet Gynecol 98:799–805.
19. The World Health Organization. (2004) Medical Eligibility Criteria for Contraceptive Use, 3rd ed. Available from: www.who.int/reproductive-health. Accessed March 27, 2006.
20. Kjos SL. (2000) Contraception for women with medical problems. Infertily Reprod Med Clin North Am 11:551–586.
21. Chapel TA, Burns RE. (1971) Oral contracpetives and exacerbations of lupus erythematosus. Am J Obstet Gynecol 110:366–369.
22. Garovich M, Agudelo C, Pisko E. (1980) Oral contraceptives and systemic lupus erythematosus. Arthritis Rhuem 23:1396–1398.
23. Travers RE, Hughes GRV. (1978) Oral contraceptive therapy and systemic lupus erythematosus. J Rheumatol 5:448–451.
24. Jungers P, Dougados M, PÈlissier C, et al. (1982) Influence of oral contraceptive therapy on the activiey of systemic lupus erthematosus. Arthritis Rheum 25:618–623.
25. Mintz G, Gutiérrez G, Delezé, Rodríguez E. (1984) Contraception with progestagens in systemic lupus erythematosus. Contraception 30:29–38.
26. Klein BEK, Moss SE, Klein R. (1990) Oral contraceptives in women with diabetes. Diabetes Care 13:895–898.
27. Gillum LA, Mamidipudi SK, Johnston SC. (2000) Ischemic stroke risk with oral contraceptives: a meta-analysis. JAMA 284:72–78.
28. Khader YS, Rice J, John L, Abueita O. (2003) Oral contraceptives use and the risk of myocardial infarction: a meta-analysis. Contraception 68:11–17.
29. Tanis BC, van den Bosch MA, Kemmeren JM, et al. (2001) Oral contraceptives and the risk of myocardial infarction. N Engl J Med 345:1787–1793.
30. Van den Bosch MA, Kemmeren JM, Tanis BC, et al. (2003) The RATIO study: oral contraceptives and the risk of peripheral arterial disease in young women. J Thromb Haemost 1:439–444.
31. World Health Organization. (1995) Venous thromboembolic disease and combined oral contraceptives: results of international multicentre case–control study. World Health Organization Collaborative Study of Cardiovascular Disease and Steroid Hormone Contraception. Lancet 346:1575–1582.
32. The National Cholesterol Education Program. Adult Treatment Panel III (NCEP-ATPIII). www.nhlbi.nih.gov/guidelines/cholesterol/. Accessed March 11, 2006.
33. Skouby SO, Jensen BM, Kuhl C, et al. (1985) Hormonal contraception in diabetic women: acceptability and influence on diabetes control of a nonaldkylated estrogen/progestogen compound. Contraception 32:23–31.
34. Skouby SO, Molsted-Pedersen, Kuhl C, et al. (1986) Oral contraceptives in diabetic women: metabolic effects of four compounds with different estrogen/progestogen profiles. Fertil Steril 46:858–864.

35. Radberg T, Gustafson A, Skryten A, et al. (1981) Oral contraception in diabetic women. Diabetes control, serum and high density lipoprotein lipids during low-dose progestogen, combined oestrogen/progestogen and non-hormonal contraception. Acta Endocrinol 98:246–251.
36. Peterson KR, Skouby SO, Sidelmann J, Molsted-Pedersen L, Jespersen J. (1994) Effects of contraceptive steroids on cardiovascular risk factors in women with insulin-dependent diabetes mellitus. Am J Obstet Gynecol 171:400–405.
37. Peterson KR, Skouby SO, Vedel P, Haaber AB. (1995) Hormonal contraception in women with IDDM. Diabetes Care 18:800–806.
38. Garg SK, Chase HP, Marshal G, Hoops S, Holmes DL, Jackson WE. (1994) Oral contraceptives and renal and retinal complications in young women with insulin-dependent diabetes mellitus. JAMA 271:1099–1102.
39. Chasan-Taber L, Willett WC, Manson JE, et al. (1996) Prospective study of oral contraceptives and hypertension among women in the United States. Circulation 94:483–489.
40. Mattson RH, Cramer JC, Caldwell BV, Siconolifi BC. (1984) Treatment of seizures with mederoxyprogesterone acetate: preliminary report. Neurology 34:1255–1258.
41. Isaac WA, Effiong CE, Ayeni D. (1973) Steriod treatment in the prevention of painful episodes in sickle cell disease. Lancet 1:570–571.
42. deCeulaer K, Hayes R, Gruber C, Serjeant GR. (1982) Medroxyprogesterone acetate and homozyguous sickle-cell disease. Lancet 2:229–231.
43. deAbood M, deCastillo Z, Guerrero F, Espino M, Austin KL. (1997) Effect of depo-provera® or Microgynon® on the painful crises of sickle cell anemia patients. Contraception 56:313–316.
44. Sinei SK, Schulz KF, Lmptey PR, et al. (1990) Preventing IUCD-related pelvic infection: the efficacy of prophylactic doxycycline at insertion. Br J Obstet Gynaecol 97:412–419.
45. Dajani AS, Bisno AL, Chung DJ, et al. (1990) Prevention of Bacterial Endocarditis. Recommendations of the American Heart Association. JAMA 264:2919–2922.
46. Abdalla MY, el Din Mostafa E. (1992) Contraception after heart surgery. Contraception 45:73–80.
47. Dajani AS, Taubert KA, Wilson W, et al. (1997) Prevention of bacterial endocarditis. Recommendations of the American Heart Association. JAMA 277:1794–1801.
48. Farley TMM, Rosenberg MJ, Rowe PJ, Chen J-H, Meirek O. (1992) Intrauterine devices and pelvic inflammatory disease: an international perspective. Lancet 339:785–788.
49. Skouby SO, Molsted-Pedersen L, Kosonen A. (1984) Consequences of intrauterine contraception in diabetic women. Fert Steril 42:568–572.
50. Kimmerle R, Weiss R, Berger M, Kurz K-H. (1993) Effectiveness, safety and acceptablity of a copper intrauterine device (CU Safe 300) in type I diabetic women. Diabetes Care 16:1227–1230.
51. Kjos SL, Ballagh SA, La Cour M, Xiang A, Mishell DR Jr. (1994) The copper T380A intrauterine device in women with type II diabetes mellitus. Obstet Gynecol 84:1006–1009.
52. Julkunen HA, Kaaja R, Friman C. (1993) Contraceptive practice in women with systemic lupus erythematosus. Br J Rheumatol 32:227–230.
53. Stewart A, Cummins C, Gold L, et al. (2001) The effectiveness of the levonorgestrel-releasing intrauterine systems in menorrhagia: a systemic review. BJOG 108:74–86.

Index

E

O

P

T